Psychiatry AND PUBLIC AFFAIRS

Psychiatry
AND
PUBLIC AFFAIRS

GROUP FOR THE ADVANCEMENT OF PSYCHIATRY

Leo H. Bartemeier, editor

Routledge
Taylor & Francis Group
New York London

First published 2012 by Transaction Publishers

Published 2017 by Routledge
711 Third Avenue, New York, NY 10017, USA
2 Park Square, Milton Park, Abingdon, Oxon OX14 4RN

First issued in hardback 2017

Routledge is an imprint of the Taylor & Francis Group, an informa business

Library of Congress Catalog Number: 2011026248

Library of Congress Cataloging-in-Publication Data

Psychiatry and public affairs / Group for the Advancement of Psychiatry; Leo H. Bartemeier, general editor.
p. ; cm.
Reprint of: Psychiatry and public affairs. Chicago : Aldine, c1966.
ISBN 978-1-4128-4283-9 (alk. paper)
1. Social psychology. I. Bartemeier, Leo H. (Leo Henry), 1895-1982. II. Group for the Advancement of Psychiatry. [DNLM: 1. Psychiatry--Collected Works. 2. Social Responsibility--Collected Works. WM 5]

HM1033.P766 2011
302--dc23

2011026248

ISBN 13: 978-1-4128-4283-9 (pbk)
ISBN 13: 978-1-1385-3100-0 (hbk)

CONTENTS

PREFACE

In "The Story of GAP," written by the noted journalist Albert Deutsch some years ago, Dr. William Menninger, one of GAP's founding members and its first President, gave a brief account of how and why the organization came into being in 1946. Dr. Menninger wrote:

> During World War II more than two and a half million soldiers, sailors and airmen were either rejected or discharged from the military service because of emotional problems. Those of us most intimately connected with the examination and treatment of these men and women were greatly harrassed and distressed. We had neither the manpower nor the knowledge to do the job that should have been done. Understandably, we looked in every possible direction for help.
>
> The frustration we experienced in attempting to practice psychiatry in the armed forces certainly was the major precipitating factor in the organization of GAP. Fortunately, many of our colleagues who had remained in civilian life were equally aware of the responsibilities that confronted us—and the opportunities.
>
> Those early years of GAP were marked by the feeling on the part of its membership that much needed to be done, and quickly. We believed that when we were faced with a problem, if we could sit down together and take time to exchange views, we could determine what we knew and did not know about the matter and could plot the course of the search for the knowledge that we lacked. Through group study we endeavored to collect and assimilate what was known about psychiatry and mental health so that it would be available when needed.

GAP is a loose federation of investigating committees, each with its own research and educational functions and goals. Each explores pertinent ideas and methods of communication in its field. At present, there are twenty-one such working committees.

Each committee is an investigative team equipped by the talent and interests of its members without regard to geography or social determinants to do a distinctive job which is highly desirable to further the progress of psychiatry and its allied disciplines.

GAP thus differs from other medical organizations in that: membership is by invitation, on the basis of special abilities; *all* members work actively on some project; the organization is not for the direct benefit of members (all of whom participate in committee work at their own expense); and the core of the organization is its committees and not its administrative officers.

In the nineteen years since its founding, GAP has published fifty-eight reports and the proceedings of ten symposia. Just a shade under a million copies of these publications have been issued in this period. But these statistics do not begin to suggest the wide-ranging influence of its recommendations and observations. To cite but one instance, the GAP report on "Confidentiality and Privileged Communication in the Practice of Psychiatry" *(Report #45)* was instrumental in securing the enactment of one of the earliest of the state statutes to be passed on this subject. The effects of this legislation, in turn, extended to other states as well.

Reports are published in the name of GAP as a whole, and represent a total group effort; in each instance a particular committee chooses the subject and carries through the writing of a draft which is then submitted to all GAP members, whose comments and suggestions are acted upon before the final report is approved. Each committee functions as a study group and formulates a report only when it thinks it is ready to say something of significance. Symposia on important topics of the day have been a regular feature of GAP's semi-annual meetings. The symposia are arranged by one or another GAP committee, with both members and invited non-member experts participating, and are followed by discussion from the floor. Upon occasion, the proceedings of these symposia are published (four have been included in this volume).

GAP's publications have been extensively reprinted in whole or in part in textbooks, manuals and professional journals. In some instances the mass media as well have given extensive coverage to its publications. This was noticeably the case with the two reports, "Psychiatric Aspects of School Desegregation" (Chapter 2 of this volume) and "Psychiatric Aspects of the Prevention of Nuclear War" (Chapter 9 of this volume).

What makes GAP live and gives it its unique character was perhaps best summed up by Dr. Dana Farnsworth, one of its former presidents, as reported by Deutsch in "The Story of GAP":

> GAP gives us all a chance to be among people who are interested in the same thing, and who are interesting people in their own right.
>
> GAP is small enough to get the real opinions of thoughtful people in the field. These opinions are not watered down by excessive caution, such as is manifested so often in larger, more formalized groups.
>
> The body of GAP represents the summation, the distillation, of what is generally the best thinking being done collectively in any specific aspect of psychiatry.
>
> GAP presents a forum for the interchange of different approaches in a "disputatious atmosphere" where individuals can disagree

> openly and frankly with their peers without the threat to reputation, friendship or self-esteem.
>
> GAP has demonstrated that it is an effective agency for harmonious inter-disciplinary collaboration leading to action on common fronts of interest. The psychiatrists and their cooperating consultants meet here as peers in a setting of equality. Nobody pulls rank, regardless of profession, position or reputation.
>
> In GAP we are continually testing ideas on the advancing edge of psychiatry.

In this volume, *Psychiatry and Public Affairs,* we seek to share with you some psychiatric insights and approaches which we hope will contribute to a better understanding of some of the social issues that concern us both here at home and aboard. We invite you to join us as we explore "the advancing edge of psychiatry."

LEO H. BARTEMEIER, M.D., *President (1963-65)*
Group for the Advancement of Psychiatry

Psychiatry and Public Affairs

1 INTRODUCTION: THE SOCIAL RESPONSIBILITY OF PSYCHIATRY

The GAP reports and symposia that comprise this volume were selected because they all concern the application of psychiatric principles to broad social problems. Despite their wide variations as to form, style and date of publication (the first two reports reprinted here appeared in 1950 and the last was written in 1964), a consistent guiding principle is discernible throughout this span of years: that of the social responsibility of psychiatry. Since this is so basic to GAP's entire program, *Report #13*, "The Social Responsibility of Psychiatry, A Statement of Orientation," can also serve as an introductory statement pertinent to all the other parts of this book. It is therefore the first of the reports to be presented here; those that follow may be viewed as a series of endeavors toward fulfilling the social responsibility of which *Report #13* is an initial declaration.

GAP's commitment to this orientation was reconfirmed when it re-evaluated *Report #13* in March, 1957, and added the following note to it:

Editor's Note. Since the writing of this report in 1949 many events in our country have further illustrated the importance of informed participation by psychiatrists in the social changes of our time. For example, before rendering its decision on the desegregation of schools in 1954, the United States Supreme Court heard testimony from social scientists bearing on the psychological aspects of segregation. This precedent has since been followed by lower courts, legislatures, and school administrators who have frequently appealed to psychological principles in support of their decisions and actions. This places on psychiatrists (among other social scientists) some of the obligation of clarifying and interpreting the psychological aspects of social issues. The growing awareness by psychiatrists of their role in the community mental health and of the ways in which social changes affect the well-being of their patients has to some extent reduced the urgency which motivated the writing of *Report #13.* Nevertheless, the need to support the principles described in this report remains.

Toward the discharge of its responsibility in this connection the Committee on Social Issues of the Group for the Advancement of Psychiatry has published two studies of psychological aspects of current social issues. These are "Considerations Regarding The Loyalty Oath as a Manifestation of Current Social Tension and Anxiety" (GAP *Symposium #1)* and "Psychiatric Aspects of School Desegregation" [chapter 2 of this volume]. Other committees of GAP have published additional reports which relate to social aspects of psychiatry.*

And so, we consider it fitting for setting the tone of this series of writings about "Psychiatry and Public Affairs" to start with our statement of orientation, written fifteen years ago, on "The Social Responsibility of Psychiatry." The continued timeliness of this report is well demonstrated by its concluding sentence: "This, in a true sense, carries psychiatry out of the hospitals and clinics and into the community." Psychiatry today is indeed engaged on an unprecedented scale, in moving into the community. September, 1965

*As of today, this 1957 "Editor's Note" needs some further updating. Thus, in 1958 the Committee on Social Issues, in cooperation with the Committee on Law and Psychiatry, arranged a symposium and exhibit on Group Opposition to Health Programs; in 1964 it formulated a report on "Psychiatric Aspects of the Prevention of Nuclear War," which is included as Chapter 9 in this volume.

THE SOCIAL RESPONSIBILITY OF PSYCHIATRY

A Statement of Orientation*

The Committee on Social Issues, since the beginning of its function as a unit of GAP, has faced the need to define its purposes more clearly and to establish a frame of reference within which those purposes could effectively be pursued. The achievement of a clear orientation to its functional position was difficult, but indispensable to progress. Two factors immediately complicated this task: (1) the tremendous role played by prejudice — individual and class prejudice — in determining attitudes toward social problems; and (2) the incompleteness of scientific knowledge regarding the relations between society and personality.

The establishment by GAP of a Committee on Social Issues carried with it the tacit admission of the principle that the psychiatrist has a pertinent role in the study of social problems. Beyond this, however, no more specific definition of this role was provided by GAP. Here and there, individual psychiatrists and other social scientists offered conjectures on the significance of that role; but no standard had as yet been formulated.

Additional impetus toward clarification came from a series of discussions in the general meetings of GAP. These discussions reinforced the conviction of the Committee on Social Issues that the mission of GAP itself in large part was a social one; that the very birth of GAP was motivated not only by the pressing need for study of mental health problems, but also by a sense of urgency in the application of valid psychiatric knowledge to the critical problems of a changing society. All the issues raised in GAP had an immediate bearing on problems of mental health, but also had a wider relevancy to problems of human welfare, as shaped by the patterns of our own social organization.

Accordingly, it seemed important for GAP to take a valid and explicit position on the social responsibility of psychiatry. At one pole, psychiatry is linked to biology and medicine; at the other pole, it is linked to the social sciences. To meet the challenge of some problems of present-day psychiatry, an implicit reference to the question of social responsibility

*Formulated by the Committee on Social Issues, and first published as Report #13, in July, 1950.

is simply not sufficient. This means that two things are needed: a clear formulation of a set of values and scientifically derived and tested principles appropriate to the task of applying the knowledge of psychiatry to the ills and shortcomings of present-day society; and, secondly, an explicit hypothesis regarding the relationship between society and personality.

GAP found it necessary to attempt a better understanding of some aspects of the relationship between mental health and certain types of social phenomena. The social phenomena which GAP considered were: the relation of prejudice and civil rights to mental health; the emotional effects of certain types of mass communication (radio, screen, press); the mental health principles disseminated through schools, books, advertising media; the problems of censorship and "loyalty" tests; trends of ill will, suspicion and other evidences of mental ill-health among those who determine public policy; universal military training; the backwardness of social and educational legislation in some parts of our country; and, finally, the whole problem of education for living.[1]

When one views this range of psycho-social phenomena, it becomes evident that any rigorous attempt to modify their pathogenic aspects would be affected not only by the large role played by prejudice and by the handicap of insufficient knowledge regarding the interaction of society and personality, but especially by the difficulty of defining the specific connections between social forces and community mental health.

In this report the Committee on Social Issues attempts to establish a working hypothesis for the relations between society and personality. In the present state of limited knowledge, we can achieve at best only a set of tentative principles, to be amended as the tested knowledge grows. Such an effort is a necessary prerequisite for delineating the social responsibility of psychiatry.

In assuming this task, the Committee on Social Issues is aware that certain trends inherent in our current social structure tend to encourage emotional sickness. It believes that many of the warps and twists of our society have significant relevance for the issues of mental health, viewed from the standpoint of both the individual and the group. It believes that certain changes in the pattern of interaction between individual and family, and individual and society, may provide a more nourishing matrix for the cultivation of mental health.

[1]Sociologists might hope that the Committee would include among the social phenomena, consideration of population pressures as these pressures affect various groups and therefore also affect the individual in terms of levels of achievement and aspiration.

Relationship Between Personality and Society

Personality and society are viewed here not as closed systems but as continuously interacting. Each influences the other selectively toward change.[2] While the intactness of personality is reflected in relatively fixed propensities of behavior, it is simultaneously in continuous interaction with, and is influenced by, the environment. Behavior is determined both by stimuli derived from the internal organization of the person and the external organization of the social environment. Constitution sets limits to behavior potentials, but structured behavior is always conditioned by social experience. The development of personality is influenced both by biological make-up at birth and by the process of internalization of elements of the social environment. All behavior, beginning with birth, therefore, is bio-psycho-social.

Individual Personality and "Social Role"

As the person matures, he achieves an identity that is at once both individual and social. Individual identity is represented in the organized behavior characteristics of the intact self, as determined by a particular set of biological dispositions and early social experience. The individual component of a person's identity reflects his specific biological tendency patterned in its expression through his total character, which is socially conditioned. It is the core of the personality; it is relatively the more personal, more private, more fixed aspect of self. On the other hand, in a strict sense, individual identity is an abstraction, highly useful, to be sure, but an abstraction nevertheless. In growth and maturation, the process of individuation is never complete or absolute. The phenomena of social dependence run parallel with those of biological dependence. The full development of individuality does not imply isolation from or immunity against social influence; rather, it connotes an increasing sense of responsibility for social participation.

The "social role"[3] of a person, or the "social self," is by contrast, more variable, less private, less personal. "Social role" is conditioned by

[2]A current point of view in sociology regards the "changes" in society in terms of homeostatic forces and uses the concepts of equilibrium and dis-equilibrium for societies rather than "change." Furthermore, change is a characteristic of our culture but not necessarily of other cultures.

[3]The sociologist's point of view on the "social role" of a person includes a multiplicity of roles—group roles, personality roles, actual role, ideal role; conflict between these roles is very important in the development of social disturbance. This same point of view is applicable to the aspect of social reality discussed in the following section.

the phenomena of group belongingness and by temporal factors. "Social role" represents a component of the total identity of a person brought into action at a given time by a special set of group phenomena. At a given time, certain aspects of the total self are mobilized into action by the elements which prevail in a given social situation, while other aspects of the total self are temporarily subordinated. Thus it is possible for a particular person to express himself in a variety of "social roles." This is a phase of the phenomenon of social adaptation, involving compliance with some group forces and protest against others. Inevitably, this process of social adaptation activates changing patterns of defense against anxiety, which have variable expedient value. The vicissitudes of a particular group situation determine whether one or another "social role" will be activated, within which the more individual aspects of self are called into play in greater or lesser part.

These principles apply to each phase of individual development, first within the family group, and, after that, the school, the neighborhood, and finally, in the relations of the adult person with wider society. In this sense, the dynamics of personality are conceived in terms of a bio-psycho-social continuum, beginning with birth and continuing through all the vicissitudes of social conditioning throughout the course of life. In each phase of personality maturation, the pattern of interaction between biological and social forces varies, thus imparting certain unique characteristics to social behavior in each era of development.

"Social Reality"

By "social reality" we mean the prevailing social institutions and the standards of interpersonal relationship which shape the adaptive efforts of each individual growing up in this society.

"Social reality" patterns the opportunity either for satisfaction or frustration of individual need. It influences the kind and degree of possible self-expression and self-fulfillment. It plays a critical role in determining the balance between self-expression and conformity to social compulsion. It conditions the capacities of persons for recognition and respect of the needs of others. Finally, it determines the specific content of dangers which the individual must face in his struggle for successful adaptation.

Social institutions are the expression of group customs, standards and goals. These provide avenues along which the individual can adapt to the group. They determine selectively the channels into which individuals may release emotion, as well as those standards which determine the inhibition of emotion. Within the frame of these social institutions, the person succeeds or fails in the assertion of his mastery drives. Within the frame of these social institutions, unconscious drives may be irrationally "acted out." A continuous impact with group experience (family, school, civic, others) is the experiential matrix in which the person grows and develops his sense of reality. In a similar manner, the individual tests and assimilates selectively the moral and ethical standards of his environment, through a process of observing responses of environmental approval or dissapproval to the spontaneous expression of his urges.

When a person feels unequal to the situation with which he must cope, anxiety is aroused. The degree of anxiety activated is in inverse proportion to the degree of skill acquired in understanding and mastering reality.

"Social reality" not only influences channels chosen for release of inner drives and the quantity of anxiety generated with that release, but also exercises a selective influence on the choice of defense against anxiety (projection, reaction-formation, symptom formation, sublimation and others).[4]

"Social reality" is the matrix in which the individual identity of all persons is strengthened or weakened. A "give and take" process characterizes the individual's relatedness to his group. Social participation of a responsible kind is one measure of maturity of personality. This implies the capacity of the healthy person to contribute to his group. Conversely, he requires from his group a measure of emotional support. On the negative side, the weaker a person's sense of individual identity, the greater the need for support of the self from the group. Identification with groups, an extension of the childhood identification with parents, is a necessary part of healthy adaptation. Acceptance by the group, vital for emotional security, should not be achieved at the prohibitive price of excessive tension, self-destructive conformity, or denial of the opportunity for maturation of personality.

Opportunity for Self-Fulfillment

The patterns of self-expression and self-fulfillment are shaped by the coincidence of social opportunity and the individual's inner disposition to fulfill a given "social role." Choice of mate, occupation, membership in a variety of social groups, all contribute to shaping the "social role" of the

[4]Some members believed that this point should be expanded with the discussion of social group defenses and individual defenses, recognizing that social reality is not the only agent which exercises a select influence on the choice of defenses against anxiety.

individual in the manner indicated. Conflict between social opportunity and inner disposition is one ready source of anxiety. Instability or unpredictability of the patterns of social opportunity have the same anxiety-provoking effects. Under unfavorable circumstances, conflict between the person and the environment may become progressively internalized and thus contribute quantitatively to the intensification of psychopathological dispositions.

The Role of Social Danger

"Social reality" patterns the dangers against which the forces of personality must be mobilized. These dangers may be direct threats to life or limb, or they may represent economic privation, or frustration of basic personality needs. These needs may relate to security strivings, pleasure drives, sexual expression, or they may represent aspects of the striving for self-fulfillment in society. If such dangers and frustrations are excessive, the adaptive energies of the person may be absorbed in the negative task of counteracting such threats. In such instances, the pathological defense reactions of the personality may be so strongly mobilized as to leave the positive aspects of emotional living and self-fulfillment relatively impoverished. The greater the psychic energy required for this negative aspect of the task of adaptation, the less the emotional capacity to enjoy the positive aspects of living. Thus, the constructive drives become progressively subordinated to the compulsory need to counteract anxiety. The sicker the personality, the more do these defensive responses to external danger correspond to the symbolic context of inner psychic threats. One result of this process is the production of rigid, constricted personalities who in turn inflict on their environment the same rigid restrictions, or else the loss of hope and of feelings of self-worth and confidence seriously impairs the capacity for constructive mastery of reality.

The opposite form of danger in the social environment is what is spoken of as the "over-protective" situation. There are two kinds of over-protective environment. In the one, the over-protection may be reflected in actual over-indulgence of the individual. If this takes place in the crucial phases of personality maturation, it may weaken the personality, discourage growth and reinforce psychopathic conduct. In the other type of over-protective environment, alleged symbols of security and indulgence are offered to the individual, but they are false, and actually represent denial and disguise of a hostile rejection. In such instances, the over-protection is simply a device for the denial of hate.

For the healthy maturation of personality, a proper balance between environmental protection and the free opportunity to test out one's strength for dealing with and mastering new experience is a prime requisite. "Neurotic over-protection" smothers the growing personality. However camouflaged in its intentions such over-protection may be, it weakens and infantilizes the person.

Those forms of social danger which involve economic privation and frustration of basic human needs may exert their efforts on personality either directly or indirectly, or both. If such dangers are imposed on an individual during the crucial era of childhood, the child may suffer directly through actual want and may be harmed psychologically in an indirect way through the insecurity and defensive hostility reflected in the parental attitudes. At later stages in growth, the harm imposed on the individual through actual want and the corresponding psychological injury may be quite direct.

Social Environment, Healthy or "Sick"

It is thus evident that the understanding of human behavior and human relations, both healthy and sick, requires not only a concept of individual development, but a unitary concept of social organization as well. Psychiatrists are increasingly aware of the sociological implications of mental health problems. They are aware that the concept of "normal" behavior, based on the statistical average of behavior in our culture, is distinct from the psychiatrist's hypothesis of a "healthy" or "normal" personality. While practicing psychiatrists have a working concept of what is "normal" in human behavior, an ideal, if you like, of "normal" personality functioning, we tend, as a group, to be less cognizant of the need for criteria for an ideal of "normal" for social structure as well. Whether we admit it or not, in our everyday psychotherapeutic work with patients, we are continuously applying both an ideal of "normal" for the individual and "normal" for the social environment. This immediately makes explicit the emotionally-weighted and elusive problem of what constitutes a "normal" environment.

Here we enter unfamiliar territory, and the fear of what we do not yet know constrains us. A science of social psychopathology is still to be developed, though the beginnings of such a science are already evident. It is exactly at this point that we feel the need for tangible help from the fields of sociology, social psychology, and cultural anthropology. Scientific data from these specialized fields demonstrate that the qualitative content of mental illness varies with the character of the given culture. From one culture to another, the content of what is repressed in the developing personality varies and, parallel with this, the content of neuroses and psychoses varies. But in every society, the quantitative aspects of mental illness, both in frequency and intensity, are conditioned by the prevailing patterns of social organization and the corresponding forces of suppression of the individual.[5] It need hardly be said that this begins with the organization of the family group and the patterns of childrearing that characterize that group.

While the specificity of emotional disability is determined primarily by the internal dynamics of the personality, this inner balance itself is continuously affected from birth on by the vicissitudes of the social environment. In general, a nourishing, supportive environment tends to strengthen the integrative powers of the personality, provided the environment contains also a challenge to the maturing capacities of the personality; likewise, in general, a harsh, restrictive environment in the formative stages of personality tends to weaken those powers and thus indirectly undermines the individual's capacity for coping with conflict. In special circumstances, a harsh environment may mobilize in an adult, a higher potential of integrative powers, provided such capacities have been earlier induced by a favorable emotional environment. Psychodynamic considerations such as these are of immediate relevance to the critical problem which presses upon us all; namely, the defective control of aggression in individuals and between groups, which imminently threatens a new World War.

The Basis of Evidence for Concepts Concerning Society and Personality

All types of challenging questions may be raised regarding the scientific validity of the ideas herein suggested. The only suitable answer one can make at this stage is that many critical objections will be clearly justified. The evidence derived from psychiatry and the related sciences is by no means complete, but the only sensible approach is to test the adequacy of such hypotheses in the actual field of everyday psychiatric investigation and social living.

The evidence we do possess derives from several levels of experience: (1) experimental data collected in the fields of psychiatry, sociology, social psychology, social statistics, economic and cultural anthropology; (2) empirical data derived from clinical practice.

Research in the field of human behavior has demonstrated the difficulty of devising controlled experiments in the more limited traditional scientific sense. We do not yet have reliable methods for scientific

[5]The Committee statement on this point was questioned in that it may be true for a large number of mental illnesses but might not be true for all such illnesses.

validation of the laws of human behavior. While endeavoring to improve such methods, we must, for the present, rely largely on empirical data derived from the direct observation of personality function in the fields of psychiatry and psychotherapy.

In particular, the largest body of evidence on which the practicing psychiatrist relies is really empirical in nature. It comes from the accumulated body of experience based on observations in psychotherapeutic situations. The subjective reactions of suffering patients registered in such situations are widely accepted as clinical evidence. It must, of course, be plain to everyone that a psychiatrist treating a person struggling toward healthy living in this society is motivated by his own personal values; these are partly derived from his own position in society, and from his wisdom built up from his scientific training and empirical experience. Thus, empirically-derived evidence with a reasonable probability of correctness grows in importance when we attempt to translate knowledge of human behavior into social action.

Once more, it must be stressed that the application of such evidence in the social field is qualified by what are generally described as value judgments. Value judgments serve as the motivational base for the execution of social responsibility. They are the immediate incentive for social action. They represent the person's orientation to the organization of society, and its attitude toward human relations and welfare.

Concepts Concerning Mental Illness and Mental Health

This view of the fluidity of the interaction of the individual with society tends inevitably to broaden the concepts of mental illness and mental health. It necessitates a more elastic view of illness as a qualitative and quantitative deviation from a hypothetical norm of bio-social adaptation. Such a concept of mental illness differs from previous definitions in that the earlier tendency was to make a dichotomy between biological and social causation. Illnesses were either organic or functional. The biological and social components of causation were dissociated, whereas in the present concept these elements represent partial facets of a continuous unified process.

Social Psychiatry and Social Action

At the time of Robert Koch, it was enough for the medical researcher to locate the tubercule bacillus, to fixate it, stain it, study its morphology under the microscope. But soon it became imperative to study the environmental conditions under which the noxious agent could thrive. The pathologist became an ecologist and eventually a public health officer who, together with other public agents, strove to eliminate dust, dirt and darkness from the environment.

The frame of reference for psycho-social phenomena which we have given above would suggest that concepts of psychiatry should be broadened in the following directions:

1. Redefinition of the concept of mental illness, emphasizing those dynamic principles which pertain to the person's interaction with society.
2. Examination of the social factors which contribute to the causation of mental illness, and also influence its course and outcome.
3. Consideration of the dynamic processes in intra- and inter-group relations.
4. Consideration of the specific group-psychological phenomena which are relevant, in a positive sense, to community mental health.
5. The development of criteria for healthy and pathological patterns of social organization.
6. The development of criteria for social action, relevant to the promotion of individual and communal mental health.

Perhaps the most problematic aspect of this whole question is the implementation of such social-psychiatric concepts in the field of social action. The Committee on Social Issues has the conviction that social action, in this context, implies a conscious and deliberate wish to foster those social developments which could promote mental health on a community-wide scale.

Within all the reasonable limits appropriate to the status of our profession, we advocate those changes in social organization which have a positive relevance to the mental health of individuals and groups.

Specifically, we favor the most intensive study of the psycho-social factors influencing human welfare. We favor the application of psychiatric principles to all those problems which have to do with family welfare, child rearing, child and adult education, social and economic factors which influence the community status of individuals and families, intergroup tensions, civil rights and personal liberty.

The social crisis which confronts us today is menacing; we would surely be guilty of dereliction of duty did we not make a conscientious effort to apply whatever partial knowledge we now possess in the interests of counteracting social danger and promoting healthier being, both for individuals and groups.

This, in a true sense, carries psychiatry out of the hospitals and clinics and into the community.

P A R T   O N E

Psychiatry and Desegregation

2

PSYCHIATRIC ASPECTS OF SCHOOL DESEGREGATION

Editor's Note. **In 1957, three years after the United States Supreme Court rendered its momentous decision on school desegregation, GAP published the following document as *Report #37*, "Psychiatric Aspects of School Desegregation." A less technical condensation was issued in 1960 in order to enlarge the Report's usefulness to more categories of readers. In the abbreviated version, entitled "Emotional Aspects of School Desegregation *(Report #37A)*, references were added to several developments that had occurred during the three years that followed publication of the original Report, such as the crisis in Little Rock, the protracted shutting of schools in Prince Edward County, Virginia, and the early Negro student "sit-ins" in southern states.**

Since then so much has happened—and is taking place daily—in the accelerated struggle for civil rights in general, and for school desegregation in particular, that the question arises as to whether these publications are still timely. From the perspective of 1965, however, psychological principles discussed in the Report eight years ago do indeed seem applicable to the complex specifics of the current revolution in race relations.

The psychosocial change process of school desegregation is in motion throughout the nation—though at different stages in different locales—and is catalyzing change in the other forms of injustice that the myth of white supremacy also serves to maintain. Between the extremes of continuing official segregation (in some school districts in the South) and of full school integration, in attitude as well as behavior, intermediate stages of the process include: desegregation in policy but not in practice, *de facto* but non-legal desegregation (related to racial discrimination in housing, as in many cities in the North), and various gradations of token and partial school desegregation.

As pointed out in our Report, conflict, tension, non-compliance and even violence in a community can represent dynamic elements of the particular phase and tempo of the desegregation process it is undergoing. For example, in reaction to an increasingly effective and resolute non-violent Negro protest movement, joined in by whites from all parts of the country, there have been intensified acts of brutal repression of Negroes, of bombings and shootings by southern white extremists. But these acts in turn have increased public awareness and gained support

for federal legislative reform. Thus the use of dogs and electric cattle prods by Birmingham police against Negro protest marchers in 1963 probably hastened the Civil Rights Act of 1964. Similarly, the 1965 brutalities in Selma by local law enforcement authorities, and the murders there, accelerated the passage of the Voting Rights Bill.

There have been four major United States Civil Rights laws enacted since the 1954 decision: the Civil Rights Acts of 1957 and 1960, the omnibus Civil Rights Act of 1964, and the Voting Rights Bill of 1965. Although in our Report we emphasized the subjective difference between behavioral compliance with laws against discrimination and the dissolving of intergroup prejudice, we also recognized the psychological importance of law and of conflicting authorities (including conflict between local, state and federal authorities) in influencing the behavior and attitudes involved in desegregation. The actualities of school desegregation so far would seem to bear out not only that laws against discrimination are not enough to overcome it, but also that without these federal laws, as was said by Lewis and his co-authors*, "There could have been nothing.... This country is at least on the right course.... The law put it there."

Thus, in 1963, the United States Commission on Civil Rights reported that "the determination of most southern school boards to employ every contrivance to evade or avoid desegregation continues to thwart implementation of the School Desegregation Cases." In the school year 1964-65, according to the Southern Reporting Service, 2.14 per cent of the Negro pupils in the eleven southern states attended school with whites. Now, in the fall of 1965, the pace of desegregation in the south, as schools open, is increasing sharply, with more Negroes entering previously all-white schools than in all the eleven years since the Supreme Court Decision. This is due to provisions in Title VI of the Civil Rights Act of 1964 whereby school districts that refuse to comply with desegregation are not eligible for federal educational grants.

The effectiveness of this kind of leverage for compliance illustrates another point that was stressed in our Report: that mixtures and varied kinds of feelings and motives, some only indirectly related to race, underlie overt reactions to both segregation and desegregation.

In our Report we discounted efforts of the day to picture the southern Negro as contented with segregation; instead we related his relative voicelessness to his oppression and political subordination. By now his voice rings out unmistakably: "Freedom now," and "We shall overcome."

*Lewis, Anthony, and *The New York Times, Portrait of a Decade, The Second American Revolution* (New York: Random House, 1964).

Two hundred thousand Negroes, with many white companions, "spoke" by marching on Washington, D. C., in August, 1963, when President Kennedy praised them for the "deep fervor and quiet dignity" of their demonstration. Twenty-five thousand spoke out again through the five-day walk for freedom from Selma to Montgomery in March, 1965. But in addition to the language of non-violent protest, there is the angry message of the Black Muslims and black supremacists, whose aims are not integration but separation of the races. And in the slums of big cities in the North and West the Negro has also made himself heard through the fury, chaos and bloodshed of riots—as in Harlem, in the summer of 1964, and in the Watts district of Los Angeles, in the summer of 1965. In sharp contrast, though, has been the eloquence in action of Negro children and their parents when they have braved the frenzied hatred of a white segregationist mob to walk into a newly desegregated school. And, of crucial importance, an inconspicuous but powerful statement of purpose is being made, day after day, by the growing number of Negro youngsters who, without fanfare, are uneventfully going to school with white children.

Psychological aspects of various kinds of leadership, and of group process were discussed in our Report, in terms of their pivotal roles in shaping the nature and extent of change in Negro-white relations. Since then, as the Negro movement has grown so markedly in scope and power, additional types of organizations and patterns of leadership have come into being that reflect and give impetus to greater diversity within the movement, psychologically as well as politically.

Now, in the fall of 1965, we seem to have reached a turning point in the inter-racial readjustments in our national life, of which school desegregation is a part. This was expressed by President Johnson in his June, 1965, speech at Howard University; he stressed that the legal gains in civil rights of Negroes, achieved by federal legislation, are not enough to undo the consequences of their prolonged oppression, so that the next and more profound stage of the struggle must concern "not just equality as a right and a theory but equality as a fact and a result."

For the socioeconomic status of most Negro Americans is still far below that of the white population. In fact, paradoxically, while accelerated gains in civil rights have helped the emergence of a small Negro middle class, disproportionate poverty, unemployment, under-education and general under-privilege not only persist for the vast majority of Negroes but have even worsened. Due to the legacy of discrimination, for instance, they are largely limited to the unskilled jobs which are being wiped out by automation.

For great numbers of these Negroes, emotionally remote from Negro middle class advances, despair, frustration and racial bitterness are intensified by continuing disparities between the conditions of their lives and those of affluent "White America."† The urban Negro riots have been regarded as explosive expressions of these tensions, not only resulting from years of prejudice, but in turn re-enforcing racial antagonisms to some extent. Another factor in some hardening of anti-Negro feeling has been the so-called "white back-lash" reaction to stepped-up Negro pressure tactics for full equality. On the other hand, among large numbers of white people there has been a marked lessening of racial bias and for many, active participation in the common struggle to overcome its damage. Instances of improved communication, understanding and feelings of genuine warmth have become much more frequent between Negroes and whites.

Within this overall context, the process of school desegregation is also moving into another phase. For example, the Southern Education Reporting Service‡ announced a shift in its program, as of June, 1965, with the explanation that "some desegregation has taken place in every state in the South and the patterns of future compliance are fairly well established.... The agency will now focus its attention on creative experiments to improve education for the culturally disadvantaged in the 17 Southern and border states."

In the rest of the country, too, the focus is shifting from the issue of desegregating the schools as an end in itself to that of the quality of education that goes on within them. Dilemmas, such as how to decrease racial imbalance of schools in cities with Negro ghettos but still retain the value of neighborhood schooling, are complicated by prejudice and fraught with inter-racial tension. But there is also a marked upsurge of innovation and progress underway in improving the educational opportunity—and with it a better chance for healthy psychosocial development—of all children in America. September, 1965

†The federal anti-poverty program, with its job-retraining, pre-school education and many other components, is part of the current effort to correct causes of this unrest.

‡*Southern School News*, April, 1965.

PSYCHIATRIC ASPECTS OF SCHOOL DESEGREGATION*

I. INTRODUCTION

> *"A social revolution with profound implications for domestic accord and world leadership confronts this country today.*
>
> *"The problem involves the dramatic legal and social adjustments facing the South as a result of the Supreme Court decision that public school racial segregation laws are unconstitutional.*
>
> *"However, the tensions that have arisen in the region underscore the fact that the problem has national dimensions. And they show that the problem must be resolved in terms of the actions, attitudes and behavior of the entire country."*[1]

Desegregation is not merely a legal problem; it is also a social problem, an economic one, and above all, a psychological one. Were it not for the irrational fears and prejudice associated with it in the minds of many Americans both in the North and in the South, the legal, economic, and social difficulties accompanying admission of Negroes to full equality of citizenship would be possible of solution. In approaching this particular problem, however, cooperative efforts at arriving at a solution are handicapped by the violent feelings which are involved.

This report is written for the purpose of discussing some of the psychological aspects of desegregation with special attention to the problems of adjustment for both races in the hope that better understanding will facilitate use of our intellectual and social skills in their solution. We cannot hope to speak with equal clarity and relevant detail to all those who are involved in this big social undertaking. Because of our own specialized professional training and experience, it seems appropriate to address ourselves primarily to

---

*Formulated by the Committee on Social Issues, and first published as Report #37, in May, 1957.

[1]*New York Times*, March 13, 1956, Article by John N. Popham.

those who have professional responsibility for carrying out the Supreme Court's decision—the educators, counselors, social workers, psychologists, and administrators of the schools. More specifically, we are writing this report mainly for those members of these professions of whom we can assume familiarity with psychological concepts and their assimilation into practice. We hope that psychiatrists and other physicians in communities that are struggling with the emotional and practical problems attendant upon desegregation will also read and make use of this report. Those parents who have been roused by the present critical issue to reconsider their own attitudes and to decide how they will participate with the schools may also find it useful.

Emphasis on psychiatric principles

In general, our emphasis will be on relevant psychiatric principles rather than on their practical application. We leave that task to those of our readers who are better qualified for it by virtue of their direct on-the-job contact with the concrete situations to be met. Nor is this a report of a research study. It represents, rather, the pooled experience of an interracial group of psychiatrists from different parts of the country, aided by consultant social scientists, who have worked over the years in a variety of ways in the general area of intergroup relations.[2]

---

[2]*The members of the Committee wish to express their great indebtedness to Drs. Stuart Cook, Marie Jahoda, and Fritz Redl who, as consultants, have been full participants with the group in preparing this report. Our thanks are also due to Dr. Gordon Hamilton and to Dr. Robert Johnson whom we have consulted during the course of the work.*

Most of the members of the Committee preparing this report have treated both Negro and white patients from both the North and South by psychoanalysis and psychotherapy. Many have served as psychiatric consultants to interracial clinics, social agencies, and educational institutions. Dr. Lief, with assistance from Drs. Stevens and Handler, is engaged in an inter-disciplinary research study at Tulane University of Negro personality structure in New Orleans, and a follow-up study of "Children of Bondage." Dr. Babcock, while on the staff of the Chicago Institute for Psychoanalysis, was a member of a multidiscipline group which studied problems of a minority group (Japanese Americans) in the process of acculturation. Other Committee members and consultants have participated in various research projects involving race relations.

Publications in this general field by the authors of this Report include: Ackerman, "The Psychology of Prejudice," presented at the New York Academy of Medicine, November 18, 1954; Ackerman and Jahoda, *Antisemitism and Emotional Disorder*, Harper & Bros., 1950; Jahoda is also co-author with Cook and Deutsch of a two-volume work, *Research Methods in Social Relations with Especial Reference to Prejudice.* The Dryden Press, 1951; Cook is co-author with Wilner

In our view psychiatry concerns itself with the study of all human behavior, not merely with the study and treatment of the maladjusted. Such activities as community psychiatry and preventive psychiatry must be based upon knowledge of normal human development and behavior.

Before undertaking this report the authors assigned themselves to study certain desegregating situations for preparatory orientation; in a few cases the preparation was carried out as part of a systematic research project.[3]

Desegregation as a process

School segregation has been declared illegal throughout the country. There is thus no question of whether or not desegregation will occur. It is already occurring. The authors of the report are in general agreement as to the wisdom and justice of discontinuing segregation practices of all kinds in this country. What we observe in various parts of the country are different stages in the occurrence of desegregation. In some communities changes have already taken place and the population is in the process of adapting itself to the new circumstances. More than 300,000 Negro children who form-

[3]Several Committee members interviewed school officials in the South. Others held discussions with teachers and principals and observed in a newly desegregated school in a Northern suburb. One member worked with groups of Washington, D.C. school teachers on classroom problems during the change to desegregation. Another member studied the group processes and activities of school authorities and parent-teacher groups in a Maryland county. Two members studied attitudes and reactions in Hoxie, Arkansas after protests arose against recently started desegregation; Marie Jahoda, of the Research Center for Human Relations, New York University, designed and directed a study on "The Status of the Public School Education of Negro and Puerto Rican Children in New York City" for the Public Education Association which reported on it in October 1955 to the Board of Education Commission on Integration. S. W. Cook presented his Presidential Address to the New York State Psychological Association on January 28, 1956 on "Desegregation: A Psychological Analysis."

and Walkley of *Human Relations in Interracial Housing: A Study of the Contact Hypothesis*, University of Minnesota Press, 1955; Bernard, "Psychoanalysis and Members of Minority Groups," *Journal American Psychoanalytic Association*, Vol. 1, #2, April 1953, and "Some Psychodynamic Aspects of Desegregation," *American Journal of Orthopsychiatry*, Vol. 26, #2, p. 256, July 1956; Marmor, 4 case studies, in *Psychotherapy and Culture Conflict*, Georgene Seward, Ronald Press, 1956; McLean, "Psychodynamic Factors in Race Relations," *Annals American Academy Political and Social Science*, 244; 159-166, 1946; Redl co-author with David Wineman, *Children Who Hate*, Free Press, 1951 and *Controls from Within*, Free Press, 1952; Stevens' "Interracial Practices in Mental Hospitals," *Mental Hygiene*, Vol. 36, #1, 1952; Stevenson, "A Psychiatrist Looks At Segregation," *New Republic*, Vol. 134, p. 22, 1956.

erly attended segregated schools have already entered mixed classes or have become eligible to do so since the Supreme Court decision.[4] Since Negro children are usually in the minority in desegregating schools, several times that many white children have therefore recently had their first contacts with Negroes in school. In communities where the changes are still seen as remote, or even impossible, adjustments nevertheless are being made to the new situation created by the Supreme Court's decision. Even in their opposition to desegregation, members of some communities may actually be working through one phase of the whole process. Thus, much of what will be said in the following pages should be considered in relation to the fact that different communities have different problems created by the particular stages of desegregation through which they are passing.

Many social changes in Negro-white relations had occurred in this country before the Supreme Court's decisions on segregation. In many areas trends toward "voluntary" desegregation had appeared. State and local anti-segregation legislation of various kinds had been enacted throughout sections of the North. Negroes were asserting their rights as a group. For many years they had largely followed the advice of Booker T. Washington to advance themselves individually, but not as a group. Referring to his address in 1884 before the National Educational Association, Washington writes: ". . . I said that any individual who . . . learned to do a common thing in an uncommon manner had solved his problem, regardless of the colour of his skin. . . . That the whole future of the Negro rested largely upon the question as to whether or not he should make himself, through his skill, intelligence and character, of such undeniable value to the community in which he lived that the community could not dispense with his presence. . . ."[5] Negroes came to learn that this wisdom was compatible with efforts for group betterment and were increasingly helping each other toward the equality of opportunity to which they felt entitled. Meanwhile, among a growing proportion of the nation's white population, opposition to segregation was gaining strength. Thus it happened that the Supreme Court's decision voiced a trend as much as it caused one. It hastened the march of events by accelerating processes which began long ago.

[4] *Southern School News*, September, 1956. *New York Times*, October 1, 1956.

[5] Washington, Booker T. *Up From Slavery*, Bantam Books, Inc., New York, 1956. Copyright 1901, Doubleday & Co. p. 142.

There is undeniably strong personal involvement on the part of those favoring and opposing desegregation. One index, although by no means the only one, to the significance of the subject of desegregation is provided by the strength of feelings aroused by the issue. What seems to an objective observer to be the immediate realistic personal interests of an involved individual may be sacrificed irrationally in the service of one or another position on the issue. Some have taken strong stands for desegregation even when this incurred economic sanctions and ensuing hardships. Conversely, others have openly defied the laws and thereby risked arrest and punishment. Moreover, people everywhere are aroused to the strongest emotions when the matter is discussed. The heat which has been engendered is not a simple, rational reaction to the desegregation issue. As usually happens with social issues, a single "cause" has served as a focus and rallying point for many kinds of grievances. These range from states' rights and the relative economic deprivation of the South, through a gamut of actual or fancied personal, social, and political inequities.

On the other hand, it would be in error to regard desegregation as a purely sectional issue with uniform sectional attitudes. Laws and customs affecting racial relationships vary in different parts of the country. But the basic issue of equal rights for Negroes and whites exists everywhere, although the related local problems to be solved vary in kind and in urgency. To speak of a Southern attitude as against a Northern attitude is incorrect. Anti-Negro discrimination and prejudice of course exist among northerners, and there are many segregated schools in the North.[6] In the South there are many elements with many opinions. Among those opposed to desegregation there are many different degrees of opposition. And opponents of desegregation form only a portion of the Southern communities. Many white people in the South favor desegregation, though they may vary in how openly they express this. Southern Negroes, even though not always so acknowledged, comprise a big part of the Southern citizenry, largely in favor of desegregation. Therefore, Negro sentiment about desegregation must be included in any assessment of Southern opinion on the subject. As the late President

[6]In some northern areas where public school segregation is prohibited by law, *de facto* school segregation persists nonetheless—linked to segregated housing patterns or sometimes covertly maintained by gerrymandering. As desegregation and integration progress and become more general, it is to be expected that these problems in the North will command greater attention from both Negro and white people.

of Fisk University has said: "Of all the voices raised in this crisis the one most ignored has been that of the Southern Negro."[7] Similarly, communities throughout the rest of the nation are composed of a number of different subgroups with differing attitudes and behavior with regard to desegregation.

Psychosocial ills arising from segregation

What are the psychosocial ills springing from the maintenance of segregation in the United States? They can be considered on three levels: that of the individual, that of the community group and its institutions, and that of the country as a whole.

The individual. Wherever segregation occurs, one group, in this instance the Negroes, always suffers from inferior social status. The damaging effects of this are reflected in unrealistic inferiority feelings, a sense of humiliation, and constriction of potentialities for self-development. This often results in a pattern of self-hatred and rejection of one's own group, sometimes expressed by antisocial action toward one's own group or the dominant group. These attitudes seriously affect the levels of aspiration, the capacity to learn, and the capacity to relate in interpersonal situations.[8]

For the segregating group, in this case the whites, the reactions, though less obvious, are nonetheless serious. A feeling of superior personal worth may be gained merely from the existence of a downgraded group. This leads to an unrealistic and unadaptive kind of self-appraisal based on invidious comparison rather than on solid personal growth and achievement. Further, socially sanctioned segregation is based on unproven concepts of superiority and permits and even encourages the expression of hostile or aggressive feelings against whole groups of people. It fosters a distortion of reality and provides a target in the lower status group for the projection of painful feelings from one's self or from significant people

---

[7]Charles S. Johnson, "A Southern Negro's View of the South," *New York Times Magazine*, September 23, 1956.

[8](A). Appendix to Appellant's Briefs "The Effects of Segregation and the Consequences of Desegregation: A Social Science Statement" (United States Supreme Court, October 1952).

(B). Davis, Allison and Dollard, John, *Children of Bondage*, American Council on Education, Washington, D.C., 1940.

(C). Myrdal, Gunnar, *An American Dilemma*, Harper & Bros., New York, 1944.

(D). McLean, *op. cit.*, 159-166.

(E). Kardiner, Abram and Ovesey, Lionel, *The Mark of Oppression*, W. W. Norton & Co., New York, 1951.

in the immediate environment onto the members of the segregated group. Anxiety springing from unrelated personal problems may thus be combatted by inappropriate displacement of the conflictful feelings to the area of race relations. Such displacement impedes more direct and mature facing and dealing with the actual anxiety-arousing conflicts.

The community. The social circumstances from which segregation developed produce a vicious cycle. The cultural consequences of segregation in turn serve to maintain segregation. Thus, the institution of separate schools for Negroes is both an expression of their lower cultural status and a factor in further depressing their economic and educational level as compared to whites.[9] Similarly, such aspects of social disorganization as high disease and death rates, some types of crime and delinquency, poor housing, substandard living conditions, and disrupted or poorly organized family life are directly related to segregation, lack of social prestige, and restriction of educational and economic opportunities.

These social ills, however, do not remain confined to the segregated segment of a population; they inevitably lower the level of well-being for the community as a whole. For example, where a local government must provide duplicate sets of "separate but equal" health, welfare, and educational services, the budget for each must be lowered by the expense of the other. If disease-conducive housing and poor health services lead to high rates of communicable disease among a town's Negroes, the white group is jeopardized as well since contact between social unequals, such as menial and boss, is just as infectious as between schoolmates. Contagiousness does not discriminate. Furthermore, segregation limits communication between the two groups. Rigid stereotypes are thus perpetuated and may promote a social climate leading to violent outbreaks of racial tension. Although some transitional intensification of racial tension is to be expected in certain quarters from the change to desegregation, it seems socially safer, in the long run, to undergo some rela-

[9]The Supreme Court decision cites evidence that schools which require racial separation cannot be equal, psychologically. Educational inferiority of facilities for most Negro schools as compared to white schools in the same locality is widely recognized. Evidence may be found in *The Negro and the Schools*, by Harry S. Ashmore, University of South Carolina Press, 1954, and "The Status of the Public School Education of Negro and Puerto Rican Children in New York City," October 1955, presented to the Board of Education Commission on Integration; prepared by the Public Education Association, assisted by the New York University Research Center for Human Relations.

tively limited and temporary stress than to endure a chronic state of widespread racial tension. It is important, of course, that the community use all possible means to circumscribe and reduce such stress reactions as they arise so as to prevent their extension and secondary complications.

The country. For the country as a whole, the existence of segregation as an unsolved conflict leads to a chronic state of tension. The consequent ill feeling and disunity drain off energies that might otherwise be applied to more constructive activities, both at home and abroad. The situation resembles that of a person in the throes of a neurotic conflict who is consequently hampered in productive living. In a psychiatric sense, the existence of segregation entails disintegration for the nation. The existence of a large proportion of our population in an economically, educationally, and socially underdeveloped state robs the country as a whole of a substantial part of its human resources.[10] And segregation looms large in other countries' view of the United States. It is extremely damaging to our prestige and friendships abroad, especially among the non-white people of the world.

Yet it would be a serious error to suppose that the only emotional forces between white and Negro in our country are hostile ones. There are also very strong positive attachments between the members of the two races. The fostering of such attachments may eventually release energy now wasted in conflict for use in the betterment of both races.

Attitudes not necessarily pathological

To conceive of segregation as pathogenic—that is, contributing to maladjustment—is by no means to imply that all those who believe in and advocate segregation are themselves maladjusted or otherwise psychiatrically abnormal. Obviously, many persons in the United States who are free from psychiatric disorders strongly favor segregation for many kinds of reasons. These range from desires for economic and political power, to sincere conviction that continued segregation is the soundest solution to the problem of Negro-white relations. There are also people who manipulate forces for segregation, not from conviction, but for deliberately calculated

[10]Ginzberg, Eli, Anderson, James K., Bray, Douglas W. and Smuts, Robert W., *The Negro Potential*, Columbia University Press, New York, 1956.
Plant, Richard L., "Blueprint for Talent Searching," National Scholarship Service and Fund for Negro Students, New York, 1957.

reasons of material gain. The approach to such motivations is outside the reach of this report. When pro-segregation opinion is based on reasoning and experience, it is up to the integrationist to show why such conclusions are in error, and to point out how some inevitable short-term stresses occurring in the transition from segregation to desegregation should not be taken as evidence against the social feasibility or desirability of desegregation in the long run. It has been demonstrated that continuance of segregation creates more social ills than it cures.[11] If such evidence can be brought to the attention of the socially-minded segregationists, it should help to modify some opinions which are not too fixed by emotional conflicts and early conditioning.

However, there is in all of us an element of the irrational. We continue as adults to hold to the prejudices with which we have been raised, and we resort to them with increased intensity under certain sets of psychological conditions. This report will discuss such psychiatric aspects of prejudice in a later section.

Finally, there are a certain number of maladjusted, seriously insecure or anxiety-ridden people who are much more completely in the grip of prejudiced thinking than the average, and who need to retain their prejudices to serve as defenses against their own inner feelings of lack of worth. From this group, on the whole, come the more irrational and violent denunciations and threats regarding the consequences of desegregation. From a psychiatric point of view, the prejudiced attitudes of this group of segregationists reflect emotional disorder, for which the most appropriate remedy would be psychotherapy.

While the existence of prejudice may be a symptom of emotional disorder and should then be treated as such, our main emphasis in this report is rather on what contributions the dynamic understanding of behavior—of individuals and groups—can make to desegregation as a part of daily living. In this context it is well to point out that desegregation problems are by no means confined to Negro-white relationships. In many regions of the country parts of the population are endeavoring to integrate with other groups in school and community living, as in California with Asians and Mexicans, or

[11]Perhaps not since the Declaration of Independence has a public federal document stressed the importance of personal feelings as an item of political consideration. The Supreme Court decision was in part based on personal, psychological, and sociological data showing that segregation constitutes a psychological and personal handicap.

in Alaska with Eskimos. In some such situations language differences provide an additional handicap.[12] Our other main point of emphasis will be the discussion of the difficulties standing in the way of solution of such problems, together with some consideration of possible psychiatric contributions to dealing with them.

Throughout this report we address ourselves to two different kinds of attitudinal situations, with respect to public school desegregation. In order to avoid confusion it seems desirable that the distinction be made explicit. On the one hand, where desegregation has not yet begun, we attempt to analyze some of the psychological barriers and how they may be reduced, in order that desegregation can get underway. In such communities, where actual experience with racially mixed public schooling is lacking, the reactions that stir the Negro and white residents so deeply are essentially anticipatory. On the other hand, in those situations where school desegregation has been started, although at different rates and in different ways, our focus is on the psychological problems that arise in the carrying out of such programs, and on their resolution. In these circumstances, the reactions of Negroes and whites are essentially influenced by their actual experience with some form of school desegregation.

Both sets of reactions—to the prospect of desegregation and to its actual occurrence—affect each other, however, and may be conceived of as really stages of a single process. For fearful and unrealistic anticipation, carried over into the new experience of school desegregation, accounts for many of the psychological problems that arise among children and adults of both races when desegregation actually begins. And conversely, initial expectations can be altered by intergroup experience in the preparatory stages even before any classroom integration has started. This is evident in those Southern communities which have decided to comply with the

[12]A fellow-member of GAP, Dr. Bryant Wedge of Yale University recalls his observations, a few years ago, of the educational mixing of races in Hawaii. "There, at all levels of education, from nursery school through the university, and from the smallest country school to the fanciest private school, there existed no racial bar of any kind. The classes were mixed in most of the schools, with Caucasians, Japanese, Hawaiians and part-Hawaiians, Chinese, Filipinos, East Indians, and a few Negroes. I had considerable experience with some of these schools, both on the public school and university level, in both of which I lectured, and I can unequivocally say that the general level of school mental health compared favorably with that in any uni-racially populated school system with which I have had acquaintance."

Court's decision but where local opinion has been too divided for agreement on how and when to start. In such localities, the pre-desegregation activities of organizations, individuals, special interest groups, and official bodies—thrown into new and intensive forms of intergroup contact—bring about psychological movement within the participants as they push and strive to fuse a school integration program out of the heat and struggle of active social process. This psychological movement is a vital step in desegregation itself.

We shall largely limit our discussion of desegregation to those aspects which involve the roles white and Negro persons adopt toward each other and toward members of their own groups. This means that many other areas of desegregation in general and many other important topics in the lives of Negroes and white persons which are indirectly, although perhaps significantly, affected by desegregration, must be neglected entirely or mentioned only in passing.

II. PSYCHODYNAMICS OF RESPONSES TO DESEGREGATION

A. Functions of Racial Myths and Prejudices

To better understand the problems of adjustment to desegregation which confront previously segregated white and Negro persons, it is helpful to examine some of the implications of their having lived under conditions of enforced segregation. People bring with them to the desegregation experience many beliefs and feelings that are, in part, a consequence of the type of society in which they have spent their childhoods and in which they have formed the social relationships that characterize their adult lives. Some of these beliefs and feelings are related to the real social and economic differences between Negroes and whites which have prevailed in the previously segregated community. Others are associated with the racial myths that have grown up under such conditions.

In dealing with Negroes, white Americans by and large react as an in-group to an out-group; a mythology has sprung up to rationalize and justify disparaging attitudes which, in turn, are derived from diverse sources not clearly recognized and understood. Such myths are not limited to beliefs about Negroes. For instance there are the beliefs that all French are lascivious, all Englishmen are stuffed shirts, all Jews are greedy for money, and all Scots are misers, or, from the point of view of a European, all Americans are immature. Perhaps some Americans displace on to the race issue, or the stranger, an indirect protest (which they would be ashamed to acknowledge openly even to themselves) against what they misinterpret as a requirement of democratic culture, i.e., that they must make friends equally with all neighbors, classmates, etc. on that basis alone, regardless of whether they have anything in common or not. Such people need reassurance that, of course, the choice of personal friendships is consistent with the democratic form of living, but that the selection does not depend on racial but on other qualities.

Myths as a defense

In the developmental history of the individual, and in the history of groups and larger social entities, conflictful and highly complicated situations occur which may appear insoluble. As these threaten individual or group security, they create anxiety. They then stimulate defensive reactions intended to diminish the anxiety. One common type of defensive reaction is myth formation. In the psychic economy a myth provides an apparently rational answer to an apparently insoluble problem. Such myths are maintained without regard to any demonstrable validity. Resisting change, they have deep roots in individual childhood experience and are sustained by ongoing social and economic forces.

It is a commonly observed fact, both in the psychiatric consulting room and in daily life, that a person's prejudiced attitudes and their accompanying myths may fluctuate in degree of belief and in emotional intensity with his level of anxiety, latent or overt. During times of ease or inner peace, prejudices lie quiescent, only to burst forth with renewed intensity when security is disturbed. There are many sources of anxiety, both in the individual and in the group: a feeling of helplessness, of conflict, of not knowing how to go about solving a problem, or being unable either to approach the problem because of inner defenses which forbid it, or even to acknowledge the existence of a problem because of still deeper defensive reactions.

In terms of racial myths, the Negro is often depicted as little better than a savage animal, intellectually and morally inferior, childish and irresponsible, and supposedly unable to control allegedly excessive sexual and aggressive impulses.

Effect on Negro-white relationships

These concepts both originate in and secondarily give rise to fears which then affect the relationship between Negroes and whites on three main levels. First, they affect the structure and arrangements for intergroup living with all the attendant socio-economic and political realities that these entail. Second, they enter into the dealings with each other in one-to-one relationships. Thirdly, they affect the thoughts and feelings experienced by individuals.

Group relationships. Enforced segregation of Negro and white Americans has been accompanied by a generally recognized difference in the social status of the two groups. Merely by reason of his membership in the white group, an individual is accorded certain social privileges, and experiences the sense of being "better" or higher class. Conversely, by mere reason of membership in (or assignment to) the Negro group, one is deprived of these privileges and experiences the sense of being "second class."

This is of particular interest as it relates to the other sources of social status within the community. For example, a highly educated Negro, accustomed to the respect of the Negro section of his community, must at times show deference on the basis of color alone to white persons who in other ways are socially inferior to him. By contrast, the white person with no special grounds for meriting the respect of his fellows other than his skin color, may still experience a sense of heightened worth in his interaction with Negroes. This is really a pseudo-feeling for the white, and there is no depth or security in it since neither the deference of the Negro nor his own superiority are entirely believable.

This difference in social status is paralleled by differences in political power and economic status, although the economic disparity is now less than it was in the past. Negroes have constituted a source of low-paid unskilled labor of particular importance in farming, domestic service, and industry. Often the use of this labor has had beneficial effects on the living standards of the white employing group. Also because, as employer or foreman (and sometimes as unskilled strawboss), the white person typically has supervised the work of Negroes, there has been a second consequence of the economic relationship: it has augmented the difference in social status. Similarly, racial mythology supports and is supported by political subordination of Negroes. Curtailment of their right to vote and the related exclusion from elective and other governmental positions of authority is rationalized by the stereotype of the inferior Negro. Their consequent inferior share of political power then helps to perpetuate the conception of their inferiority. Such a relationship between a myth and the social reality has been aptly termed by Merton "a self-fulfilling prophecy."[1]

As a result of these differences in social, economic, and political status, the white members of our segregated society have filled practically all of the positions of leadership. To the extent that such positions bring to their occupants the social approval of their fel-

[1]Merton, Robert K., *Social Theory and Social Structures;* Chapter 7, "The Self-Fulfilling Prophecy," Free Press, Glencoe, Ill., p. 179.

lows and confer upon them a degree of social influence they might not otherwise have, this feature of enforced segregation becomes still another source of either self-esteem or, conversely its deprivation.

Interpersonal relationships. In one-to-one relationships between Negroes and whites certain roles are implied by the components of the myth. The Negro person should be fun-loving, improvident, deferential, deeply loyal, dependent, fearful toward whites, and capable of hard physical labor with little need for rest or relaxation. (In certain versions of the myth, this entails obligations on the part of the white person analogous to caring for beloved pets or useful farm animals). Conversely, the white person should enjoy pleasure but not love it, plan for the future, accept the role of leader, be independent and unafraid, and utilize Negroes for hard labor and menial tasks.

Because in fact, as contrasted to the myth, Negroes are human, possessing the same potentialities and capacities as do whites, and experiencing the same basic emotional needs and reactions, such a relationship is inherently strained. In order to maintain it without gross disharmony or open conflict, certain psychological adjustments on the part of both the Negro person and the white person are required. The Negro is expected to repress his drives toward self-realization and development, and the white must either force the Negro to continue in the mythical roles through implicit or explicit threats and punishments, or make it attractive for him to do so by offering such advantages as freedom from responsibility at the price of low status, and paternalistic protectiveness in exchange for dependent servility. Some of the types of accommodation to this situation are well known: the benevolent master, the overseer, the Negro mistress, the Uncle Tom figure, the Negro who steps off the sidewalk to let the white man pass, expresses humble gratitude for discarded clothing, expects to be addressed by a first name, not necessarily his own, and to reply with such titles of respect as Sir, Captain, or Mister.

No matter how well Negro-white relationships may appear to function in the context of the myth, beneath the apparent compliance and conformity are anger, resentment, and fear which are defended against by such unconscious psychological mechanisms as reaction formation, denial, somatization, and projection. In settings where the myth is most firmly believed, relationships are role-stereotyped and thus minimally expressive of genuine feelings or perception, taking on aspects of ritual. Even in relationships between Negroes and whites where the myth is consciously rejected, there are often subtle anxious elements inhibiting genuine closeness and acceptance. Perhaps the myths must be destroyed before interpersonal relationships between Negroes and whites will be possible on the same terms as those of Negroes with Negroes and whites with whites. This should not imply, of course, that various forms of status difference and social role, with their own psychodynamic implications, are not part of Negro-Negro and white-white relations.

Intrapsychic processes. On the deepest personal level, prejudices and their supporting myths can be understood as a means of maintaining feelings of self-esteem and security. In this sense they serve a defensive function. Many people of any race have acute doubts about their own worth, their adequacy in their sexual roles, and their acceptability as members of their groups. Turning attention to others' deficiencies permits one to remove the focus from fears and misgivings about oneself. Relief from intolerable feelings of self-contempt may be sought unconsciously by turning the hatred away from the despised part of oneself onto another person or group who, by the distortion of racial mythology, can represent the bad self. A down-graded minority, then, can become the source of a somewhat illusory security about oneself . . . the basis that "I am better than they are. . . ." But guilt feelings with associated anxiety are a frequent price for whatever psychological gains may come from such defensive dealing with inner conflicts. The use of the myth as a defense against insecurity, therefore, is self-defeating for it not only fails to reach a realistic solution of the original difficulty but also increases the original burden of guilt. The well-known vicious circle of anxiety, defense, increased anxiety, and increased defensiveness may then ensue.

It is an often unrecognized fact that the Negro may come to believe in the prejudicial myths about him and frequently be as unaware as the white person that he is reacting defensively to inner impulses in an irrational, self-destructive manner. If a child is repeatedly addressed or treated as if he were no better than a dirty, savage, stupid animal, he will accordingly react either in conformance with this belief or develop psychological defenses against it. In this way a group that is discriminated against can develop a devalued concept of itself as inferior to the dominant group (which frequently stands for parental authority). This explains the reaction of some Negroes who feel dirty because of their skin color, who feel dependent on the good graces of the white parental authority figures, and who are disturbed by attempts of Negro leaders to gain full adult democratic privileges for them. (Such anti-Negro feelings by Negroes also entail guilt feelings that set up psychological vicious circles).

Through lifelong association of specific meanings to certain colors, there is an automatic tendency to impute to those presenting a particular color, psychological qualities which they may or may not possess. These imputed qualities then serve as a very unreliable basis of evaluation and action. The emotional content of reactions to color differences are patterned differently in different cultures, and within our own culture vary with emotional conditioning within particular subgroups.

Some knowledge of the meanings of different skin colors in our society is helpful in understanding the division of concepts regarding Negro and white. For example, several studies carried out in this country[2] have indicated that most small children of both groups preferred light dolls to dark ones, even though there is little or no antagonism discernible toward the dark ones. Attractiveness was often associated with the light dolls, and ugliness or dirtiness with the dark ones.

Skin contacts form an essential part of the important relationships from infancy through childhood, and a variety of emotional attitudes come to be associated with particular colors, forms, and textures of the skin. Dunbar[3] describes several studies of blushing and other skin reactions which elicit specific emotional responses in interpersonal relationships. Some psychoanalytic studies show that many persons equate roughness and darkness of the skin with "wrong" or with "masculinity," while smoothness and whiteness of the skin are equated, in fantasies, with "right" or with "femininity."[4]

---

[2]Goodman, Mary E., *Race Awareness in Young Children*, Addison-Wesley, Cambridge, Mass., 1952.

Clark, Kenneth B. and Mamie P., "Racial Identification and Preference of Negro Children." In T. M. Wentworth and E. L. Hartley (eds.), *Readings in Social Psychology*, Holt, New York, 1947, 169-178.

[3]Dunbar, Flanders, *Emotions and Bodily Changes*, Columbia University Press, New York, 3rd Ed.

[4]Deutsch, Felix and Nadell, Raymond, "Psychosomatic Aspects of Dermatology with Special Consideration of Allergic Phenomena," *The Nervous Child*, Vol. 5, No. 4, October 1946.

In this culture, yellow, brown, or black tend to be associated with ideas of dirtiness or destructiveness or unpleasant smell, while light colors, especially white and pink, tend to be associated with ideas of cleanliness, purity, innocence, and chastity. Since the skin and its extensions—the hair and nails—cloak the entire body, it becomes that part of a person most quickly accessible to superficial perception and evaluation. Consequently, the association of particular meanings to certain colors and textures of skin often determines the manner in which one person relates to another. It would seem that negative associations to their skin color combine with the other reasons we have considered so far in accounting for the disesteem of Negroes in this country. That it cannot be the sole factor is shown, for instance, by the high social value placed on sun tan by many white people.

Negroes are often as frightened by the mythical image of the dirty, sexually aggressive Negro as many a white person and may become severely restricted and inhibited in their development as adults.[5] Psychiatrists and social scientists are aware that Negroes develop their own hierarchies of status based on how close skin color approaches white and how close social and sexual customs approach the supposed white middle-class standards. It is well known how much money and time many Negroes feel driven to spend on cosmetics, deodorants, clothes, and automobiles in efforts to break away from the destructive, devaluing self-concept which they have developed as the result of childhood guilt and shame. Paradoxically, even this is used as propaganda against them. The complaint is voiced that they have become "uppity," that they do not know their place. Even some Negro leaders preach against these attempts to secure some measure of comparable status. However, such upwardly-mobile efforts are not only a defense against the negative Negro myth; they also express a positive effort toward social participation. The extra intensity of pressure toward this particular form of participation by Negroes stems from the fact that so many other channels which are open to the white population are closed to them.

Fears related to sex

Processes of desegregation are complicated and handicapped by widespread fears of the breaking down of traditional barriers

[5]Kardiner and Ovesey, *op. cit.*

against sexual relationships between the two groups. We have been examining the significance of racial mythology and prejudice to desegregation. Unrealistic emotions and fantasies also abound in the many conflict areas of psychosexual development and sex relations in general in our culture, quite aside from questions of race. We can therefore appreciate how acutely emotional intensity can be compounded by interconnections between these two myth-laden areas, sex relations and race relations.

In general our attitudes towards sexuality are split; sex represents the culmination of love and tenderness, but because it is also regarded in our society as dirty and degraded, it may be used as an avenue for the expression of aggressive defiling and retaliative impulses as well. By those who look upon another group as inferior or exploitative, sex relations with members of that group are felt to express aggression rather than love.

A higher social status group commonly stereotypes a lower status group as sexually more violently primitive. This holds true for group relationships other than Negro-white, as between various class levels, for instance. Such an attitude towards members of the lower-status group is closely linked to attributing greater sexual prowess to them. Thus, according to a prevailing sort of folklore, all Negro males are thought of as extremely potent and Negro females as invariably responsive. This is unsupported by fact.

The fusion of the misconception of superior sexual potency with notions of the primitive aggressive nature also imputed to the Negro makes for a myth which has become tenaciously woven—and with formidable repercussions—into the fantasy life surrounding sex in our culture. The upbringing of every American child and the process of maturation include the conflictual tasks of harmonizing sexual and aggressive drives with social prohibitions. This always involves some repression and relinquishment of strong childhood wishes and direct forms of impulse release. How completely and in what ways individuals accomplish this—regardless of race—is highly variable, depending on complex psychological and social interacting factors within their specific life experience. Residuals of these basic sexual and aggressive conflicts persist in adulthood in varying degrees as conscious or unconscious fantasies with their related anxieties and defenses.

As a part of such sexual fantasy-life, the myth of the primitively aggressive, potency-excelling Negro is central to the attitudes and emotions surrounding interracial sex relations. It provides a focus for displacement through which old repressed urges may seek covert fantasy expression, while the terror of unleashing all that was learned as bad, forbidden, and disastrous, demands even stronger defensive taboos. When dominated by such fantasies, it is understandable why interracial sex relations, for both the Negro and white person, are more expressive of hostility than tenderness.

The pattern of segregation, through suppression of all aspects of mature social interaction between Negroes and whites, does much to create the very results its fearful proponents suppose it can ward off: it converts interracial relationships into just the kind of immoral, prohibited wrongdoing that seems to carry out the fantasies so that more guilt results, for which even stronger intergroup barricades are sought.

Unacknowledged white male jealousy of the Negro male's fantasied advantage as a sexual rival for the white female is an emotional source of power behind the extreme taboo, maintained by the white-supremacy code, ostensibly to protect white womanhood. This code sanctions the most savage reprisals for Negro male violation, or even the most realistically flimsy suspicion of it, as in the Emmett Till "wolf whistle" case. The irrational emotionality of a lynch mob reveals the terrible antisocial power of racial myth. The white-supremacy code also provides immunity to the white male from Negro resistance or retaliation for the white's sexual freedom with Negro females. And so, fear and hate, founded and maintained by racial sex mythology, breeds ever more fear and hate within members of both races.

The stereotype of the sexual Negro which we have been describing has entered deeply into the emotions of many people, especially among Southern whites, to form a psychological barrier against Negroes; this is so strong that it would outlast any sudden removal of the physical barriers of segregation. To such people this image of the Negro has intense psychological reality, although in objective reality it is groundless. This subjective reality is all the harder to correct because certain surface facts do seem to make it agree with objective reality.

From psychiatric experience and delinquency studies there is reason to believe that antisocial, precocious, and impulsive sexual behavior is more prevalent among those raised under conditions of socio-economic deprivation and disorganized family and community living. When those whites for whom the Negro sexual myth feels real cite statistical evidence of comparatively poor sexual restraint among Negroes to support their thesis, they may be right about the figures but wrong about what the figures mean. Correct interpretation of the evidence hinges on the question of cause. Such figures are actually a clue to social, not racial, differences between certain Negro and white groups. Conditions of cultural disorganization correlate with similar sexual patterns for any racial group, but in this country discrimination has caused a greater proportion of Negroes to live under such conditions. Many Negroes, whose individual life experience has not been socially damaging in these ways, not only disprove this sexual stereotype by their adherence to middle-class standards of sexual behavior but, in reaction to the myth, quite a number have developed over-compensatory psychosexual inhibitions of such magnitude that these constitute psychiatric disability.

The actuality of segregation-fostered isolation, emotional and social—as well as certain kinds of disorganized group relations—promote the very kind of sexual behavior many people fear; but greater social justice for the Negro would tend to lessen this kind of sexual activity.

Of course many psychological patterns and mechanisms are involved in the psychosexual aspect of race relations. It is not within the scope of this report to attempt a full discussion of them. We have pointed out how fear and aggression predominate over affection under conditions of segregation, and how sexual attitudes and behavior between the races are based on racial myth in displaced attempts to solve personal problems. We do not conclude from this that white and Negro individuals are incapable of emotionally healthy love relationships, including its sexual component, when freed from the effects of racial mythology. We do conclude that such mythology, especially destructive in the psychosexual area, is promoted by segregation and is, therefore, a false basis on which to maintain further segregation. While the difficulties and complexities of dealing with antisocial sex behavior must not be minimized, its sources should not be falsely attributed to mythological folk tales rather than to the social, economic, and psychological forces which can be observed, understood, and constructively dealt with.

Interracial unions—marital and extramarital

The fear of intermarriage and the desire for "preservation of racial purity" against the threat of "mongrelization" are central to white arguments in defense of segregation. Let us test these fears against the facts; do they stem from objective reality or from morbid elements disguised within rationalizations? The very word "mongrelization" defines biological events in terms of white prejudiced attitudes. Its implied assumption of the genetic inferiority of Negro stock is unsubstantiated by available biological evidence[6] so that the use of the term in this context reflects racial mythology. There are, however, many white people throughout the North, as well as the South, with deep feelings of opposition to the idea of Negro-white amalgamation. Such opposition may, of course, be claimed to be due to biological ideas about heredity. But if that were the whole story, two curious aspects of this opposition would seem inexplicable: first, the great disparity in social attitude towards marital and extramarital relations between the races; and second, the profound contrast in social attitude towards sex relations of white men with Negro women, on the one hand, and of Negro men and white women, on the other. Intermarriage challenges powerful emotional prohibitions which are enforced by law in some states and by severe social penalties in the rest. Out-of-wedlock and casual relations between the races, on the other hand, are relatively condoned in most sections and even generally expected in some. This social acceptability is rigidly limited, however, to the white male-Negro female combination, while the Negro male-white female contact arouses maximum punitive fury. How could one account for these significant distinctions if the fear of racially mixed progeny were a realistic, rather than a rationalized, basis for segregation? The mingling of Caucasian and Negro genes occurs without regard to whether the man is white and the woman Negro, or vice versa, so that emotionally-laden fantasies, rather than rational thought, seem predominant in this fear.

Since the baby's genetic endowment depends, in an interracial union as in any other, on the sum of the parental contributions, there would be no difference, genetically, between the infant born

---

[6]Boyd, William C., *Genetics and the Races of Man. An Introduction to Modern Physical Anthropology*, Little, Brown and Co., Boston, 1950.

Lewis, Julian H., *The Biology of the Negro*, University of Chicago Press, Chicago, 1942.

to a Negro mother by a white father, or to a white mother by a Negro father. Each would reflect hybridization to an equal extent. But segregationists regard the one with relative acceptance and the other with horror and condemnation. The one child can become part of its Negro mother's household, but the other must be excluded from its white mother's world on penalty of severe reprisal. The difference is not intrinsic to the child but to what the child symbolizes in terms of racial myth. The skin color of the interracial child is closely linked to these fears and attitudes, bearing visible proof, as it were, of the parent's social transgression. According to the racial myth in this country, skin color correlates with personal worth on a descending scale from white to dark.

A common form of miscenegation fear is the fear of "throwback," i.e., that the offspring of light-skinned parents may revert to a much darker skin color inherited from some Negro forebear. This fear seems to be another instance of mythical distortion and exaggeration elaborated around a kernel of fact. As far back as 1913, Charles Davenport published a study of "Heredity of Skin Color in Negro-White Crosses" and could find no cases nor theoretical evidence for throwbacks. He concluded that the idea of throwbacks was probably a myth.[7] Davenport's study, limited by its small sample, remains a scientific classic in this relatively unexplored area. Because, however, recognizably Negroid traits, such as hair texture, facial feature, and skin color are genetically transmitted independently of each other, it is theoretically possible, due to different genetic combinations, that an offspring may appear somewhat more Negroid, in one or another respect, than either of its Caucasian-appearing parents. This is far from the popular concept of throwback, however, and the fear that might be recognizable as Negroid because of the negative social connotations. The biological questions surrounding throwback raise a false issue that obscures the real issue: because of the severe social penalties for being a Negro, which their own white prejudice has imposed, white people dread the appearance of any recognizable Negro-ness in their own kin.

The Supreme Court decision against school segregation is opposed by many on the grounds that it will remove existing barriers to racial amalgamation. But in actuality, it was the importation of Negro slaves more than two hundred and fifty years ago,

[7]Boyd, *op. cit.*, p. 311.

rather than the Court's recent action, that was responsible for "deciding" this country on the course of racial intermingling which has been under way, for better or worse, ever since. Thus Herskovits[8] found that 78% of the U. S. Negroes who were interviewed in his sample of 1500 testified to some Caucasian or Indian ancestry, and only 22% to exclusively African background. These figures were recently confirmed by Stern,[9] who found that the proportion of mixed ancestry for American Negroes had even risen since Herskovits' study over twenty-five years earlier. Those who oppose school desegregation as a prelude to racial admixture often fail to recognize that this is already an accomplished fact, to a large extent, and—as Stern has pointed out—to the same degree in regions with legal segregation as elsewhere.[10]

The counterargument by white segregationists might be made, however, that their fear is not so much concerned with the white genetic contribution to the Negro population, but with the protection of the whites from African admixture, because of its assumed inferiority. Realistically, however, it is not possible for considerable cohabitation to go on for over two and a half centuries, as has been true in this country, with only uni-directional results. One way in which the white genetic pool has been augmented over the years by African genes is through the steadily increased rate of "passing" by light-skinned individuals of Caucasian appearance who have some fraction of Negro ancestry but who do not identify themselves socially as Negroes. "Passing" is made possible by the increased white admixture to the Negro population. The intensity of the desire "to pass" is due to the Negro's inferior place in American life. An individual's skin color and facial appearance, which permit his "passing," are by no means reliable indicators of his genetic endowment. Therefore, "passing" establishes a

---

[8]Herskovits, Melville J., *The American Negro; A Study in Racial Crossing*, Alfred A. Knopf, New York, 1928.

[9]Stern, Curt, "The Biology of the Negro," *Scientific American*, October 1954.

[10]The ancestry of the Negro is mixed, and substantially so, as Stern and others point out. Without such corroboration however, the reliability of the Herskovits data could be subject to question since it was based on testimony rather than physical examination at a period when Negro subjects were eager to claim non-Negro ancestry as socially more acceptable.

According to a distinguished authority, Th. Dobzhansky, "Race mixture has been going on during the whole of recorded history. . . . Mankind has always been, and still is, a mongrel lot." (Dunn and Dobzhansky, *Heredity, Race and Society*, 1952, 115).

medium for the dispersal of Negro genes into the general white genetic pool. Since discrimination stimulates the incentive for passing, and passing augments amalgamation, the segregationists actually defeat their ostensible goal of preserving racial purity. This is another indication of the irrationality inherent in these attitudes.

The fear of increased intermarriage, as a consequence of desegregation, is often expressed interchangeably with the fear of genetic fusion. These are related but far from identical. The expectation, voiced by many people, that school desegregation will result in a great rise in the rate of intermarriage, seems to be an expression of their bias and fear, rather than a reliable prediction. As a matter of fact, the information on which to base predictions with regard to racial intermarriage rates is extremely sparse and rather confusing. The most authoritative current work on the subject opens with the statement: "Only limited and unsatisfactory data are available on Negro-white intermarriage in the United States."[11] The many factors that determine fluctuations in the rate of racial intermarriage are far from clear. In Boston, where legal school desegregation has been in effect for decades, there was a relatively high rate in the years immediately after 1900, and a marked decrease in the next decades despite a constant ratio of Negroes to the total population. In urban New York State (other than New York City) the rate climbed between 1916-24 and then dropped steadily for the next ten years. No satisfactory explanations for these shifts have been established. The facts indicate that legal school desegregation per se does not influence the rate of intermarriage in ways that are as yet predictable.

As Merton points out, "the term interracial marriage is an insufficiently analytic statement of a complex kind of event. It fails to bring out the fact that such intermarriage involves intercaste, and sometimes interclass, as well as interracial marriage."[12] In the light of available experience we cannot venture an opinion as to if, how, and when school desegregation will affect interracial marriage rates. We do recognize that those who so readily offer

[11]Wirth, Louis and Goldhamer, Herbert, "Negro-White Intermarriage in Recent Times," Chap. IV of Part V, "The Hybrid and the Problem of Miscegenation," in *Characteristics of the American Negro*, ed. by Otto Klineberg, Harper & Bros., New York, 1944.

[12]Merton, Robert K., "Intermarriage and the Social Structure: Fact and Theory," *Psychiatry*, Vol. 4 #3, 1941.

predictions on the subject do so for emotional reasons or from ignorance. Many complicated psychodynamic and social factors determine marital choice, but for many people, similarity of social and economic backgrounds is an influence in the choice of partner. Under the psychosocial conditions of American race relations today, such commonality between Negro and white is rare.

Integration

Perhaps the effects of desegregation should be regarded less from the standpoint of the frequency of intermarriage and more in terms of shifts in the quality of close relationships between Negroes and whites. School desegregation as a behavioral change may in the long run lead to attitude changes which can be called integration, that is, to a much greater degree of equal interaction between the races. If and when there is a shift in the direction of integration, this would show itself as a shift toward greater mutuality and breadth of shared experience between whites and Negroes in their total relationships, including psychosexual components. One might expect, therefore, that if there were eventual Negro-white integration, there would also be a shift from a preponderance of illicit interracial unions to the fuller, more enduring legalized unions of marriage. Should this occur, it would not necessarily alter the present course of biological mixing of the population, but would rather bring about a psychosocial realignment. Psychosocial realignment, then, is a foreseeable consequence of desegregation, whereas biological admixture is already in process and is not dependent on desegregation.

B. Psychodynamics of Changing Attitudes

1. SOME ASPECTS OF ATTITUDE CHANGES

The desegregation decision of the Supreme Court has met with a wide range of responses throughout the country.[1] In many communities the new law of the land has been implemented in a matter-of-fact way, proceeding with little upheaval, while in a few, problems and opposition have arisen some time after a smooth initial phase.[2] In other communities the very suggestion of following the

[1]Fleming, Harold C. and Constable, John, "What's Happening in School Integration?" *Public Affairs* Pamphlet #244, New York, 1956.

[2]When Washington schools integrated in 1954, there were student strikes at three high schools (out of the 116 desegregated schools) which were quickly aborted by prompt and firm action by school and municipal authorities. (*see page* 31)

Supreme Court's order has met with violent feelings among otherwise apparently law-abiding citizens. Important as the difference between these opposed reactions is, it would be wrong to assume that an equally marked difference has come about in the attitudes of people in these varied types of situations.

Behavior change can be induced by the application of many kinds of external pressure, ranging from legal enforcement to neighborhood custom. But a genuine translation of such behavior into an enduring change in attitude is a long process involving important psychological processes.

Goals of attitude change

Ideally, one may suggest that the goal of this process is an attitude between Negroes and whites which is based on acceptance of a fundamental right of human beings to be judged as individuals and not as members of this or that ethnic group. But it would be unrealistic to expect that such a fundamental change in attitude can take place among the majority of the current adult generation. While working towards this goal, by all appropriate means, it nevertheless seems likely that the progress possible in the next few years will be more limited: change in attitude based upon acceptance by both white and Negro parents of the fact that their children are exposed to an experience fundamentally different from the one they have had themselves in regard to growing up in relation to the other group.

Carl F. Hansen, Asst. Supt. in charge of District of Columbia senior high schools, has reported on the Washington integration program, now in its third academic year, as a miracle of social adjustment. (See "Miracle of Social Adjustment: Desegregation in the Washington, D. C. Schools," Carl F. Hansen, 1957. Freedom Pamphlet Series, Anti-Defamation League of B'nai Brith, New York.)

In September 1956, a Congressional Subcommittee investigated D. C. schools. The hearings brought out evidence of greater academic retardation among Negroes than whites. The Subcommittee majority of 4 Southern members issued a report recommending that the Capitol schools be resegregated, but the other two opposing Subcommittee members contended the majority report was biased. A three-month study of the Washington schools, initiated during the Congressional hearings by the Washington Committee for the Public Schools, a 31-member group of public leaders, found, as does the Hansen report, that the worst educational problems were caused by the old system of segregation and were being gradually solved by integration. This is supported by even more recent reports of the rate at which the Negro children are making up their academic achievement deficit. Since the Supreme Court rules that all public school children should be desegregated, the question of achievement level differences is a separate, though important, issue. Confusion of these issues is one of the mistakes of some of those who oppose desegregation.

Why is it Utopian to expect more radical change in many adults of the current generation? The reason for this has to do with the meaning of Negro-white relations for the psychic economy of many who have grown up in a situation where segregation was the rule. It is important to distinguish between attitude and behavior. Even when an individual strives to change a deep-seated attitude because of more recently acquired intellectual or moral conviction, he may be unable to, due to the hold of early conditioning. However, if he can admit and accept this as his limitation he can control his behavior to accord with his convictions rather than with the repudiated though retained attitude.

Psychiatric experience as well as theories of human behavior suggest that the way a person thinks and feels about himself is intimately linked to the way he feels about others. The way he thinks and feels about others depends on the place these others are assigned in the world, a set of facts which the growing child first learns from his parents and later from his own experience outside the family.

The greatest task in growing up consists of coming to terms with oneself, of learning to know who one is, what one can do, and how one stands in relation to others. Any help that the environment offers toward obtaining an answer to these questions is seized upon. In a community where there is segregation between dominant and subordinate groups, the existence of this external distinction is used by both Negro and white children in defining themselves to themselves. They learn, as one early answer to the central questions about their own selves, that they are *not* members of the other group. This knowledge can have both gratifying and frustrating aspects. The Negro child might feel relief in realizing that he need not make great efforts to succeed, since he is not meant to succeed. But on the other hand, he may be frustrated to realize that many opportunities are closed to him. The white child might feel gratified about at least not being a member of the inferior group and frustrated by realizing that the official assignment of inferiority carries for the Negro child some rewards unattainable by him, such as protection and less need for the same kind and degree of control.

To the extent that the adults of the current generation have used the now obsolescent pattern of segregation in coming to an understanding of their own selves, their attitudes toward the other group have become deeply ingrained in their personalities. As adults, the psychological uses they have earlier made of segregation are often kept out of conscious awareness. Instead, the justification of their attitudes appears to lie in other rational or rationalized facts. Yet the balance they have found with regard to themselves and the world rests upon these earlier processes. A radical attitude change would presuppose a restructuring of their entire personalities, a task which very few adults can perform without individual psychological help.

Intensification of hostility

Even the more limited goal of attitude change in the current adult generation meets with considerable psychological opposition in many persons. In many communities the Supreme Court decision has led to an apparent intensification of anti-Negro hostility and has evoked violent emotions, occasionally turning into violent action.

One important reason for such strong feelings among white persons lies in their fear of Negro retaliation, physical aggression, and even role reversal of the two groups in the event of Negro acquisition of power from the outlawing of segregation. The facts, however, point otherwise. Out of several historically proposed roads in the course of American Negro movements, the road that has prevailed under Negro leadership and by Negro organization—the N.A.A.C.P.—has been that of legal and social action through due process of law and peaceful, democratic principles.

Of special significance to the white fear of role reversal is the new Negro movement through the churches which is supplementing, not supplanting, the legal and political methods. This Negro movement of Gandhi-type non-violent, passive resistance has been dramatically demonstrated by the 50,000 Negroes of Montgomery, Alabama, from all walks of life, in their effective year-long boycott of segregated buses under the leadership of the Rev. Martin Luther King, Jr.[3] This movement and this type of responsible leadership are extending beyond Montgomery to other Southern areas. These Negro masses are determined to get rid of Jim Crow, but, in accord-

[3]Barrett, George, "Jim Crow, He's Real Tired," *New York Times Magazine*, March 3, 1957.

Lerner, Max, "Negro Roads and Blind Alleys," *New York Post*, March 11, 1957.

ance with Dr. King's preaching of Christian faith, and with steady self-discipline, they have refrained from retaliating to provocations ranging from insult to dynamite by white segregationists. In an address at the First Annual Institute on Non-Violence and Social Change, under the auspices of the Montgomery Improvement Association in December 1956, Dr. King said, "But if we retaliate with hate and bitterness, the new age will be nothing but a duplication of the old age. We must blot out the hate and injustice of the old age with the love and justice of the new. This is why I believe so firmly in non-violence."

There is no evidence to indicate that ideas of Negro-white social role reversal are any more than fantasies which individual Negroes and whites may engage in under conditions of segregation. Most persons are able to learn from experience. A great psychological value of the desegregation decision in initiating the process of attitude change (even in localities which have so far resisted the law) lies in the fact that it has provided a chance to learn from the experience of other communities. To be sure, some serious problems have arisen for children and teachers where desegregation has been introduced. And, certainly, serious problems also ensue where communities try to resist desegregation by mob action. But in none of these situations has role reversal occurred. This fact has not remained hidden. It should constitute an essential turning point in the process of attitude change.

Whether or not a person is able to learn from experience depends largely on the degree of his inner tensions and insecurities. Those who are ridden by irrational fears will learn less than those who can master their anxiety in constructive ways. It is the latter group—undoubtedly stronger in number and prestige—who will carry on the process of learning from experience. It should be pointed out, however, that the new experience need not be the result of a firm sentiment in favor of Negro-white equality. Repeatedly, civic and educational officials from Southern communities that embark on desegregation declare their continued belief in white supremacy and segregation, but state that they will implement desegregation to obey the law. Sometimes the financial factor involved in having to send Negro children by bus to the nearest Negro school in another town has tipped the balance in favor of desegregation. Political or other economic motives have had the same result in other communities. Thus exposure to new learning situations coming from experience with school desegregation has in some cases been brought about from motives which have little to do with favorable attitudes towards desegregation itself.

Stages in attitude change

Learning from experience starts a new series of stages in attitude change which need not follow a simple course of gradual improvement. The nature of the experience as well as inner forces in a person will combine to create many ups-and-downs and in-between stages. We do not yet know well enough all the possible stages that can occur. A few, however, have been observed and studied and deserve to be identified.

Compartmentalization. There is, first, the stage of compartmentalization. In Northern public housing projects it has been observed that Negro and white persons living as next-door neighbors have learned to get along with one another. One white woman, for example, describing how deeply prejudiced she had originally been against Negroes and how she had changed so that Negroes now called her by her first name when she met them in the project, added: "but of course I'd faint if they did this to me in the main street of town." A study of a mining community showed that the easy companionship of Negro and white miners on the job ended abruptly when they came to the surface.[4] With school desegregation this compartmentalization may express itself in a variety of ways. In faculty or parent meetings people may still feel more at ease with segregated seating arrangements or may recoil from sharing a meal or toilet facilities. Mixed classrooms may be accepted by parents who would not permit a child of the other group to visit their home. Such compartmentalization may be deliberately and consciously established, or may just "happen" without anybody planning it. Whatever the case, it is clearly an in-between stage in the acceptance of desegregation.

Denial of differences. Another in-between attitudinal stage consists of denying all difference between the two groups and of completely ignoring the special historical, psychological and social conditions under which Negroes live throughout the United States. In practice, this attitude seems to be quite widespread in various

[4]Cook, Stuart W., *Desegregation: A Psychological Analysis*, Research Center for Human Relations, New York University, 1956.

school systems in the North, to the detriment of many deprived Negro children who may need but do not receive the special care and attention from school authorities to which their precarious social and economic position entitles them. This attitude is actually fostered by many minority group organizations which have for a long time insisted, as a defense against the crudest forms of discrimination, that no public record be kept of whether a school child is white or colored. Knowing the child's race, like other factual information about him, such as his age, sex, and health, can enable schools to better recognize and meet whatever his special educational needs may be; this should be an educational goal for both Negro and white children. Constructive acceptance of realistic differences between individuals is by no means the same as the use of differences to justify disparagement or inferior treatment.

"Mascot" attitude. A third in-between stage has been observed in the North as well as in the South. White people in this stage will often overdo their admiration for the cuteness of minority-group children; they will emphasize the Negro's gift for music and dance, his gaiety, carefreeness, and the like. They will feel proud about having once invited one Negro to their home, etc. We may call this stage the "mascot" attitude to Negroes. There is a parallel to this attitude on the part of the Negro who may regard the white person as magically over-endowed with glamour or power and who may draw some spurious self-esteem from acceptance by such a being which is as false and unreliable as the white person's sense of worth for his "tolerance."

In this stage beliefs and action orientation have apparently changed. For practical purposes this means a step forward. But the attitude still overlooks the real attributes of members of the other group, both positive and negative ones, and implies a fantasied acceptance of the other, or the taking of a position which is in accord with one's ideals of tolerance, without real-life experience to back it up.

What we have referred to as the realistic, though limited, prospect of constructive attitude change for the current adult generation differs in an essential way from this "mascot" attitude: it is free from the compulsive pretense of acceptance. The attitude change will be completed only when the adults genuinely accept the fact of a fundamental difference in the life experience of their own generation compared to that of the new one.

When one identifies an individual or a group as being at any one of these mentioned in-between stages in the process of attitude change, the question arises of how to handle these stages so as to promote further changes.

Essentially, there are two routes open: to aim at increased awareness of the transitory nature of the in-between stage, by drawing attention to it in individual or group discussion; or to leave matters as they are, on the assumption that each stage has its own specific function in the process and needs to run its course before people are ready to move further. In other words, are non-directive or directive approaches more indicated? Non-directive or directive methods are applied by group leaders who have theoretical convictions on the point and professional experience to support them. A change from one method to the other is dictated by a full understanding of the balance of forces at play at any moment, and timing of the change is the result of careful examination of the needs of the group.

Examples are available of the success or failure of either method. Drawing attention to the fact of segregated seating arrangements, for example, may lead to a disturbing extent of self-consciousness about it which can interfere with the learning experience. On the other hand, pointing out in a different group that a common snack at a meeting might help to break the ice may turn out to be an acceptable step forward.

Factor of timing

No hard and fast rules can be established about the more promising method, which will always depend on the concrete situation and the persons in it. All that can be done is to point out in a rather general way, that the right thing done at the wrong time will lead to failure as much as the wrong thing done at any time. As a guide, then, to this extremely important factor of timing one will do well to consider whether the group is solidly committed to common goals or in danger of breaking up at a slight provocation; whether its leading individuals are the more stable or the more shaky members with regard to attitudes toward the other group. One must consider these and similar problems before deciding on interference with the established adaptations. In each of the in-between stages identified here, there is a certain amount of readiness to move toward the limited realistic goal we have here suggested for the process of attitude change. The speed and thoroughness with which adults reach it will then affect the manner in which their children absorb their entirely different experience of developing a new orientation toward the other ethnic group rather than changing an old one.

2. EFFECT OF GROUP PROCESSES ON ATTITUDES

In addition to the more specifically personal forces and dynamisms which play a role in acquiring and in changing attitudes, other important factors that enter into the choice of sides in an issue come from the influences of various groups in the community. Each person belongs to many groups, which are of varying importance to him, for instance, a political party, a church, a trade or professional organization, a social group, a family, and so on. These may differ greatly from each other in their attitudes on any important local or national issue. Moreover, even the groups to which a person does not belong exert an influence upon him, both in terms of possible reprisal from an opposing group and in terms of his wish for approval by a group in which he may desire membership.

Need to belong

A sense of belongingness is of crucial importance to the average person's sense of well-being. Such extreme types as the genius, the reformer, and the seriously maladjusted may live in apparent independence of family and community group pressures. Yet even here there is often a somewhat hidden need for approval which is expressed in a roundabout manner. The reformer may be making great efforts to carry group opinion with him in a new direction; the creative genius may be dependent on the appreciation of his audience for recognition and encouragement of his creativity; the maladjusted person may have withdrawn from group relationships in despair of acceptance. But for most of us, the attitudes and opinions of those groups which are of importance to us exert powerful influences in shaping our own.

At the present time, many groups split on the issue of desegregation. For example, the ruling element in a given community may be resisting the general trend toward desegregation which the nation as a whole has begun. But within the same community there may be other, perhaps smaller or less vocal, groups, such as a church group, which favor it. In the members of these smaller groups conflicts may arise between attitudes toward desegregation and the wish to be identified with the entire local community; equally in the dominant group there may be conflicts between national and local values.

Taking a stand

What determines why some people take a stand which supports the national and opposes the dissenting values of the dominant local group while others do not? The ability to take an independent position is often equated with personal maturity. However, the completely mature man possessed of total independence of judgment, is a somewhat illusory ideal. At best the independence is relative—that is, a mature person may be more resistant to group opinions, or he may be more selective of the groups whose opinions he accepts, or he may be less inclined to adopt group opinions without criticism. He may be more aware of the ways in which he adapts to group pressures, or he may be more able to tolerate without too much insecurity a certain degree of difference from the group. On the other hand, personalities who are exceedingly immature can often be seen to take positions that are dissident from the majority opinion in the local group. Such examples as the criminal or the eccentric or the childish rebel may be used as illustrations. It is necessary, therefore, to recognize that a person's agreement or disagreement with a group cannot by itself be made a criterion of maturity. An attitude must be viewed in the context of the functioning of the total personality before such an appraisal is legitimate.

In addition to the question of what degree of independence of judgment is possible for a given person, other factors which enter into decisions may be mentioned. First, an inability to conceptualize the nation with its larger purposes and goals may make it difficult for a person to identify himself with national values. Poorly educated people usually have a more constricted view of the nation, and identification with national attitude and policies becomes difficult because these are meaningless abstractions without impact. Second, a person making up his mind on an issue will often be more influenced by the wish to gain or preserve the approval of those with whom he is in actual contact than to gain or preserve the approval of distant and depersonalized authorities. Similarly, those who fear reprisals from opposition groups are likely to be more influenced by fear of persons in the local community than they are by the support coming from remote sources, even when this support may express national values and federal authority.

Those who reach beyond the values of the dominant group in the local community to accept the values of the region or of the nation usually have a higher education and a wider interest in regional and national affairs than their fellow citizens whose attachments are more local. In addition, such persons must also derive some support from a group of like-minded people inside the community. This group may be as small as a family, or may include a substantial band of firm enthusiasts for a particular point of view. The members of this smaller group are fortified by the support which they give each other as well as by their adherence to what they believe to be the goals and ideals of the larger group, such as the region or the nation. The attachment to these larger goals and ideals in the abstract without some support from people close at hand is rarely enough to sustain a heresy against the doctrines of the dominant local group. It seems to be extremely difficult, if not impossible, for most individuals to take sides on an issue against the overwhelming majority of the local community unless they have some direct personal support from at least one or more members of the local community.

Mixed motives

In considering motivations underlying attitudes and behavior toward desegregation, what needs emphasis is the almost universal existence of mixed motives. In different persons there will be various mixtures of rational and irrational motives, of self-interested and group-interested motives, and of conscious and unconscious motives. Many people may resist changes in the social institutions because of the discomfort evoked when they are called upon to relate to members of another group in a different way. Frequently, reluctance to change social roles may contribute to the attitudes toward desegregation on the part of many members of Southern communities, both white and Negro. Each group has something to gain and something to give in the traditional relationship. Each may be loath to risk the loss of present security by trying to adjust to a new relationship. And in both groups, this reluctance to change may exist alongside a realization of the advantages and fairness of desegregation and a wish to bring it about.

Motivations quite unrelated to the issue of desegregation may influence the adoption of a particular position on desegregation to an extent rarely realized by the person himself, or even by most untrained observers. For example, a person unable to adjust to the customs and authority of his community may adopt the values and attitudes toward desegregation of a group outside the community and thus satisfy a vengeful motive against the local community. Or someone who believes himself to be an underdog in his own family may vigorously take up the side of the underdogs in the community when he is really mainly serving his own needs.

Private and public attitudes

Personal motivations influence also the important distinction between the private attitudes of a person on the issue and his public statements of his attitudes, as well as the equally important distinction between his expressed attitudes and his behavior when confronted with a new situation. A number of studies have demonstrated wide discrepancies between a person's public avowals, his private sentiments, and his actual behavior.[5] In situations, for instance, where prevailing local feeling against desegregation has been whipped up, people who feel desegregation to be morally right are afraid to claim this publicly and dare only support it on grounds of upholding the law. Comparably, in Northern circles, many people typically feel under social pressure to conceal whatever prosegregation feelings they may have, from public utterance, or even from themselves. Or to cite another example, many of those who beforehand express strong opposition to desegregation may actually do nothing to interfere with it when it takes place in the schools. Indeed, they may even come to endorse it after a time. A person's public avowals are influenced by his perception of his immediate interests. These perceptions will naturally change with the situation. He may see that it is in his own interest to abide by the law or adhere to a new attitude taken up by the majority of a group. Such factors account to some extent for the influence of one com-

[5]Cook, Stewart W., *op. cit.*

"A Tentative Description and Analysis of the School Desegregation Crisis in Clinton, Tennessee." Anna Holden, Bonita Valien, Preston Valien (with the assistance of Frances Manis). Fisk University, Nashville, Tennessee. Published by the Anti-Defamation League of B'nai Brith in cooperation with The Society for the Study of Social Problems, December 1, 1956.

munity on another and for the occurrence of "bandwagon effects" in changing patterns of behavior.

When one person presents his attitudes on the issue to another person, he is influenced by a wish to appear rational. To this end, he assembles ostensibly plausible arguments which seem to him to justify his decision and which he hopes will make his decision appear sensible to his listener. Such arguments may have little relation to the sentiments and values underlying the decision. Nor are they usually related to the more rational reasons that might be given for adopting a particular side of the issue. Thus many of those who oppose desegregation voice dire predictions of the far-fetched disasters it will bring, in an effort to account for their opposition. Fewer people discuss in a commonsense fashion the handling of the real difficulties which must be anticipated in the transition phase.

Besides wishing to appear rational, the person explaining his attitude usually seeks approval by appearing altruistic, and he disclaims personal benefit from his decision. According to his point of view, he may appeal to ideals, to the law, to Christianity, to the facts of human nature, to the good of the community, etc. Rarely does he acknowledge that he has acted for what he believes to be his own good. Nor is he usually even willing to attribute selfish motives to the group he joins. To do so would implicate himself in some of that corruption. So he also attributes to the group unselfish, rational behavior serving the interests of great ideals or still larger groups.

Finally, the presentation of reasons for a decision is strongly influenced by the speaker's perception of the person to whom he is talking. He wishes to appear rational and laudable not only in the eyes of the members of the local group to which he adheres, but also in the eyes of the opposition. The wish to convert or raise doubts in the mind of the opposition is reinforced by his human wish to be well thought of by everyone. Accordingly, the speaker will adapt his arguments to suit his current audience. For example, if he perceives the listener as an educated person, he may advance arguments based on "scientific evidence" seeming to justify the decision, which has actually been made on entirely different grounds. If he sees the listener as a religious person, he may cite arguments that try to reconcile his choice with the ideals represented by the listener.

When the issue of desegregation is brought close to a community, the opinions of the groups within it crystallize gradually as the issue grows in significance. What eventually forms as the attitude of a particular group may begin as an inchoate collection of poorly defined individual attitudes. As the members of the group clarify their attitudes and announce their decisions, more and more people find it possible to take a definite stand on the issue. There results a "bandwagon effect" in that the rate of joining a side accelerates.

A great many persons, motivated by a desire for group approval or perhaps by fear of reprisals, base their decisions on what they imagine to be the attitude of a given group. The attitude which they attribute to the group may in fact reflect very inaccurately the real opinions of its members. A person's perception of the group may be markedly distorted by his lack of information and by his unverbalized wishes. The result of these distortions may be that the person responds to his conception of the group will rather than to the actual wishes of the majority. A false picture of the group will may stem from outmoded wishes of the group or from wishes of comparable groups in other places.

Reinforcing convictions

Once a person has made his decision, the mere fact of having done so severs his connections with the other side. Now he stands to lose face by the failure of his side in the issue. Thus a personal investment in being on the winning side tends to reinforce convictions. Moreover, the wish to win or the fear of losing may distort perceptions of the situation so that the strength of a particular side is quite unrealistically evaluated.

Other events besides the act of taking a definite stand on the issue may reinforce convictions. Of these the most important is probably the crystallization and expression of opposition. Such opposition reminds the partisan that his side may ultimately lose. It also reminds him that his side may be wrong. Both of these thoughts may arouse doubts in his mind about the wisdom of his attitude, and these doubts may be suppressed by a strengthening of original convictions and a more vigorous combatting of the opposition. These factors are relevant to the problem of "outside interference" which is frequently complained about in communities grappling with the problem of desegregation.

Whatever people's anticipatory feelings and behavior may be, it is important to note that reports from those areas which have already desegregated their schools are generally favorable. There has been a minimum of substantial or sustained opposition, and many fears and predictions of dire consequences have proven groundless. As of May 1956, desegregation in public elementary and high schools had occurred in nine Southern states and the District of Columbia, but not in eight states of the South.[6] However, the Southern Regional Council's inventory of the seventeen Southern and border states for the two-year period since the Supreme Court decision (May 1954-May 1956) reports that Negro children began attending additional Catholic grammar and high schools, formerly all-white, throughout the South, including three of these eight resisting or defiant states, and that the merging of most of the remaining white and Negro schools on military bases in the South—including "Deep South" states—proceeded smoothly.[7] Reports have indicated that desegregating the schools has engendered a more accepting attitude toward it among many people. It has also been demonstrated by experience that many of the difficulties which were anticipated did not occur. Nevertheless, there have been many real problems. On these, many school officials have expressed themselves as feeling that they were not of such kind and degree as to appear insoluble.

In those communities where there has been violent opposition after desegregation has been started, the instigation seems to have had multiple determinants, many of which were unrelated to desegregation. In one such place—Hoxie, Arkansas—studied by members of this committee and also reported in the *Southern School News*,[8] the violent opposition to the onset of desegregation was led by a farmer—himself relatively uneducated—who seemed to be driven to assume leadership by personal motivations extraneous to the issue. The emotions he played upon in winning a following

[6]Loth, David and Fleming, Harold, *Integration North and South*, New York: The Fund For The Republic, 1956, p. 51.

[7]*Ibid.*, pp. 57-58; 97-98.

[8]*Southern School News*, September 1955 and November 1956. A suit springing from the Hoxie situation has recently been heard by the U.S. Court of Appeals. The School Board was granted by the U.S. District Court a permanent restraining order enjoining the defendants (some citizens of the community) from interfering with the desegregation of the schools. The restraining order was appealed, but the U.S. 8th Circuit Court of Appeals upheld the injunction, ruling on October 25, 1956 that administrators of desegrating public schools had a right to be free of "direct and deliberate interference."

among many of the white residents were largely unrelated to convictions about desegregation. In addition he was strongly supported by a barrage of propaganda from professional white supremacists in other states, augmenting his poorly conceived religious and "scientific" biases and other rationalizations.

Parallels are to be found in the Clinton, Tennessee situation. Desegregation there had been a subject of litigation and a topic for discussion for several years prior to the fall of 1956. At this time, as a result of a court order, the high school was integrated, peaceably, if not enthusiastically. The arrival of an out-of-state, pro-segregation agitator sparked explosions of violence which required the use of the National Guard.[9]

As in Hoxie, the inflammatory role of a single pro-segregation crusader was conspicuous, in this instance John Kasper, who too was reinforced by out-of-state extremists. The likelihood that Kasper's activity is also driven by contradictory personal motives—unrelated to the social realities of school desegregation—is suggested by apparently documented accounts of his active participation in Negro-white socializing only one-and-a-half years before.[10] This has been corroborated by Kasper's own testimony elicited at a Florida Legislative Committee hearing.[11]

Where there has been minimal turmoil in the preparatory and early phases of school desegregation, there has been maximum acceptance of it and an increased community pride. Such has been the case in Louisville, Kentucky, where intelligent preparation of the community has resulted in a system of voluntary desegregation which has been accepted peaceably and cooperatively by those involved.[12] In Washington, D.C., school superintendent Corning's desegregation plan was formed out of group process, including inviting suggestions from the community, planning-meetings by school system staff, and an in-service program for intercultural education.[13]

---

[9]*Southern School News*, September 1956 and January 1957.

"A Tentative Description and Analysis of the School Desegregation Crisis in Clinton, Tennessee," *ibid.*

[10]*New York Herald Tribune*, Series by Robert S. Bird on John Kasper, February 1957.

[11]*New York Times*, March 12, 1957.

[12]*U.S. News and World Report*, September 21, 1956.

[13]Miracle of Social Adjustment, Hansen, *op. cit.*

When there has been maximum turmoil at the outset, as in Hoxie and the University of Alabama, there has been a continuation of increased resistance, intensified hostility diffusely expressed to anyone even remotely connected with the issue, and consolidation of the opposition on the basis of shared hostility. When leadership has been divided or has failed to cope with the confusion and uncertainty which is a natural expectation of the initial phase, more anxiety and defensive anger are bred in a vicious circle. To formulate this principle more positively: available studies agree that firm, clear-cut policies by educational leadership and careful planning that includes all levels of the school system and general community play a major role in effecting smooth transitions from segregated to desegregated schools.[14]

3. ROLE OF AUTHORITY IN CHANGING ATTITUDES AND BEHAVIOR

Conflicts regarding types of authority

The citizens of those states where school segregation has been required and enforced by the authority of law are now confronted by the reverse situation, whereby the highest governmental authority of the land has ruled that segregated schooling be abolished. The Southern citizen—Negro or white—especially in the deep South, is thus caught up in an open conflict between these two types of authority, both of which he traditionally recognizes. Now he is faced with the dilemma of choosing which to obey or defy by the position he takes on desegregation. This inevitably entails some

[14](A). Ashmore, Harry S., *The Negro and the Schools*, University of North Carolina Press, Chapel Hill, 1954.

Miracle of Social Adjustment, *ibid.*

Williams, Robert M., Jr. and Ryan, Margaret F., *Schools in Transition*, University of North Carolina Press, Chapel Hill, 1954.

Everett, Samuel, "A Community School Ends Segregation," *The School Executive*, July 1954, pp. 52-53.

(B). The Fisk University team of social scientists who studied the first Clinton crisis included three suggestions about preparation as "Lessons from Clinton's Experience": 1) Preparation should take in the functional community or the total area affected by desegregation. (Preparation had been focussed on one school and one town, whereas the court order to desegregate was county-wide; 50% of Clinton High School pupils came from outside Clinton, and Kasper's responsive audience was from the whole county.) 2) Community preparation should reach groups at all economic, educational, and social levels. (The lower socio-economic and educational level groups were left out of Clinton's preparatory planning. Much of the trouble came from people in these groups.) 3) Preparation of students and faculty proved to be very valuable and important. (Students responded excellently to being given responsibility.)

degree of personal conflict, since whatever stands he adopts will involve him in real difficulties with at least some of the important people in his life, as well as with opposing psychic elements within himself. Because these authority conflicts have intense emotional bearing on the grave problems posed by the violence and vehemence of some protests against desegregation, it is important to try and understand their psychodynamic implications.

Levels and radius of authority

For individuals and for groups a close connection exists, psychologically, between their ways of response to desegregation and their characteristic attitudes and reactions to authority in general. Authority relationships are maintained on several levels of experience: political, social, intrafamilial, and intrapsychic; dynamically, these levels of authority relationships have interconnections. There is also a distance factor in attitudes toward authority. Everyone is subject to control and regulation by multiple authorities in a successively widening radius out from himself, beginning in the home and extending on to those who exert immediate power over his daily life, such as the "boss" and beyond to the local and then state officials, and thence to the more distant federal government. The emotional meaningfulness of governmental authority, for many people, varies with its perceived closeness and remoteness, so that when the commands of the near and the far authorities clash, many individuals obey the near because it feels more compellingly real for them. Some of the factors that influence whether federal government is perceived as an abstraction or a vital component of one's own felt world have been discussed above (B-2). An additional factor is the degree to which a sense of political participation is experienced with its accompanying feeling of identification with one's own government. According to Dr. Johnson,[15] for instance, "The Southern Negro viewpoint is more broadly national than regional. . . . In philosophy the Southern Negro identification is with the nation and not with the Southern region, which is, in spirit, separatist."

Responses to implied coercion

Legislative control over the interracial schooling of children entails enforcement, whether for legal segregation or desegregation.

[15]Johnson, Charles S., *op. cit.*

And enforcement implies authoritative coercion. Parenthetically, it it might be pointed out (because it is so frequently overlooked) that it has been just as coercive to legislate into segregated schools those Southern Negro and white citizens who were opposed to segregation, as it is now to legislate into desegregation those other Southern white and Negro citizens who are opposed to desegregation.[16] The public's responses to such authoritative coercion can include a wide range of alternative variations and combinations of willing or unwilling compliance or disguised and open defiance.

Factors in authority acceptance

But an oversimplified view of the citizen's psychic conflict as due to opposing local and federal mandates fails to take into account sufficiently the following four factors: the intricate and conflicted nature of everyone's authority alignments, at least in this society; the universality of conflicting motives and attitudes pertaining to desegregation, and the relationship of these to conflict-solving by means of authority; variables of leadership; the question of the citizen's own participation in the authority of government through the democratic processes.

Conflicting authority alignments

If the law forces a citizen into segregated behavior despite his conscious or unconscious objections, his response will involve the dynamic interaction of his whole particular and complex system of external and internalized authorities. Perhaps this accounts for his heightened susceptibility to the influence of leadership, either for or against desegregation, at such a juncture, since the authority of the leader may be so timed and of such a nature as to tip the scales of a precariously balanced equilibrium of the other forces of authority operating within and upon him. All of us have developed some of our attitudes toward authority out of a conflictful series of life events. As adults we have not neatly abolished those conflicts; instead we normally evolve a working balance of psychic forces.

---

[16]Supt. of Schools Omer Carmichael bases the Louisville plan of "voluntary integration" on the view that compulsory racial segregation is what the Supreme Court has ruled as unconstitutional, an interpretation in line with a July 15, 1955 ruling by a Federal Court in South Carolina. (*U.S. News and World Report*, October 5 1956).

Development of attitudes to authority

An explanation for this is to be found in the psychology of development. The foundation of conscience, values, and ideals is formed in early childhood on the basis of the need for love and approval and the fear of punishment from the parents or parent substitutes who are the primary authority figures. At this stage the child does not accept or reject parental values and standards because of how reasonable they may or may not be, but because of his emotional needs and fears. The mixture of loving and hostile feelings which a small child normally develops towards his parents out of his dependency and their power to protect and to harm him is felt towards their power of authority over him as well. These double feelings affect and cling to the values and attitudes he assimilates from them. This process of authority-derived attitude-formation continues on through childhood and adolescence for similar emotional reasons, although the range of influential authorities progressively widens to include such persons as ministers, gang-leaders, etc. Only with maturity can the rational and intellectual content of an attitude become the main basis for its adoption and repudiation. Even then the attitudes acquired through the operation of fact and reason must always struggle against residual, unconscious emotional attitudes formed in our childhood relations with authority figures. This stems from the nature of our child-rearing, even when the parents themselves are normally reasonable individuals.

Vicissitudes of responses to authority

These buried irrational attitudes are present throughout a person's life, ready, if reactivated, to overthrow or encroach on his rational attitudes in unexpected and disguised ways. We can not expect, therefore, an absence of conflict in our attitudes toward authority, but rather at most, preponderant attitudes which are the resultant of contradictory feelings. These general principles apply significantly to the desegregation situation, where the individual must cope not only with the conflict in his relations with various social and governmental authorities, which may themselves be in conflict, but also with his internalized amalgam of parental and other authorities who were significant in forming his racial attitudes.

Authority and conflict-solving

Closely related to the universality of conflictful authority feelings is the universality of some degree of mixed motives and conflicting attitudes toward desegregation. We have already emphasized how mistaken it is to ascribe undivided feelings on this issue to individuals or to blocs of people (Northern, Southern, white or Negro). Therefore, people's reactions, both in attitude and behavior, to authoritative enforcement of desegregated schooling largely depend on the varying reasons for their manifest and latent feelings on the subject, as well as on the intensity and relative proportions of their mixed feelings which may not be apparent, even to themselves. Maslow[17] has pointed out, for example, that prejudice and discrimination are differently motivated and therefore respond to different social treatment. Many people conform to the discriminatory practice of segregation, not because of prejudicial attitudes, primarily, but from their compelling need to conform to dominant group patterns. Such individuals can smoothly readjust themselves to desegregation when this is the course firmly prescribed by authorities whose protection and approval they require. Perhaps this is illustrated by the impressive success of desegregation in institutions with a strong authority tradition like the army and the Catholic church. The effects of these instances of military and religious authority, however, entail other psychological considerations as well.

As explained above, the manifest position of an individual with respect to his system of authorities is maintained as the preponderance of continuously opposed psychic forces. Similarly, his overt position about desegregation depends on the balance of conflicts: between his sense of what is right and what is wrong—of what is safe and what is dangerous—between his more mature rationality and his more childish irrationality. When the march of events, as at present, pushes these latent conflict constellations closer to the surface, the individual is especially receptive to authoritative influence on two counts: the external authority can free him from the deadlock of his opposing inner authority forces, as well as help tip the balance of his conflicts about desegregation.

---

[17] Maslow, Will, "Prejudice, Discrimination and the Law," *Annals of the American Academy of Political and Social Science*, May 1951.

Timing, surfacing of conflicts and trust

The factors of timing, surfacing of the conflicts, and confidence in the authority are significant to its role of shifting attitudes about desegregation: the Supreme Court decision came at a time when nation-wide gains in public opinion against segregation had been well underway as a sizeable encroachment on pro-segregation sentiment. The moral and legal authoritative impact of the decision has driven the segregation controversy to the foreground and shaken up established patterns regarding it. It would seem as though conditions were present that are conducive to leadership by those authorities in whom the public has confidence for improving the patterns of race relations in this country. The effectiveness and timeliness of such authoritative action is not refuted by its evoking some transitional turbulence if measures are taken to keep it within tolerable bounds. This is part of the process of change and is socially healthier than the calm maintained at the price of harmful suppression. By way of concrete illustration: many white Americans have to keep fighting down their own ideals of brotherly love and fair play in order to feel themselves in the right about segregation. External authority, in the form of church, or military establishment, or through a body of social law, or a respected leader, can provide extensive support to bolster these existent latent ideals and share the responsibility for them, while the security and satisfactions obtainable from such authorities may replace some of the psychological need to segregate. Thus the individual's own psychic pressure against segregation can become stronger and his emotional impetus to segregate weaker, bringing about a shift in his previous position. According to this concept, the Supreme Court decision does not force an allegedly homogeneously opposed segment of the population to behave against its will and conviction, but rather provides reinforcement to those ingredients of public attitude which, though entangled and smothered by conflict, are prevalent throughout this land and are in accordance with its professed ideals, as well as with fact rather than myth.

As we have already seen in some instances in the South, this principle can work in either direction, depending on whether the accepted external authority takes its stand in the conflict for or against desegregation, although the latent attitudes and wishes supported by the pro- and anti-segregation leaders are opposite. In either case a timely shift in the position of the external authority sets psychodynamic realignments in motion whereby attitudes and behavior may be modified. Like any other form of power, this can be constructive or destructive depending on how well the process is understood, to what purpose it is used, and the extent of safeguards against abuses of power.

Leadership

The dynamics of leadership, so important to all phases of social organization, are far too complicated for any attempt at full discussion here. However, the functions and role of leadership have such relevance to the social change-over to desegregation that some remarks, at least, are in order.

There are many kinds of leadership, varying as to aims, results, and modes of operation. Some of the differentiating factors between effective and poor leadership for enhancing group efficiency and morale, include the type of relationship patterns between group and leader, the leader's motivations and values, his attributes and abilities, and how these fit the needs and character of the group.

Leader-group relationship patterns

Manifold and complex patterns of relationship are possible between leader and group. For instance, leadership may be carried out on an authoritarian basis[18] or on reciprocal terms with the group. In the authoritarian type, the leader's role fulfills for the group an unrealistic father-image—whether benevolent, stern, or tyrannical —misperceived as all-wise and/or all-powerful. This form of leadership is maintained by fear, and the leader is separated from his group by the height of his position above it. But the leader, who as focal point for his group is in front of it rather than above it, remains part of its membership on terms of mutual respect and interchange. Such a leader can serve as catalyst for mobilizing group strengths and as synthesizer and channel for their expression and implementation. The feedback between the leader and the group in this type of leadership, which is lacking in the authoritarian form, constitutes a critical difference between the two patterns. Other

[18]The term "authoritarian" connotes dictatorial power over people, entailing irrationality, such as magical awe for the leader. It should not be confused with rational authority based on competence. (See Erich Fromm, *Man for Himself,* Rinehart & Co., New York, 1947, p. 9.)

decisive differences between leader-group interaction patterns lie in the extent to which it is the socially cohesive or socially disruptive tendencies and purposes within the group that are selectively reinforced and implemented by the leader, as well as how closely the leadership meets the realistic needs of the group.

Comparison of two types of leader-group situations arising out of the desegregation issue, which have been referred to in this report, may serve to illustrate these points. Kasper and White Citizens Council leadership came into Clinton as outsiders. As self-appointed town leaders they played on dormant local fears, fantasies and hostilities to the point of mob violence and social chaos. By contrast, Rev. King and other leaders of the Montgomery Negro bus boycott were pulled into the leadership by the activation in process within their group and its need for direction. The group members' feelings against segregation, which Dr. King voiced and strengthened, were not "stirred up" by him but had been astir among them for a long time.[19] His influence not only reinforced the group urge for social justice but also the group morality of brotherly love and control of violence and retaliation. The result has been group unity and stability, with perseverance for group goals by orderly social means.

Motivations and attributes of leaders

The leader's own values and mixed motivations, conscious and unconscious, for assuming leadership and using it for or against desegregation, affect his mode of leadership and consequently his impact on social action and public opinion. The motives in this area seem to range from the most socially altruistic to the crudest personal aggrandizing, with many forms, gradations, and combinations of these. Leaders, like all individuals as stressed throughout this report, may fool themselves as well as other people by the gap between the ostensible and actual reasons for their attitudes and behavior.

Leadership varies too with the attributes and abilities of the leader. Leaders are persons who are actually or apparently endowed with qualities which the follower admires and would like to add to himself. Leaders generally make up their minds on an issue ahead of the majority, which waits for cues from them. They have the drive and the know-how to map and carry out a course of

---

19Barrett, George, *New York Times Magazine, op cit.*

action. They are usually also more articulate in the expression of their views and have acquired more of the available avenues for such expression than are open to the average citizen. The ability of leaders to move ahead of others in making decisions and acting on them, or in being more vocal, may be prompted by judgment and foresight, by their wish for the profits of leadership, by the need to defend and maintain leadership, by a strong sense of responsibility, and by firm convictions on the issue. They are apt to have the vision to see broader implications beyond the immediate.

Although we can identify many of the personal motives and values and personal attributes and abilities that make for leadership, whether constructive or destructive, there are personality intangibles, as yet unstudied, or that elude study, which enter into the talent for leadership. In any case, leaders depend on the group's acceptance and approval for maintaining their power, while the group relies on the authority and support of the leader.

The participation of citizens in government

We may extend the last statement regarding the interdependence of leader and group to government and the citizenry. The psychological position of an individual with respect to governmental authority is basically different in a dictatorship than in a democracy, because the latter provides for his political participation through the franchise and other means. As one of the authors of this report has previously stated,[20] "Our body of laws and judicial institutions, devised by common consent and agreement, may be conceived of as our society's methods of self-regulation by carrying out functions of group conscience. Thus, they provide instrumentalities whereby citizens can reach collective decisions between right and wrong on the basis of as much fact, reason and justice as they are capable of at any given period. These judicial decisions that regulate social behavior, then, stem basically from the citizenry from whom they also derive the delegated power for enforcement." But when we consider the use of governmental authority in enforcing segregation or desegregation we must take into account at least two highly relevant features of the situation.

One has to do with the disenfranchisement for the most part of Negroes in the deep South, so that despite the Fourteenth and Fif-

[20]Bernard, Viola W., "Some Psychodynamic Aspects of Desegregation," *American Journal of Orthopsychiatry*, Vol. 26, #3, p. 459, July 1956.

teenth Amendments they do not share in the wielding of political authority, the power of which is retained by white people. As one of the gaps between American political theory and practice, Negro citizens in the deep South live under an undemocratic regime and are excluded from holding governmental positions of authority. They have been subject to coercive segregation laws without political voice or representation in their enactment. Although it has often been said of them that they prefer this, such occasions for the direct expression of their opinion as the past year's Montgomery bus strike belie this. The southern Negroes, therefore, have been denied the psychologically important sense of control, through legal means, over their governmental authorities whose regulations for intergroup behavior they are compelled to obey.

The other important point is the need to identify the political and social units under discussion when attempting to think through some of the psychosocial implications of legally enforced desegregation. Do we refer to the whole nation or to one of the states or counties in the deep South?

For some white Southerners, the authority conflict implicit in the issue of states' rights versus federal rights has a significance which is not easily understood by the average Northerner. The vigorous defense of states' rights has, since before the Civil War, carried the meaning of self-assertion, independence, and self-respect to many Southerners, who have seen in this position a way of combatting domination by the North through its greater economic resources, larger population, and consequent superior political power. Disregarding the rights and wrongs of this philosophic position from the point of view of the welfare of the country as a whole and its regional subgroups, the fact remains that self-respect has become intricately tied up with the philosophy of states' rights for many white Southerners. While it may, then, do violence to their self-respect from one point of view to relegate the Negro to a deprived and subservient position, it also does violence to feelings of self-respect to be (as they view it) "given orders" by a dictatorial or self-righteous North. In this situation many white Southerners can not look at the human rights issue with regard to the Negro because they are too immersed in the human rights issue which they feel exists with regard to their own status as second-class citizens of the United States who must not be dictated to by an arrogant majority. This is related to the reactions of some white

Southerners, as expressed by the Southern novelist William Faulkner[21], who have worked hard to improve Negro-white relationships but when "told to do so" by outsiders feel impelled to take a defiant position.

Many apparently reasonable defenders of segregation cite an unquestioned psychological truth when they state that authoritative decisions are better accepted when they have been arrived at by some citizenry participation than when imposed. They feel that race relations were gradually improving so that it would have been better psychologically to wait than to have desegregation imposed upon the South. The applicability of this psychological truth to the desegregation situation depends on one's interpretation of the social unit concerned, and in political terms, on the states' rights issue. For the United States as a whole, the Supreme Court's decision was made through the democratic machinery of self-government at a time when it reflected the country's gradually changing mores and the wishes of the overwhelming majority of the population. It was made in the light of increasing reports, from both the North and the South, of successful experiences of integration. From the standpoint of the deep South, however, the decision was contrary to the most conspicuous views of the white Southern majority. The decision was out of keeping, therefore, with the majority wish of a segment of the nation's population, i.e., some white citizens of some Southern states. An important question of democratic process relates to what limitations should be placed upon majority coercion of a minority, in this instance, the majority of Americans and the minority of segregationists. In recent times we have all seen the monstrous example of denial of rights to component minorities by totalitarian states. A big difference between this, however, and the exercise of federal judicial authority by the Supreme Court decision is not only that the decision was made in accordance with the democratic principle of timely legalizing of changes in majority mores, but that the minority "right" in question entails injury to others. If, in the name of safeguarding minority rights, the segregationists should remain legally empowered to go on damaging their fellow citizens—and the evidence of psychological damage from school segregation is considerable[22]—it would seem as absurd and

[21]Faulkner, William, "A Letter to the North," *Life*, March 5, 1956.

[22]U. S. Supreme Court opinion, May 17, 1954 (see footnote eleven of the decision).

unthinkable, socially, as guaranteeing the freedom to kill or steal.

Closely related to this distinction between the socio-political units under discussion is the need to differentiate between the levels of governmental authority—national, state, and local—when considering their application to desegregation in the South from the standpoint of their subjective effects. Local and state authority in the deep South is in the control of those who have vested political and power interest in the segregationist status quo. Many public officials and civic leaders in that region feel obliged, for fear of reprisal from those on whose power the preservation of their own power and personal safety depends, to oppose desegregation even when they might privately prefer to lend the authority of their office to implementing it. The danger of such reprisal is indeed real. Economic pressure, threats and acts of violence, and various forms of personal harassment have been used against those considered insufficiently segregationist. Political penalties to candidates for elective office for opposing segregation are too conspicuous to require documentation. Negro school teachers are being discharged in some Southern communities for failing to sign statements that they do not advocate mixed schools.[23] A white woman physician was discharged from a Southern State Department of Health for lunching with a Negro woman staff member. Resignations of state and municipal white professional employees are being forced, through the creation of untenable working conditions in order to circumvent tenure, as punishment for suspected traces of pro-desegregation sympathies. The known and unknown instances of reprisal could be multiplied many times over.

Many of the citizens of the deep South, and many of the local officials, school superintendents, and members of school boards who feel their hands are tied by the local white power situations, welcome with a sense of relief whatever authority the federal government can bring to bear in the situation. Since for the most part, those who feel this relief dare not openly express it, their attitude is seldom recognized, concealed as it is behind the more vocal protests of the segregationists against "outside intervention."[24] Actu-

---

[23]*U.S. News and World Report,* September 21, 1956, p. 50.

[24]The term "outside intervention" has often been used as a slogan to stir up anti-Negro violence in the South and to displace the blame for it. This technique of agitation plays on the deep feelings of Southern pride and defensiveness which we have referred to earlier.

ally, federal and state authority can greatly support the morale and strengthen the hand of many local authorities who dare not otherwise act in accordance with their own convictions as to their responsibilities. In a number of situations of mob violence around desegregation in the South, federal authority has been appealed to. In such instances it has been regarded as an aid to local authority rather than a threat to it. Thus, in the two Clinton crises, within a few months of each other, responsible officials and citizens sought and obtained needed help from the Federal District County Judge in Knoxville for restoring and maintaining law and order. On the second occasion Clinton citizens and officials also called upon the federal District Attorney in Knoxville for assistance, and the School Board wrote to the United States Attorney General for aid. Action by these federal authorities enabled the state and town authorities, and the local educational authorities, to reopen the school under orderly conditions.

C. *Responses of Various Groups to Desegregation*

What are the psychological consequences of school desegregation for the various groups most immediately involved? Of primary concern, of course, are the children themselves. What is the impact upon them of this new experience? What are the positive experiences and what are the new conflicts aroused? How do the changes in school and community affect the educators who are in charge and upon whom, therefore, much of the responsibility for success or failure lies? And how are parents affected, both via the changes in the community at large and the changed attitudes in their children? Much of what will be said in this section is grounded in experience with mixed racial groups in the North and in those Southern communities where desegregation is now under way.

1. THE CHILDREN

In many communities it has happened that a relatively small number of Negro children have appeared in some originally white classrooms, or that a small number of white children have found themselves in a school which is predominantly Negro. Desegregation also means that, irrespective of racial proportions, many children find themselves in new groups. In all these instances the reactions of the individual who finds himself a stranger in a group, as well as the reactions of the group as it tries to cope with the newcomers, assume great importance.

The newcomer and the group

Some students will experience an increase of actual rejection. The student previously sensitized to rejection may re-experience the pain of former rejection as well as the new one, and old patterns of handling such feelings may reappear. Any marked disparity in cultural backgrounds will also fortify such feelings. In line with the distinction between desegregation and integration referred to earlier, some evidence suggests that at first, friendship ties and social interactions of a minority group of newcomers will be greater on a within-group than between-group basis.[1] However, as soon as educators achieve a favorable school climate through resolution of their own conflicting attitudes and provision of strong objective leadership, the children's racial loyalties can be expected to give way to school, team, and class identifications and loyalties.

Projection of family role

There will, in the initial stages of new-group adjustment, be a number of possible individual reactions depending on a particular child's specific personal history. For example, a child who feels unloved and unjustly dealt with in its family will often identify strongly with children in the larger "school-family" whom it perceives as also unloved and unjustly dealt with. Thus unconscious feelings and conflicts associated with emotion-laden family relationships may underlie marked tensions and conflicts over racial problems. On the other hand, a child who is striving toward identification with parents perceived as highly principled and assertive may identify with those teachers who are similarly perceived and then will actively take sides in school with such teachers.

The child takes a role in social issues in a manner which parallels the tendencies shown in the home but which also strives toward resolution of problems in the larger social-family which were not satisfactorily solved in the home-family unit. New experiences with the important adult figures at school may do much toward putting a child on the pathway toward resolving old conflicts and developing a better integrated concept of his self.

---

[1] "Cognitive and Affective Factors in Sociometric Reactions of Negroes and Whites," Bryant Wedge, Robert R. Blake, Clifton C. Rhead, and Jane Srygley Mouton (to be published).

Adjustment mechanisms under stress

Becoming a member of a new group often stirs up in the newcomer a whole sequence of behavior mechanisms by which he tries to cope with this experience. Under the impact of such experiences, even otherwise normal and well adjusted individuals will often suffer temporarily a distortion of their social perception, and processes similar to those described under the term "emigration neurosis" will often occur. Some individuals react to the impact of their newness in the group by overexpectation of acceptance, thus making many mistakes in group behavior which they would not have made in their old groups. Others tend to develop near-paranoid interpretations of the behavior of the members of their new group, expecting rejection even where none occurs, or producing fantasies of being mistreated by the new group because their own need to accept the new group threatens their inner loyalty to the old. At the same time, under the impact of newness and stress, many individuals use already existent defense mechanisms such as overtalking, excessive assertiveness, overcompliance to the wrong subgroup demands, or producing such a strong cloak of shyness, isolation, withdrawal, that even friendly gestures toward participation by the new group fall on non-perceptive ears. The adults on the staff of desegregated schools will benefit in their own adjustment to the new staff-group situation by being aware of these processes in themselves, and they need also to be aware of, in order to be able to help, the same problems when they affect the *children* in their classrooms.

The conscious and unconscious fantasies of each educator and of each pupil will be important determinants of individual attitudes and emotional reactions. Individual problems in relating and communicating with each other usually have such a basis. A teacher or pupil may fantasy a loss of status with the home social group through "fraternizing" with a different racial group at school. All too frequently such fantasies, when verbalized, are regarded as though they were founded in reality, which they are not. An educator at a planning level may find his work complicated by fantasies of threatening mass response or unfavorable publicity.

The group's reception of the stranger

In addition to the adjustments required of the individual when coming into a new group, the group itself reacts to the stranger with a variety of responses, and must eventually reintegrate itself to make a place for the new addition. Among the more common and important responses of groups in general to newcomers the following can be mentioned:

The group may temporarily exclude a newcomer, banding together to ignore him. After some time—a sort of initiation period—he then may be accepted as a part of the group. This behavior can be seen whenever a child moves into a new neighborhood, or even, though less blatantly, when an adult becomes a member of a new group.

There may be an overacceptance of the newcomer, with temporarily a great deal of special attention being given to him, and a corresponding overexpectation of exceptional behavior from him. This may be followed by a rejection phase, initiated after the newness has worn off, because the newcomer has not lived up to the grandiose expectations focused upon him.

In a group which is already under pressure because of some previously existing tensions—such as, for example, the pressure of a feared autocratic leader—the new member may be cast for a role on the basis of the group's pathology whether he fits in the role or not. A new child can then be cast as rebel, enemy, or suspected teacher's pet, depending on the specific tensions already existing in the group, irrespective of how the group actually feels about the newcomer.

The group may accept a newcomer easily and socialize with him amicably, and yet his newness may continue to be a fact remembered about him for a prolonged period. There may be a withholding of complete trust and acceptance shown by the fact that he is not elected as officer or selected as representative by the group. Or he may be assigned jobs or roles that the old members of the group would prefer to avoid, a condition of the acceptance then being his taking on an undesirable job.

These few illustrations of the dynamics of group reaction toward the "newcomer" or the "stranger" may suffice to remind ourselves how important it is for teachers and parents in desegregating schools to become aware of these processes.[2] Many such group processes

[2]Educators do have long experience with situations in which all the children are new to the school at the same time, i.e., kindergarten and the entering class of Junior High School. When everyone is a stranger, aside from groups or pairs who have been friends in prior settings, the interactions between group and individual will doubtless differ in some respects from what has been described. Educators can bring to newly formed interracial classes their familiarity with the initial group insecurities of these entering classes.

occur without becoming conscious to the individuals involved. Neither the bully who pesters a new child in order to protect the old group from his intrusion, nor the new child who is suddenly up against rejective behavior—even though he had little reason to expect it—knows what is motivating him. In interracial camping it has long been known that one of the most important skills of a counselor is the ability to umpire wisely in fights among children in the early days. For many such fights have nothing to do with real hostility or even racial issues, but are merely the customary neighborhood ritual in which a newcomer is tested. Far from being a sign of rejection of a new child, challenges to this type of fight are often the very signal of potential acceptability. The differentiation between a personal squabble, an incident of scapegoating against a minority group, and a ritualistic test is one of the most important tasks of the adult in charge.

The development of attitudes and behavior patterns

Under the impetus of a wide variety of pressures and motivations, people of all ages are constantly modifying their attitudes and behavior patterns. Such modifications have been discussed in section B of this report. With children, the more immature the child, the more completely the goals of gaining immediate pleasure and avoiding pain govern the development of patterns. With maturation considerations of current and future reality increasingly influence attitude and behavior. A child at the age of four may assume a specific attitude and behavior in a social situation in order to gain the approval and love of those around him, or, if he feels rejected and hostile, may assume attitudes and behavior in opposition to those desired. The same child at a later stage in his development, say at the age of seven, may adopt the attitudes and behavior patterns of a revered adult by a process of incorporating them into his own character, and in so doing may have quite different goals and use quite different psychological processes than at the earlier age. The direct one-to-one correspondence between attitude and behavior which is found in small children also changes with development, until at the adult level behavior patterns may be quite different—even diametrically opposite to—conscious or unconscious attitudes. It is necessary, then, in dealing with children's behavior and in planning learning experiences for them, to take cognizance of their stage of emotional maturation. Methods of presenting new material as well as recognition of underlying attitudes which affect learning will vary according to developmental level.

Practical problems

On a practical level, the adults in charge of newly desegregated groups of children encounter innumerable specific situations which are the resultant of all the pressures impinging on the new group. Elements in the final behavior come from each member's character make-up, the attitudes and actions of the school adults, and the various influences of the parents and the wider community. Some of the problems in behavior which can be expected to arise are discussed below.

Racial conflict as a screen

In areas where desegregation occurs without too great resistance and parental objection, the first results may be astonishingly good. The children accept each other and begin working and playing together without untoward incident. Yet as the novelty wears off and the daily routine sets in, a variety of difficulties may occur. The children may experience hostile and aggressive impulses toward each other. After an early stage of smooth sailing, groups of children may gang up against each other in aggressive warfare. The fighting itself may reinforce prejudiced attitudes, as well as affect the adults—parents or teachers—with disappointment and discouragement as to the workability of desegregation. They may fail to remember that children are characteristically prone to gang up in groups and to regard others as strangers and enemies. Even among children of the same ethnic group it frequently occurs that similar children in the next block are stereotyped as "outsiders." Differences in skin color may provide a convenient focal point for such ganging up and may for a time suggest to the more inexperienced that prejudiced attitudes are unchangeable.

Prejudices can also be used by children, as well as adults, as serviceable rationalizations for other difficulties. In some summer camps, for instance, it was noted that Negro and white children cooperated amicably in activities together, but that when difficulties arose the reasons given by the children for the trouble would draw in the racial difference, whereas in similar trouble between two children of the same race, resort would be made to some other characteristic as an explanation. This easy use by children of racial rationalizations for their quarrels may lead many of the adults to the unjustified conclusion that prejudice is the primary motivation for all of them. In a similar vein, it should be remembered that racial invectives are often used in everyday conflicts among children in anger. Such use is frequently based on the perception by the angry child of a sensitive spot in his opponent, rather than being an indicator of specific racial hostility on his part.

The impact of the surrounding atmosphere

Further disillusionment may arise if one does not recognize that the ability of children to be free from the prejudices with which they were originally imbued depends to a large degree on the support they get from the atmosphere of the immediate environment in which they live. Thus, in some camps with a high degree of racial integration, it was observed that even children who came from neighborhoods with heavy racial tensions were quite capable of living happily with each other without having to resort to the display of prejudicial behavior. Some of these children, however, upon return to their old neighborhoods and under the impact of environmental pressures, resumed their old patterns of prejudiced action. The same observation has been made with soldiers who worked and fought together harmoniously but who returned to old stereotypes when they resumed civilian life.

Does this then mean that people—both children and adults—will aways return to such attitudes when the setting demands it and when psychological stress rises beyond a certain threshold? Perhaps there is a critical level of stress for each person, beyond which he will revert to defensive processes, such as calling upon prejudicial attitudes to boost his own security. It is for this very reason that the moral support of the law of the land, as well as its more obvious enforcement power, plays such an important role in actually making real and workable a social change. It strengthens and supports the other social forces which initiated the change and which still operate to make it effectual. It also must be realized that in a sufficient period of time—and under certain favorable conditions—children's new experience of the others as persons like themselves will render prejudiced attitudes obsolete. That is, the others will be taken for granted.

Another challenge which may have to be met in the early phase of desegregation is that of helping children with some problems of loyalty conflicts that may arise. A child may, for instance, be happily included as a member in a mixed group. In consequence of this he may, however, find himself reproached for being a renegade, or he may come into conflict with parental attitudes. This is not too dissimilar to some of the conflicts that children of immigrant parents are known to go through.

Since local community standards and values influence the behavior of the children, it is to be anticipated that with the existence of a desegregated school environment and the co-existence of a segregated community environment, conflict may arise. For instance, the same child who is expected to conform to and feel comfortable in desegregated patterns at school functions, may find himself confronted with the demand to conform to a segregated pattern in social activities outside of school. Such a double standard may well lead to confusion in the child. It will not necessarily, however, produce conflicts of unmanageable severity. Human beings quite commonly live under conditions of varying standards, as the situation of many women in our society illustrates.

The problem of "compatibility"

Unfortunately, at present the achievement levels of white and Negro children of the same age vary widely in most communities. The quality of teaching and school equipment have been inferior for the Negro child. This has been coupled with a poorer educational level of the parents, as well as less developed intellectual and cultural interests. Consequently, children in Negro schools are at a disadvantage when compared with children of the same grade from white schools. I.Q. levels in the two groups may also be different. Proponents of segregation point to this as evidence of innate inequality, while integrationists attribute it to inferior opportunity. The consensus of expert opinion, as expressed by leading scientific organizations and the vast majority of recognized social science authorities, is that there is no scientific evidence of inborn difference in intelligence between Negroes and whites.[3] There is general recognition that the school achievement of Negro children, especially from segregated schools, is lower on the average than white

[3]Recently a psychologist took a different position in a magazine article. This article was widely publicized. A statement was issued shortly thereafter, signed by eighteen of the country's leading psychologists and other social scientists, restating the more widely accepted scientific thinking. See: "Does Race Really Make a Difference in Intelligence?" *U. S. News and World Report,* October 26, 1956.

children, although some Negro children do better than the average white child. The fact of the difference brings still another problem both to the children and the adults in a desegregated school system. Since the lower I.Q.[4] and achievement levels seem due to life circumstances, a transition period of varying length will be expected in the resolution of these differences. Louisville's Superintendent of Schools Omer Carmichael, when interviewed on TV in September 1956, agreed that the one-and-a-half year educational gap between Negro and white sixth graders presented a problem, but "not as great as many people feel. For example, if you will take any standard test you please, the spread of children from high to low on that standard test will be much greater than the spread between the median for the Negro and the Median for the white." In the meantime, both the stress involved for the slower child and the handicaps to the faster child must be taken into account in the organization and management of classes from the points of view of size, scholastic goals, methods of teaching, and so forth.

A final source of difficulty which may be mentioned is the fact that in some desegregated schools groups of children may be thrown together who, because of socio-economic differences and incompatibilities of personality type, would not mix regardless of their ethnic origin. For instance, middle-class, conforming children, whether white or Negro, will have trouble integrating with pre-delinquent, aggressive children from an underprivileged group. Such troubles may be falsely explained as racial when they are primarily social and psychological.

2. THE EDUCATOR

The creation of a desegregated school where there previously was segregation offers the educator a rich inventory of new opportunities. Many of the problems which have been created or accentuated through the pathogenic impact of the segregated atmosphere will no longer hamper him in the pursuit of educational ideals.

There is moreover a strong probability of increased enthusiasm and vigor in educational programs with increased pride and com-

[4]I.Q. values are vastly overrated as measures of intelligence in general and in particular with regard to these measures of Negro intelligence. Florence Goodenough and Dale Harris have stated that "the search for a culture-free test, whether of intelligence, artistic ability, personal-social characteristics, or any other measurable trait, is illustory." "Studies in the Psychology of Children's Drawings: II, 1928-1949," *Psychological Bulletin*, 1950, 47: 369-433.

petition in achievement. Currently, there is a stronger focus of interest on educational systems than has ever occurred in the past. Community interest and activity, although motivated by the emotion-laden desegregation issue in some areas, will certainly uncover many areas of inadequacy and complacency and result in effective pressure for improvement.

On the other hand, it is obvious that while transitional periods have in them the blessings of a gradual liberation from what was pathogenic before, they also force all people involved to go through the difficulties of transition. During the breaking up of previously ingrained patterns, and before new ones are firmly established, not only individuals but whole groups, too, develop symptoms of tension, insecurity, and confusion and call forth all available normal or pathological mechanisms in order to cope with them.

Educators must face new challenges in two directions in a newly desegregated school system. They must themselves integrate with colleagues of the other race and, while forming themselves into a harmoniously functioning organization, must concurrently recognize and deal with the adaptation problems of their pupils.

Much of what has been said as to processes in Negro-white adaptations (Section B) has relevance here. Certainly teachers are not immune from the conflicted attitudes which beset the rest of the population in regard to race relations and desegregation. It is particularly important to emphasize that well-intentioned efforts to overlook the problems for the sake of surface harmony are likely to prove harmful in the long run. Children are particularly sensitive to conflicts in basic attitudes between adults. In the home, such conflicts between parents are observed by a child and lead to disturbed behavior even when the parents fondly believe they have concealed them by "never quarreling in front of the children." So, too, in school, conflicting attitudes in a teacher, or opposing attitudes between teachers, even when kept from open expression, may cause loyalty struggles in the children which will interfere with learning. Wise leadership in the school must, therefore, provide opportunities for airing and resolving the inevitable differences which realistically can be expected to arise. To reach this goal open channels of communication are essential. Although frankness about mutual sensitivities and criticisms may lead to transiently increased tension between educators, it can be expected to facilitate the achievement of a really integrated working relationship in the long run.

Troubles during the transitional phase

In dealing with the children, educators will encounter special problems in the transitional phase. There is danger that many problems which arise from other sources will be thought of as due to the desegregation process itself. It is a human weakness, in times of social change, to be on the one hand overly optimistic about the disappearance of old sores, or on the other, to ascribe old problems which continue, to the process of change itself. Among the more obvious sources of such confusion the following should be mentioned:

Desegregation, like any other change in a school, will provide opportunities for rationalizing deficiencies. The teacher who has perpetually experienced difficulty in handling the task of group leadership and in developing a child-oriented atmosphere of discipline in the classroom, will continue to have problems during desegregation and may find it convenient and popular to point to desegregation as the cause of troubles she would have had anyway.

Classrooms which are badly composed—e.g., those with distance between achievement levels much too great, age range of children way beyond what a given group can take, ill-advised mixtures of types of children which would create trouble in any case, and tensions on the basis of socio-economic class, etc.—will automatically produce severe teaching and behavior problems. Where desegregation occurs without anything being done about the already pathogenic group composition of such a classroom, all the so-called predictions of problems made by the opponents of desegregation may very well come to pass. The problems were already there to begin with. It is important for the educator to be skillful in his recognition of the sources of these problems, and it is his task as well as that of the community to do away with pathogenic grouping—including wrong size of groups—if desegregation is expected to work.

Lack of auxiliary services which classrooms need, especially in underprivileged areas or in neighborhoods where social tension is rampant anyway, such as leisure-time clubs, adequate group life experience for teenagers, psychological counseling and guidance work, will always create additional casualties in learning as well as in personality development. Lack of social services to work on pathological home conditions, of foster homes and institutional placements for children with disrupted families, will, of course, produce child behavior in schools which will negate many of the otherwise well-developed school-and curriculum-designs. Disruption of the learning process and the failure of the educational tasks in terms of character education, etc., will remain a problem of such schools, segregated or not. It is important that communities keep this in mind, instead of viewing as potential desegregation dangers what in reality were problems of unmet social service needs to begin with.

Constant community pressures, publicity, and controversies outside of school are apt to keep teachers temporarily overly sensitive and reactive to differences in appearance and performance of children. This, while present, may limit individual teachers in their capacity for free and comfortable work with students in mixed classes.

Unconscious extraneous motivations, such as the devaluation of a superior or of a rival, may strongly influence the behavior of an individual teacher in adopting an attitude and taking a stand. None of these reactions will be new for the teachers using them. They will most frequently be the habitual unconsciously employed, built-in personality patterns which have been used by the individual teacher for years.

Another frequent temptation to which human beings are known to fall victim under the impact of social change is that of exchanging one set of prejudicial stereotypes for another more acceptable one. In the area of racial integration, the most frequent form this takes is the exchange of racial prejudices for prejudicial attitudes toward socio-economic classes, or neighborhood styles of behavior. It frequently occurs that the white as well as the Negro teacher, when surrendering his original prejudicial defenses, increases his demands for middle-class behavior and conformity to social mores from both the children of his own group as well as those of the other race. From this some of the Negro children visibly gain. If they come from educated homes or socially upward mobile families, they will find themselves free of the great amount of previously experienced discrimination because their "Negro-ness" will now not count. Their less economically privileged or less well brought up contemporaries, however, will find themselves in double jeopardy, for they will not only remain unacceptable to the whole school population because of their unacceptable social forms, but they experience an additional conflict. They may discover that even other Negro children of more middle-class background may be embarrassed by their behavior, or that even "their own" Negro teachers will feel the same way. In fact, the teachers may even put increased pressure of expectations on them because they have to prove how wrong the pessimistic expectations of the segregationists had been to begin with. The same Negro child with a learning problem in a mixed class may present a completely different problem to different teachers. A white or colored teacher might reject the child simply because he serves as a roadblock to his efforts at progress for the class as a whole; or he may reject the child as a verification of strong feelings of Negro inferiority; or he might identify with the child as an underdog and devote more effort and sympathy to that child than to others. No generalization would cover all cases. The reaction will be that which is characteristic for the individual teacher.

To broaden the point, it can be said that in general both white and Negro teachers will interact with some students in a manner designed to confirm their personal opinions or will push certain children to achieve lofty goals inspired by personal wishes. The destructive effects of this on the children are just as great when the behavior is to all intents and purposes benign and friendly as when it is overtly hostile and critical, since in either case it overlooks the child's needs. This kind of teacher approach can be expected to yield to efforts at teacher training and consultation, since a major step in learning to cope with it is developing the insight to recognize the presence of such attitudes.

Among the most clearcut forms of confusion the educator may fall prey to is the phenomenon referred to as "mascot" cultivation in Section B. This is experienced by the educator himself as a benign attempt to be especially nice to the poor kid of the minority group and is therefore expected to produce all the signs of gratitude and positive response in the victim. In reality, such singling out of the special merits, advantages, and good sides of the discriminated-against minority group is still only the reverse side of a prejudicial coin, and is experienced as such by the group of children involved. For, while benign in intent, it still tells the children: "I am not looking at you as persons. To me you are primarily something that reminds me of your race." Whatever good things are then said of this race, the fact that the child involved finds himself shorn of his individual personality and seen only as a symbol of a group remains deeply disturbing.

Complications in professional life

For many educators, there are emotional similarities between their own childhood family structure and the hierarchy of authority and the relationships between colleagues in the school system. Devaluation or overvaluation of the principals or supervisors is common, as are rivalrous feelings toward colleagues on the same status level. Administrators and supervisors, too, are confronted with the obligation to be fair and not play favorites. In situations of emotional stress or crisis it will be easy to ascribe the success of some educators and the failure of others to favoritism based on race. Additionally, where separate school systems with duplicated jobs for white and Negro teachers must be fused into a single system, many persons will be relegated to assistant roles in departments which they previously headed. There will in such instances inevitably be feelings of reduced status and a revival of old sibling rivalry conflicts. Some members of the group may feel initially threatened by working with outstanding people of the other race.[5] It is a further strain on Negro teachers' stability to distinguish truly unavoidable administrative problems of transition from administrative pretexts for discrimination. Both are taking place. In Maryland, desegregation has proceeded in Baltimore and other parts of the state without incurring the dismissal of any Negro teachers. In some other states desegregation has brought about discharges of Negro teachers.[6] There are localities said to employ large numbers of untrained and inexperienced white teachers and to leave vacancies unfilled rather than employ available experienced trained Negro teachers. Such practices not only do injury to the Negro teachers, but in depriving children of good teachers, reduce their opportunities for sound adjustment to desegregation.

The demand of the present period of transition on the patience, insight, and skills of school personnel cannot be overemphasized. For all present school personnel as well as for those responsible for teacher training and school counselor training, increased exposure to the techniques and insights developed in the field of

[5]Educators may find some useful guidance through reviewing the experiences of social workers in interracial agencies. See Inabel Burns Lindsay, "Race as a Factor in the Caseworker's Role," *Journal of Social Casework,* 1947, 28, pp. 101-107.

[6]*New York Times,* October 14, 1956.

group dynamics seems important. Much insight into the processes that go on in groups and their impact on individuals is available and should begin to contribute an important part of teacher training as well as of in-service training of personnel on all levels.[7]

3. THE PARENTS

Although children are the direct participants in the process of school desegregation, their attitudes and behavior are largely affected by parental attitudes. There is little doubt that where the parents as a group approved of desegregation, the problem of transition has been uneventful. However, an individual's role as a parent is not isolated from his role as an adult member of a community. Many negative attitudes toward desegregation have been gained by the parent as an individual and have little, if any, bearing on his role as a parent. Certainly there is no reason to believe that the fact of parenthood changes an individual's personality in any way which causes a significant lessening of his social prejudice.

Parents in our society are immensely concerned about the welfare and future of their children. According to the general mores, almost no sacrifice is too great to make for their benefit. Even in families with modest means, money is often saved from marginal incomes for college education; life and endowment insurances are purchased; and much social scheming takes place—for the benefit of the children. Certainly parental love and fear are most powerful psychological forces. It is this very dedication of parents to their children that has been utilized as a major force against desegregation. The threat of damage to children implicit in the alleged dangers of intermarriage effectively prevents a realistic appraisal of the evidence for and against segregation by many parents. Such fears

---

[7](A). Allport, Gordon W., *The Resolution of Intergroup Tensions, A Critical Appraisal of Methods*, National Conference of Christians and Jews, New York, 1952.

(B). Cartwright, D. and Zander, A. eds., *Group Dynamics, Research and Theory*, Row, Peterson, Evanston, Ill., 1953.

(C). Guetzhow, H. ed., *Groups, Leadership and Men*, Carnegie Press, Pittsburgh, 1951.

(D). Hare, A. P., Borgatta, E. F. and Bales, R. F. eds., *Small Groups Studies in Social Interaction*, Alfred A. Knopf, New York, 1955.

(E). Lewin, K., edited by Gertrud Weiss Lewin, *Resolving Social Conflicts*, Harper and Bros., New York, 1948.

(F). Storen, Helen F., *Readings in Intergroup Relations*, National Conference of Christians and Jews, New York, rev. ed., 1956.

have been discussed in Section A of this report. Many parents are also concerned about the possible psychological damage to their children, of whichever ethnic group, by the conflicts which they fear will be engendered in the mixed group. And further, both sets of parents are apprehensive about the educational problems which must be solved in a newly desegregated school.

Concerns and anxieties

White parents may fear that academic standards will be lowered by the admission of Negro children, that the child or family will lose status in the community, that their children will be exposed to lower moral standards and to communicable diseases. White parents may also have fears in regard to relatively direct contact with Negro parents, such as at parent-teacher meetings.

Negro parents, having no less concern for the welfare and future of their children, are also affected by doubts and fears regarding desegregation. Will their children be able to compete satisfactorily in a desegregated school with higher standards? Will they receive fair and impartial treatment from the teachers? Will the white children hurt them physically or emotionally? What indignities should they, the parents, anticipate in attending a parent-teacher meeting?

Some of the apprehensions of parents are realistic, at least in part, but the evidence provided by studies of areas which have been desegregated indicates that some of these fears dissipate quickly when experience demonstrates either that they were ill-founded or that the new problems can be solved. For example, research studies of desegregated housing in previously segregated areas suggest that there is an initial feeling of loss of status on the part of white tenants which corrects itself rather quickly. After an initial sense of loss of status, the tenants' individual feelings adjusted themselves to the realities of everyday living (as had happened throughout their lives in other situations). The signs of a sense of loss of status disappeared.

White parents with fears of loss of status may also be reassured by reports from areas where school desegregation has taken place, which indicate that status problems may be lessened by making attendance at desegregated schools not a matter of personal decision, but requiring desegregation of all the schools of a given community. Partial desegregation apparently encourages resistance. When all schools are desegregated, no child has a special advantage or handicap.

The fact that many Negro children will be relatively backward academically is primarily a problem for the school teachers and administrators and is discussed in another section of this report. Educators will need strong support from parents in meeting this problem. Gifted children of either race need not suffer academically from desegregation unless overcrowding, poor teaching, or other educational handicaps are present.

Similar considerations should lessen fears of white parents that their children may suffer a lowering of moral standards or catch communicable diseases from the Negro children. Neither delinquency nor communicable diseases are primarily related to race. Both are directly related to the complex social, psychological, and economic forces that form the ingredients of the pattern of inferior status of the Negro. Positive changes in these forces should lessen delinquency and improve the health of Negro children.

Sources of support

The parent-teacher meeting is a point at which white and Negro parents come into relatively direct contact with each other in a desegregated school. The beliefs and feelings many adults bring to meetings have been discussed elsewhere. However, the fact that contact in these meetings is on a basis of equal status as parents is unusual and leads to apprehensions. The parents attending these meetings, however, have a common bond and purpose which will assert itself positively in the direction of cooperation when the parents come to realize that irrespective of race they all want the same things for their children.

Whether the fears of Negro parents are realistic will vary from community to community and will be influenced by the social climate and the quality and character of the teachers. Some teachers, even though they know that present achievement is related to past educational and living experience as well as native ability, will have difficulties. Supplementary teacher training and constructive support from the parents will lessen these difficulties.

There are, of course, many parents who, being aware of social change, will desire that their children have experiences with desegregation which they themselves missed as children. The essence of education is to equip the child with skills and experience which may be effectively utilized and drawn upon in later life, among them the ability to get along with different people. Thus, while desegregation in schools will pose new problems for some parents for a period of time, it will at the same time relieve them of other problems incident to segregation.

III. SUMMARY AND DISCUSSION

As emphasized at the outset of this report, we recognize that the ruling of segregation as unconstitutional has meant that the process of desegregation is now definitely under way, although it proceeds at very uneven rates in different localities. Indeed, the resistance is so great in some communities that desegregation is only evidenced so far in the form of intensified opposition and efforts to circumvent it.

The anticipation of school desegregation arouses many mixed reactions of relief, hope, fear, and hostility, depending on the multiple constellations of racial, social, political, and psychodynamic variables discussed in this report. We have recognized that these reactions may be centrally or tangentially concerned with desegregation per se, for the individual, and that he may express them through manifold permutations and combinations of overtly or covertly going against or with the tide (however it may run for him); of floundering in its cross-currents or adding to its swell by his own energies.

We know that those whose intransigent resistance to desegregation serves irrational or unscrupulous purposes will not react to objective evidence of its workability by a change in their opposition. But there are more psychologically flexible people at every level of most communities' preparation for desegregation, who are responsive to reality-testing as a guide for their decisions and actions, even though it may not alter very much feelings that persist from their lifelong conditioning by the mores of segregation. For such people, reliable and informative reports of successful methods and results with desegregation elsewhere can help to modify misconceptions and disprove needless fears.

As the number of areas desegregating their schools increases, the opportunities and need for large-scale systematic psychosocial research study of this dynamic change become even greater. Research designed for application to the process of desegregation could have obvious immediate value. Long-term research, as well, using the "natural laboratory" of educational desegregation holds promise of advancing the basic knowledge of behavior.[8] It is strongly advisable that both types of research be undertaken.

Incoming reports by social scientists of desegregation case histories have some admitted limitations, such as the lack of uniform methods of data collection and analysis. Nevertheless they have great value as the record of a growing body of actual experience with desegrating by some communities from which others can learn. Although no locale can wholly take over the *modus operandi* of another, because of the characteristics specific to each, certain principles and techniques, found to be useful in the desegregation process, are transposable from one setting to another, with suitable modifications to fit the special circumstances. (Many of these principles and techniques have been referred to in this report.)

In preparing this report we have tried to bring together some facts and principles drawn from general knowledge of human behavior as well as from special experience in this particular aspect of it. We have tried to show the bearing of these on the processes of behavior and attitude change which must accompany desegregation. No law can by itself bring about a fundamental alteration in personal and group attitudes and their underlying feelings. The legal regulation can change external behavior; for a lasting change in attitudes and mores there must be long-term exposure to new experiences together with opportunities to develop new insights as the result of those experiences. If one approaches a new situation with a viewpoint already determined by a deeply-ingrained prejudice, the possibilities of learning from it are greatly reduced. It is for this reason that conceptions of Negro inferiority—intellectual, moral, and social—play such a crucial role in preventing attitude change. We have pointed out that the concept of the Negro as inferior intellectually is partly derived from observations of Negroes who have lived as a deprived group, economically, socially, and politically; that educational opportunities in the schools and cultural enrichment in the home have both been lacking. Since the environment of most Negro children is so markedly different from that of most white children, there is no valid basis for comparisons of the

---

[8]Williams, R. M. Jr., Fisher, B. R. and Janis, I. L., "Educational Desegregation as a Context for Research," *American Sociological Review*, 21, 5, October 1956.

potentials of the two groups. A common fallacy is to compare achievements, for example, in school, and to assume that achievement differences mean potential differences. Even the supposedly reliable I.Q. figures do not lend themselves to simple comparison where background differs so widely.

We have also pointed out that beliefs in Negro inferiority are made a matter of intense feeling and inflexibility because of the numerous irrational emotional factors which focus around this issue. Such irrational forces range from unconscious guilt feelings springing from the long exploitation of Negroes by whites, to the use of feelings of superiority by whites to bolster up self-esteem and combat problems of insecurity or anxiety coming from other aspects of their own lives. We have discussed the general principle that conflicted feelings or wishes in all human beings may be kept out of conscious awareness and displaced onto some other, seemingly rational, issue which can then be reacted to, while the more basic, inner sources of turmoil are avoided. Conflicts survive in all of us as remainders of childhood difficulties with parental authority and the necessity of adapting our wishes and drives to life as it is. Therefore none of us is immune to the use of defensive rationalizations. Vigilant recognition of the possibilities of being misled by rationalizations is incumbent upon all who are dealing with problems of interracial relationships.

We have discussed the intensely emotional issue of intermarriage, pointing out that racial mixing has not so far been prevented by laws forbidding intermarriage. Irrational fears and superstitions are especially prevalent in this area and are particularly hampering to reasoned efforts to find a way of living and working together which suits the needs and wishes of both races.

We have also discussed the changes attendant upon desegregation from the point of view of group processes in the community. Powerful forces can be mobilized, both constructive and destructive, by the interactions of people in groups. Results of constructive group action may be seen, for example, in Louisville's carefully-planned and relatively calm transition to desegregation, while the disturbances in Clinton, Tennessee exemplify the way in which group feeling can be stirred and channelized by fanatic leadership and how such effects can snowball once the process is under way. We believe that adequate recognition of the strength and dynamics of group forces is needed in order that wise leadership may assist in channeling them constructively. In every human being, with the possible exception of seriously maladjusted persons, there is a vital need for a feeling of belonging, of recognition and acceptance by the various groups to which he belongs. Leaders, too, are not independent of the groups which they lead. Recognition, approval, and a reciprocal relationship of opinion-formation and action-taking require involvement of the leader in the group mores as fully as the group members themselves. Training leaders in recognition of the important elements in their roles can help in establishing and maintaining constructive action.

We have discussed the dynamics of people's attitude toward authority in the process of social change. In many areas of the South, citizens of both races are caught in the open conflict between local authority which forbids compliance with the Supreme Court ruling and federal authority which requires it. In most people there are quite complex attitudes towards authority based on remnants of childhood conflicting attitudes toward parental authority, conflicting attitudes toward the very inconsistent admonitions of external authority throughout life, and conflicting attitudes toward one's own inner codes of right and wrong. These personal struggles are inevitably heightened in the present intense clash between the local and federal governmental authorities. In addition, even religious authority has not been able to take an unequivocal position on the desegregation issue. These serious differences between external authorities, plus internal conflicts over attitudes toward authority, coupled with intense feelings about desegregation springing from other sources, put many Southerners into situations of conflicted loyalty and conflicted sense of right and wrong which make rational action extremely difficult. It is of vital importance that those who stand in positions of authority recognize both the existing state of conflict and their opportunity and responsibility to do something about it by exercise of leadership, wise timing, and dynamic understanding of the total situation.

And finally, we have discussed in considerable detail the various aspects of desegregation as they affect the main participants—the children, the educators, and the parents. The children's attitudes with regard to race are largely determined by those of their elders and by the mores of the group in which they live. It can be strikingly demonstrated that in a neighborhood where the mores are those of racial discrimination and strife the children will behave in a similar fashion, while in a camp setting where there is no significance given to racial differences the same children accept those of other races as being without importance differences. Disturbance in the classroom can come from hostile or fearful attitudes about desegregation brought from home. It can also come from tensions in the group or in the children individually which have sources other than racial ones. Teacher leadership here must be responsible for correct identification and handling of classroom tensions. However, the teachers too will have processes of change and adaptation to go through. In aiding in these adaptations school supervisors and principals will be most effective if they recognize the need for constructive assistance to teachers in clarifying their own viewpoints as well as in understanding the processes which are going on in the children. The school leadership must carry not only this responsibility but also that of bringing the parents into a working relationship with the school on the new problems arising out of desegregation, just as they have on other aspects of their children's education.

We have tried to avoid in this report the use of global generalizations on a problem which is experienced differently in different communities and by different individuals. As psychiatrists we know from our work with individuals the dangers and difficulty of proceeding according to oversimplified, arbitrary rules. We have tried to present a way of looking at desegregation in schools as a human problem. The principle which has governed the production of this report is our belief that insight and understanding—that is, a rational approach to the profoundly irrational forces which move man—are the only appropriate ways of dealing with the issues of desegregation. We hope that we have demonstrated that problems attendant upon desegregation require for their solution not only an understanding of the social situations in which these problems occur, but also an insight into the complex motives—rational and irrational, conscious and unconscious—which influence attitudes toward these problems. We hope that this report will prove useful to those who are professionally involved in the problems arising from desegregation and that they will be aided by it in the task of translating understanding of psychodynamic processes into practical application.

IV. ANNOTATED READING LIST

The following reading list includes literature of particular relevance to the student of desegregation and of Negro-white relations in general. It does not claim to be comprehensive. Items which are quoted in the body of the report are so identified in parentheses citing the section of this report in which reference is made to them.

BIBLIOGRAPHY

Adorno, Theodor W.; Frenkel-Brunswick, Else; Levinson, Daniel J.; and Sanford, R. Nevitt. THE AUTHORITARIAN PERSONALITY. New York: Harper & Bros., 1950. (See chapter II-B).

Describes the research and theory on which the relationship between authoritarian character structure and anti-semitism (as well as prejudice in general) was formulated.

Allport, Gordon W. THE NATURE OF PREJUDICE. Cambridge: Addison-Wesley Publ. Co., 1954.

A text giving a comprehensive treatment of the development and modification of social attitudes.

Anastasi, Anne and D'Angelo, Rita Y. A Comparison of Negro and White Preschool Children in Language Development and Good-enough Draw-a-Man I.Q. J. OF GENET. PSYCHOL., 1952, 81,147-165.

A study of 5-year-old children at Dept. of Welfare Day Care Centers in New York City. Children from white and Negro uni-racial and from bi-racial centers were the subjects.

Ashmore, Harry S. THE NEGRO AND THE SCHOOLS. Chapel Hill: Univ. of No. Carolina Press, 1954. (See chapter II-B).

A history of the development of segregated education in the South, including a review of recent trends toward integration. Statistical data are given describing Negro and white schools and the relationship of education to population trends. Foreword by Owen J. Roberts.

Bernard, Viola W. Psychoanalysis and Members of Minority Groups. J. AMER. PSYCHOANALYTIC ASSOC., 1953, 1, 2, 256-267.

Discusses the place of considerations of minority status, especially of being Negro, in the patient-analyst relationship. Points out some of the dangers inherent in either overemphasizing or underemphasizing patient-analyst differences, in maintaining inflexible attitudes about dealing with the situation, and in carrying minority group or majority group stereotypes into the analytic relationship.

Bernard, Viola W. Some Psychodynamic Aspects of Desegregation. AMER. J. ORTHOPSYCHIATRY. 1956, 26, 3, 459-466 (See chapter II-B).

A contribution to a round table on *Desegregation: Its implications to Orthopsychiatry.* Indicates some ways in which orthopsychiatry can help meet the problems that many individuals will encounter as a consequence of the changes brought by desegregation. Discusses, briefly, some broader psychodynamic implications of authority in relation to desegregation.

Bird, Charles and Monachesi, Elio D. Prejudice and Discontent. J. OF ABN. AND SOCIAL PSYCHOL., 1954, 49, 1, 29-35.

A questionnaire study, in a Northern city, of the relation between neighborhood and occupational contentment, and prejudice toward Negroes.

Bird, Charles; Monachesi, Elio D.; and Burdick, Harvey. Studies of Group Tensions: III. The effect of parental discouragement of play activities upon the attitudes of white children toward Negroes. CHILD DEVELOP., 1952, 23, 4, 295-306.

A questionnaire study on the influence of parental attitudes and play prohibitions, including parental agreements and disagreements, on the attitudes of young white children toward Negro children.

Boyd, George F. The Levels of Aspiration of White and Negro Children in a Non-segregated Elementary School. J. OF SOCIAL PSYCHOL., 1952, 36, 191-196.

An experimental and questionnaire study of the aspiration levels of 25 equated pairs of Negro and white children, age 13.

Boyd, William C. GENETICS AND THE RACES OF MAN. Boston: Little, Brown and Co., 1950. (See chapter II-A).

A summary of current thinking about the question of race based on the study of genetics. Brings technical genetic information to bear on the problem of the descent of man and the origins of human races.

Brenman, Margaret. The Relationship Between Minority-Group Membership and Group Identification in a Group of Urban Middle-Class Negro Girls. J. OF SOCIAL PSYCHOL., 1940, 11, 171-197.

A report on a series of depth-interviews with 25 older Negro middle-class girls, each of whom spent 15-30 hours with the investigator. The development of attitudes of identification with, and rejection of, both whites and Negroes is examined as they appear to arise from earlier experiences.

Brenman, Margaret. Urban Lower-class Negro Girls. PSYCHIATRY. 1943, 6, 3, 307-324.

Report on a field study of a few lower-class Negro girls with whom the investigator interacted as a participant observer and interviewer. The girls' reactions to minority group membership, interracial attitudes, sexual behavior, and morality standards were the focus of the research.

Brown, Luna B. Race as a Factor in Establishing a Casework Relationship. SOCIAL CASEWORK. 1950. 31, 3, 91-97.

Reports the results of a survey of social casework agencies on problems they may have had in assigning case workers to clients of another race.

Clark, Kenneth B. PREJUDICE AND YOUR CHILD. Boston: Beacon Press, 1955.

Deals with the ways children learn about race and the harmful effects of prejudice on children of both races. Indicates the roles that schools, social agencies, churches, and parents can play to promote integration, and discusses the rate at which desegregation can best proceed.

Clark, Kenneth B. and Clark, Mamie P. Emotional Factors in Racial Identification and Preference in Negro Children. J. OF NEGRO EDUC., 1950, 19, 3, 341-350.

A further investigation of emotional conflict involved in the racial self-identification of young Negro children. Studies 5-7-year-olds in the South and North.

Cook, Stuart W. Desegregation: A Psychological Analysis. AMER. PSYCHOL., 1957, (in press). (See chapter I, II-B).

A systematic analysis of the variables involved in (1) taking a public position on desegregation and (2) change in interracial relationships and attitudes in unsegregated social situations.

Cook, Stuart W. and Selltiz, Claire. Some Factors Which Influence the Attitudinal Outcomes of Personal Contact. INTERNAT. SOCIAL SCIENCE BULL., 1955, 7, 1, 51-58.

An analysis of the conditions which determine the attitudinal outcomes of involuntary contact between persons from different ethnic groups.

Davie, Maurice R. NEGROES IN AMERICAN SOCIETY. New York: McGraw-Hill Book Co., 1949.

A text covering the cultural history of the Negro in the United States. Beginning with importation for slavery, the development of Negro life is indicated in some 22 chapters dealing with diverse aspects of Negro-white relations.

Davis, Allison. Child Training and Social Class. In Barker, Roger G., Kounim, Jacob S. and Wright, Herbert F. CHILD BEHAVIOR AND DEVELOPMENT. New York: McGraw-Hill Book Co., 1943, 607-619.

A discussion of middle- and lower-class child-training goals and methods among Negroes in the deep South.

Davis, Allison. American Status Systems and the Socialization of the Child. In Kluckhohn, Clyde and Murray, Henry A., PERSONALITY IN NATURE, SOCIETY, AND CULTURE. New York: Alfred A. Knopf, 1952, rev., 567-576.

A discussion of socialization as it is influenced by age, sex, and social class variables which indicate the appropriate roles to be learned.

Davis, Allison and Dollard, John. CHILDREN OF BONDAGE. Wash., D.C.: American Council on Education, 1940. (See chapter I).

A case study approach to the problems which arise in the personality development of Negro children growing up in Southern urban communities. Eight cases, covering all class levels, are treated extensively, and many more are drawn upon.

Davis, Allison and Havighurst, Robert J. Social Class and Color Differences in Child-Rearing. In Kluckhohn, Clyde and Murray, Henry A., op. cit., 308-320.

A study comparing child-rearing practices as reported by four groups of parents: middle-class white, middle-class Negro, lower-class white, lower-class Negro.

Dean, John P. and Rosen, Alex. A MANUAL OF INTERGROUP RELATIONS. Chicago: Univ. of Chicago Press, 1955.

Gives suggestions for community workers interested in reducing segregation and discrimination. Based on both social research and practical experience. Foreword by Charles S. Johnson.

Deutscher, Max and Chein, Isidor. Psychological Effects of Enforced Segregation: A Survey of Social Science Opinion. J. OF PSYCHOL., 1948, 26, 259-287.

A survey of opinions of social scientists regarding the psychological impact of involuntary segregation upon both those segregated and those enforcing the segregation.

Does Race Really Make A Difference In Intelligence? U.S. NEWS AND WORLD REPORT. Oct. 26, 1956, 74-76. (See chapter II-C).

Full text of a joint statement released Oct. 16, 1956 by eighteen social scientists, most of them members of the American Psychological Association.

Drake, St. Clair and Cayton, Horace R. BLACK METROPOLIS. New York: Harcourt Brace and Co., 1945.

An exhaustive and intensive community study of the Negro in Chicago. A wealth of material is presented on Negro culture, social norms, and relations to whites.

Ellis, Albert and Beechley, Robert. Comparisons of Negro and White Children Seen at a Child Guidance Clinic. PSYCHIATRIC QUARTERLY SUPPLEMENT. 1950, 24, 1, 93-101.

Statistical comparison of 71 Negro and 1,000 white children on twenty-eight variables. These include family background, emotional adjustment, psychiatric diagnosis, and type and extent of treatment.

Everett, Samuel. A Community School Ends Segregation. THE SCHOOL EXECUTIVE, July, 1954, 52-53.

A brief description of how a developing suburban area handled its school problem by integrating its facilities. (See chapter II-B).

Frazier, E. Franklin. NEGRO YOUTH AT THE CROSSWAYS. Wash., D.C.: American Council on Education, 1940.

A study of the dilemmas and problems facing Negro youths who grow up in the middle, or border, states. The influences of various social and community factors are discussed as they affect the feelings and attitudes of the youths toward themselves as Negroes. Case history material is also presented.

Frazier, E. Franklin. THE NEGRO IN THE UNITED STATES. New York: The Macmillan Co., 1949.

A comprehensive historical analysis of the processes by which the Negro acquired American culture and has emerged as a minority group, and of the extent to which he is being integrated into American society. Twenty-eight chapters cover most sociological and political topics, each treated in historical terms.

Ginzberg, Eli, assisted by Anderson, James K.; Bray, Douglas W.; and Smuts, Robert W. THE NEGRO POTENTIAL. New York: Columbia Univ. Press, 1956. (See chapter I).

A report on a study by the Conservation of Human Resources Project. The Project, established by Dwight D. Eisenhower as President of Columbia University, studied the expanding economic opportunities for the Negro and his educational preparation. It finds Negro gains due primarily to prosperity and characterizes the nation's Negroes as "the single most underdeveloped human resource in the country." Develops the thesis that, unless accelerated, the Negro's preparation to take advantage of new occupational openings may lag behind their availability.

Goodman, Mary Ellen. RACE AWARENESS IN YOUNG CHILDREN. Cambridge: Addison-Wesley Press, 1952.

A study of the emergence of racial awareness, identification, and bias in four-year-olds at an interracial nursery. The acquisition of these attitudes in the children's social life is studied and discussed.

Hammer, Emanuel F. Negro and White Children's Personality Adjustment as Revealed by a Comparison of Their Drawings (H-T-P). J. OF CLINICAL PSYCHOL., 1953, 9, 1, 7-10.

A comparison of drawings on the House, Tree, and Person Test by Negro and white children at two segregated schools. Evidence of more "emotional disturbance" among Negro children was sought as part of the reason for lower I.Q. scores for Negro children.

Heine, Ralph W. The Negro Patient in Psychotherapy. J. OF CLINICAL PSYCHOL., 1950, 6, 4, 373-376.

A brief discussion of the interpersonal problems that may characteristically arise between Negro patients and white therapists in the psychotherapeutic relationship.

Herskovitz, Melville J. THE AMERICAN NEGRO: A STUDY IN RACIAL CROSSING. New York: Alfred A. Knopf, 1928. (See chapter II-A).

An anthropometric study, covering four years of work, of the physical form of the American Negro and of the racial mixtures of which he is the product.

Hill, Herbert and Greenberg, Jack. CITIZEN'S GUIDE TO DESEGREGATION. Boston: The Beacon Press, 1955.

A review, written for laymen, of the legal status of racial segregation and the recent challenges to it. Contains a section on suggestions for action by citizens who wish to support desegregation.

Himes, Joseph S. and Manley, A. E. The Success of Students in a Negro Liberal Arts College. J. OF NEGRO EDUC., 1950, 19, 4, 466-473.

An analysis of the reasons for ultimate withdrawal, before graduation, of two-thirds of the students who entered No. Carolina College during the years 1936-1941. Language deficiencies and psychological unpreparedness are pointed out as major contributing factors to failure.

Ireland, Ralph R. An Exploratory Study of Minority Group Membership. J. OF NEGRO EDUC., 1951, 20, 2, 164-168.

A brief general review of the results of a content analysis of 72 papers on the topic, "What it means to be a Negro," written ostensibly as a freshmen assignment by Negro students. The data suggest little homogeneity of outlook in the group studied.

James, H. E. O. and Tenen, Cora. THE TEACHER WAS BLACK. London: William Heineman Ltd., 1953.

A study of attitude change among children being taught by two visiting Negro teachers in English elementary schools.

Johnson, Charles S. GROWING UP IN THE BLACK BELT. Wash., D.C.: American Council on Education, 1941.

A study, using many research tools, of the problems faced by Negro youths growing up in the rural South. Special attention was paid to studying variations in the agricultural patterns of the rural areas, for reasons of their intrinsic interest and to provide a basis for accurate sampling for statistical measures.

Kahn, Jane; Buchmueller, A. D.; and Gildea, Margaret, C. L. Group Therapy for Parents of Behavior Problem Children in Public Schools: Failure of the Method in a Negro School. AMERICAN J. OF PSYCHIATRY, 1951, 108, 5, 351-357.

An analysis of the reasons why a group therapy program for mothers of children with behavior problems failed in a Negro school after it had succeeded in 5 white schools. Methods in mental health education to meet minority group tensions are outlined.

Kardiner, Abram and Ovesey, Lionel. THE MARK OF OPPRESSION. New York: W. W. Norton & Co., 1951. (See chapter I, II-A).

Based on the psychodynamic analyses of the life history and personality structure of 25 intensively studied Negro men and women drawn from diverse economic and social strata. Presents a psychoanalytic interpretation of the effect on the psychodynamics of Negro personality of being a member of a minority group that is the target of strong prejudice and discrimination.

Klineberg, Otto (Ed.) CHARACTERISTICS OF THE AMERICAN NEGRO. New York: Harper & Bros., 1944. (See chapter II).

Contains material initially collected for Myrdal's *An American Dilemma.* The six sections of the volume are: (1) The Stereotype of the American Negro, Guy B. Johnson (one chapter), (2) Tests of Negro Intelligence, Otto Klineberg (four chapters), (3) Experimental Studies of Negro Personality, Otto Klineberg (three chapters), (4) "Race" Attitudes, Eugene L. Horowitz (eight chapters), (5) The Hybrid and the Problem of Miscegenation, Louis Wirth and Herbert Goldhamer (nine chapters), (6) Mental Disease Among American Negroes: A Statistical Analysis, Benjamin Malzberg (one chapter).

Knobloch, Hilda and Pasamanick, Benjamin. Further Observations on the Behavioral Development of Negro Children. J. OF GENET. PSYCHOL., 1953, 83, 137-157.

44 of an original group of 53 Negro infants were examined for the third time and their developmental progress studied and correlated with various individual and environmental factors. The average New Haven Negro child between 18-31 months remains fully equal in behavioral development to his average white coeval.

Lee, Alfred McLung. FRATERNITIES WITHOUT BROTHERHOOD. Boston: Beacon Press, 1955.

A report on the status of racial, religious, and ethnic discrimination practices in social fraternities at American universities.

Lewis, Julian H. THE BIOLOGY OF THE NEGRO. Chicago: Univ. of Chicago Press, 1942. (See chapter II-A).

A compilation of reported facts about the biology of the Negro, including pathology. Chapters include anatomy, bio-chemical and physiological characteristics medical and surgical diseases, obstetrics and gynecology, diseases of the skin, eye, ear, nose and throat, and dental diseases.

Lindsay, Inabel B. Race as a Factor in the Caseworker's Role. J. OF SOCIAL CASEWORK, 1947, 28, 3, 101-107 (See chapter II-C).

A discussion of the race of the case worker as a component in his professional behavior. Considers, particularly, difficulties due to unresolved conflicts about race of the case worker and points to the need for self-awareness.

Loth, David and Fleming, Harold. INTEGRATION NORTH AND SOUTH. New York: The Fund For The Republic, 1956. (See chapter II-B).

A comprehensive listing of specific instances of desegregation in the United States during the period May 1954 to May 1956. Education, private employment, public employment, housing, organizations, public accomodations, recreation, health facilities, and religion are the activities covered.

Maslow, Will. Prejudice, Discrimination, and the Law. THE ANNALS of the American Academy of Political and Social Science. Philadelphia. 1951, 275, 9-17. (See chapter II-B).

Discussion of the role and efficacy of legislation as an instrument to counter discrimination. Refers to several relevant psychological studies on changing discriminatory attitudes. This entire volume of *The Annals* is devoted to the topic of civil rights.

McLean, Helen V. Psychodynamic Factors in Racial Relations. THE ANNALS of the American Academy of Political and Social Science. Philadelphia. 1946, 244, 159-166. (See chapter I).

A discussion of the psychological dynamics of whites and Negroes stemming from the superior-inferior social relationship that the dominant white society maintains. The aggressions, dependencies, fears, and projections of both groups are discussed. This entire issue of *The Annals* is devoted to the topic of prejudice.

Merton, Robert K. Intermarriage and the Social Structure: Fact and Theory. PSYCHIATRY, 1941, 4, 3.

A sociologist's discussion of intermarriage, with particular emphasis on why intermarriage occurs most frequently between a white man and a Negro woman.

Milner, Esther. A Study of the Relationship Between Reading Readiness in Grade One School Children and Patterns of Parent-Child Interaction. CHILD DEVELOPMENT, Vol. 22, No. 2, June 1951.

A study of the relation of reading readiness to the socio-economic status of the families of first-grade children, using, also, Negro and white children.

Myrdal, Gunnar. AN AMERICAN DILEMMA. New York: Harper & Brothers, 1944. (See chapter I).

The most complete treatment of the situation of the American Negro. Presents an interpretation based on much research and direct observation by the author and his team of collaborators. The approach considers historical, sociological, psychological, political, and philosophical factors.

Nichols, Lee. BREAKTHROUGH ON THE COLOR FRONT. New York: Random House, 1954. An account, written for laymen, describing the changeover from segregation to integration in the armed forces of the United States.

Pasamanick, Benjamin and Knobloch, Hilda. Early Language Behavior in Negro Children and the Testing of Intelligence. J. OF ABN. AND SOCIAL PSYCHOL., 1955, 50, 3, 401-402.

40 Negro children examined by a white examiner at 2 years of age gave evidence of early awareness of racial difference with loss of rapport. The authors point out that this apparent finding has serious implications in the field of ethnic group psychology.

Powdermaker, Hortense. AFTER FREEDOM. New York: Viking Press, 1939.

A study of Negro and white cultures, and their interrelations, in a cotton-growing community in the deep South. The investigator was an anthropologist who lived in the community for the equivalent of a year, functioning as a participant observer. The emphasis is primarily on the Negro in the situation.

Prothro, E. Terry. Ethnocentrism and Anti-Negro Attitudes in the Deep South. J. OF ABN. AND SOCIAL PSYCHOL., 1952, 47, 1, 105-108.

A brief article documenting the point that in areas where prejudice has strong historical and cultural support, the relationship between ethnocentrism and prejudice is lower than is otherwise the case.

Rose, Arnold. THE NEGRO IN AMERICA. New York: Harper & Bros., 1948.

A condensed edition of *An American Dilemma* by Gunnar Myrdal. Foreword by Myrdal.

Schanck, Richard L. A Study of Change in Institutional Attitudes in a Rural Community. J. OF SOCIAL PSYCHOL., 1934, 5, 121-128.

A study of the social forces that foster and maintain institutional attitudes. Differences in public and private attitudes are revealed, and the type of events that might bring them into closer agreement for many individuals are indicated.

Seward, Georgene. PSYCHOTHERAPY AND CULTURE CONFLICT, with 4 case studies by Judd Marmor. New York: The Ronald Press Co., 1956.

The book presents various cultural aspects of psychotherapy, pointing out needs for more appropriate treatment, through better understanding of members of subculture groups who suffer from culture conflict. Dr. Marmor contributes four representative cases drawn from his psychoanalytic practice.

Simpson, George E. and Yinger, J. Milton. RACIAL AND CULTURAL MINORITIES. New York: Harper & Bros., 1953.

A text synthesizing material on (1) the causes and consequences of prejudice and discrimination, (2) minorities in the social structure, (3) the reduction of prejudice and discrimination. Many minority groups are treated, with the Negro and Jewish groups getting most attention.

Stern, Curt. The Biology of the Negro. SCI. AMER., Oct., 1954, 191, 4, 81-85. (See chapter II-A).

A brief survey of current information on the racial makeup of the American Negro, further indicating the high degree of admixture of African, Caucasian, and Indian progenitors.

Stouffer, Samuel A., etc. THE AMERICAN SOLDIER. Princeton: Princeton Univ. Press, 1949, 486-599.

The final section of this work investigates the impact of interracial contact on white soldiers who have fought side by side with Negro soldiers.

Sutherland, Robert L. COLOR, CLASS, AND PERSONALITY. Wash., D.C.: American Council on Education, 1942.

A summary volume, interpreting the material collected and presented in four coordinated studies listed in this bibliography: Davis, Allison and Dollard, John. *op. cit.*, Frazier, Franklin, 1940, *op. cit.*, Johnson, Charles S. *op. cit.*, Warner, W. Lloyd, etc. *op. cit.* Part II contains suggestions for an action program to improve the position of Negroes.

Warner, W. Lloyd; Junker, Buford H.; and Adams, Walter A. COLOR AND HUMAN NATURE. Wash., D.C.: American Council on Education, 1941.

A systematic study of the effects of discrimination upon the personality of Negroes in a large Northern city. Attention is paid to the differential effects that emerge as a result of varying "shades of Negroidness" and of social position in the Negro community.

Williams, Robin M., Jr. THE REDUCTION OF INTERGROUP TENSIONS. New York: Social Science Research Council, Bull. 57, 1947.

A survey of research on problems of ethnic, racial, and religious group relations, together with a formulation of the important research issues remaining to be solved.

Williams, Robin M., Jr. and Ryan, Margaret W., Editors. SCHOOLS IN TRANSITION. Chapel Hill: Univ. of No. Carolina Press, 1954.

A series of case studies of communities along the border of the South that have changed from segregated to integrated public schools during the past few years, mostly under the compulsion of state laws. (See chapter II-B).

Wilner, Daniel M.; Walkley, Rosabelle P.; and Cook, Stuart W. HUMAN RELATIONS IN INTERRACIAL HOUSING. Minneapolis: Univ. of Minnesota Press, 1955.

A report on a controlled field experiment in several public housing projects. The purpose was to discover whether attitude changes in whites and Negroes toward each other were systematically related to their physical proximity and daily intergroup contact.

Woodward, C. Vann. THE STRANGE CAREER OF JIM CROW. New York: Oxford Univ. Press, 1955.

A historical review of the development of segregation since Reconstruction and of the more recent moves toward desegregation.

PERIODICALS

THE ANNALS, of The American Academy of Political and Social Science, Vol. 304, March, 1956. Entire volume devoted to "Racial Desegregation and Integration," consisting of a large number of papers by different authors, edited by Ira De A. Reid, Ph. D.

THE JOURNAL OF NEGRO EDUCATION, "A quarterly Review of Problems Incident to The Education of Negroes." Published for the Bureau of Educational Research, Howard University, by the Howard University Press, Howard University, Washington 1, D.C. Vol. XXI, No. 3, summer, 1952. Vol. XXIII, No. 3, Summer, 1954. Vol. XXIV, No. 3, Summer, 1955.

THE JOURNAL OF SOCIAL ISSUES, published for the Society For The Psychological Study of Social Issues, a division of The American Psychological Association. Vol. V, No. 3, 1949. A symposium on consistency and inconsistency in the area of prejudice. Vol. VIII, No. 1, 1952. Devoted to a series of studies of the effects of intergroup contact upon the attitudes of the participants. Issue Editor, John Harding. Vol. IX, No. 4, 1953. Entire volume entitled *Desegregation: An Appraisal of the Evidence*. Issue author, Kenneth B. Clark.

RACE RELATIONS LAW REPORTER, Published six times a year, starting February, 1956, by the Vanderbilt University School of Law. *Race Relations Law Reporter* describes itself as "A complete, impartial presentation of basic materials, including: court cases, legislation, orders, regulations." Vol. I, No. I, February, 1956. Vol. I, No. 2, April, 1956.

SOUTHERN SCHOOL NEWS, published monthly by Southern Education Reporting Service, 1109 19th Ave., S., Nashville, Tenn. The Southern Education Reporting Service describes itself as "an objective, fact-finding agency established by Southern newspaper editors and educators with the aim of providing accurate, unbiased information to school administrators, public officials and interested lay citizens on developments in education arising from the U. S. Supreme Court opinion of May 17, 1954 declaring segregation in the public schools unconstitutional. SERS is not an advocate, is neither pro-segregation nor anti-segregation, but simply reports the facts as it finds them, state by state."

REPORTS AND PAMPHLETS

A TENTATIVE DESCRIPTION AND ANALYSIS OF THE SCHOOL DESEGREGATION CRISIS IN CLINTON, TENNESSEE. December 1, 1956. Anna Holden, Bonita Valien, Preston Valien (with the assistance of Frances Manis) Fisk University, Nashville, Tennessee. Published by the Anti-Defamation League of B'nai B'rith in cooperation with The Society for the Study of Social Problems.

Report also includes interviews with a number of those involved in different capacities and offers recommendations on the basis of the Clinton experience. (See chapter II-B).

BLUEPRINT FOR TALENT SEARCHING. New York; 1957. National Scholarship Service and Fund for Negro Students.

An account of projects in the South and New York City to identify and stimulate able students from economically, culturally, and educationally deprived groups, and to facilitate their obtaining suitable education. (See chapter I).

DESEGREGATION IN THE BALTIMORE CITY SCHOOLS. Baltimore: July, 1955. The study sponsored by The Maryland Commission on Interracial Problems and Relations and the Baltimore Commission on Human Relations.

MIRACLE OF SOCIAL ADJUSTMENT: DESEGREGATION IN THE WASHINGTON, D.C. SCHOOLS, Carl F. Hansen. 1957. Freedom Pamphlet Series, Anti-Defamation League of B'nai B'rith, New York.

A positive evaluation and account of desegregation in Washington, D.C., including the preparatory steps involving many levels of the community and school system. (See chapter II-B).

READINGS IN INTERGROUP RELATIONS, Helen F. Storen. Revised Edition, 1956. Intergroup Education Pamphlet. National Conference of Christians and Jews, New York.

A bibliography of materials in the intergroup relations field selected on the basis of their usefulness to teachers. (See chapter II-C).

SAINT LOUIS INTEGRATES ITS SCHOOLS. January, 1955. League of Women Voters of St. Louis. A brief review of successful integration in St. Louis public schools.

THE RIGHT OF EVERY CHILD. April, 1955. American Friends Service Committee. The story of the Washington, D.C. program of school integration.

THE RESOLUTION OF INTERGROUP TENSIONS, Gordon W. Allport. January, 1952. Intergroup Education Pamphlet. National Conference of Christians and Jews, New York.

A critical appraisal of methods for reducing group tensions, based on Allport's own researches and the work of other scientists. (See chapter II-C).

THE STATUS OF THE PUBLIC SCHOOL EDUCATION OF NEGRO AND PUERTO RICAN CHILDREN IN NEW YORK CITY. October, 1955. Presented to the Board of Education Commission on Integration. Prepared by the Public Education Association, assisted by the New York University Research Center for Human Relations. A comparison of school facilities and educational achievement of white and non-white children in New York City. (See chapter I).

WHAT'S HAPPENING IN SCHOOL INTEGRATION. December, 1956. Harold C. Fleming and John Constable. Public Affairs Pamphlet #244. New York. A brief account of developments since the Supreme Court decision, based on studies conducted by the Southern Regional Council.

PART TWO

Psychiatry and International Relations

3
THE POSITION OF PSYCHIATRISTS IN THE FIELD OF INTERNATIONAL RELATIONS

Editor's Note. An account of how the work of the GAP Committee on International Relations evolved may add to the reader's perspective for considering the papers in this section.

At its inception in 1947, the Committee, under the chairmanship of Dr. Frank Fremont-Smith, was primarily engaged in preparatory activities for the Third International Congress on Mental Health which was to be held in London in August, 1948. For this Congress the Committee's focus was on the International Conference on Mental Hygiene, one of the three separate but related meetings out of which the World Federation for Mental Health came into being.

It is pertinent to note that the 1948 International Conference on Mental Hygiene was committed essentially to the task of explaining what psychiatry, in conjunction with other social sciences, could contribute to the urgent problems of mental health and human relations facing mankind at every level from the individual within his family to the individual nation within the family of nations. This credo reflected the GAP Committee's own position and has continued to guide its deliberations and studies to the present time.

Following the 1948 World Mental Health Congress, the Committee on International Relations decided to formulate a program of investigation and action for its fellow members in GAP. Published in January, 1950, as *Report #11*, this program illustrates the pioneering enthusiasm and hopefulness of the original members of the committee. It is reprinted here to recapture their mood and intentions.

The succeeding reports produced by the Committee show that the members became increasingly conscious of the difficulties in approaching vast problems and delicate political areas. The post-war reaction against an originally over-optimistic expectation from the psychiatric profession lessened the use of psychiatrists in government. The Committee on International Relations began to address itself to such matters as the nature of the relationships of psychiatrists to governmental agencies in international situations. Only then did the members feel that the Committee was ready to expand its horizon beyond the national scene in studying the psychological adaptations of citizens of one country going abroad to work and live for extended periods. These are more pragmatic approaches toward major, still unresolved problems, which the earlier members of the Committee posed for themselves and which their successors continue to study in the light of developing concepts of social psychiatry.

THE POSITION OF PSYCHIATRISTS IN THE FIELD OF INTERNATIONAL RELATIONS*

The knowledge of psychiatrists can bring much of value to the solution of group as well as individual problems. As citizens, psychiatrists, by virtue of their particular training, carry a special responsibility for utilizing this knowledge to its fullest possible extent, without claiming sole or special wisdom in settling the problems of nations or the future of society.

The specific competence of the psychiatrist is derived from his knowledge of individual motivations. Since groups are composed of individuals, this special knowledge can contribute to the understanding of group relations.

In the field of international affairs psychiatrists can at present best utilize their knowledge through such activities as:

Encouraging group conferences in which social and political scientists and other trained personnel with field experience will participate. Wherever possible, such conferences should be conducted in university settings or under other suitable auspices.

Establishing interdiscipline institutes for research and training programs, having one or more of the following purposes:

To educate younger psychiatrists and other specialists in the methods of interdiscipline collaboration.

To orient experienced individuals in the same methods.

To encourage cross-fertilization of related fields, especially between university faculties.

To develop skills for broadening the acceptance of psychiatrists and other social scientists as needed participants in the field of advisory and consultant services to government.

To prepare personnel by suitable training methods to meet calls

*Formulated by the Committee on International Relations, and first published as Report #11, in January, 1950.

from agencies of government when special knowledge of human relations is required.

To study actual problems, presented by government officials or other experts with field experience, as a basis for teaching—a method comparable to the case teaching methods in Law and Medicine.

Exploring possible contacts with leaders of government who are known to have understanding of the social sciences.

Making available to authorities in occupied countries, through collaboration with other social scientists and historians, precise knowledge of the psychological issues involved in their tasks.

Supporting in every way possible all programs sponsored by the United Nations, or its specialized agencies, for the improvement of human relations.

Making careful case studies of exiled leaders and of the problems of political refugees and displaced persons.

Studying the psychology of leaders and their followers at local, national, and international levels.

Making comparative studies of the psychology of psychopathic leaders in various countries.

Studying those factors which obstruct or delay the orderly progress of parliamentary procedures in national and international assemblies and thus interfere with the attainment of reasonable compromises.

Examining public statements by national leaders, with a view to achieving a more accurate evaluation of their content.

Assisting in the preparation of manuals of information for government officials and commercial agents sent on missions to other countries, so designed as to insure an intelligent orientation to the principal historical and traditional attitudes prevalent in these countries.

Emphasizing through appropriate channels the importance of psychological considerations in the planning and implementation of international policies, which are often considered solely from the economic viewpoint.

Particular emphasis should be laid on the following considerations if psychiatrists are to develop their full usefulness in the field of international relations:

They should be cautious in making sugestions or recommendations until:

They have had sufficient field experience to become adequately acquainted with given problems;

They have had sufficient contact with the administrators and others concerned to have achieved mutual understanding.

They should consider it their primary function to focus their efforts on problems of urgent concern to those responsible for their solution. Wherever possible, the officials concerned should be invited to participate in the discussions. The scientific personnel of such conferences should in all cases include individuals who have had some field experience in the area under discussion.

4

APPLICATION OF PSYCHIATRIC INSIGHTS TO CROSS-CULTURAL COMMUNICATION*

INTRODUCTION

Mottram Torre, M.D.
Chairman Committee on International Relations

The Committee on International Relations accepted with enthusiasm the request of our President and of the Steering Committee to present a symposium during World Mental Health Year which we are observing in 1960. As members through GAP of the World Federation for Mental Health, many of you are already familiar with the various World Mental Health Year activities and studies that are being conducted in many parts of the world. We would like to direct the symposium to a discussion of one important specific area of research—that of the role of the psychiatrist in furthering international understanding.

You and your committees and GAP have already significantly contributed to the advancement of psychiatry internationally. By generously making the GAP reports available to the World Federation for Mental Health for distribution to the various professionals working in the mental health field in various parts of the world, you have stimulated and assisted our colleagues in the underdeveloped countries in their professional growth and development.

Our committee would like to see GAP and GAP members make a similar contribution to the less defined but equally important field of international relations. Much of the committee's time has been spent just trying to define the specific areas in which psychiatrists can make a contribution and how this can best be done.

Our first report, GAP report No. 11, The Position of Psychiatrists in the Field of International Relations, *is simply an enumeration of the areas of international relations in which psychiatrists have some interest and some knowledge.*

---

*The papers that follow were presented at the meeting of GAP in April, 1960, and were first published as Symposium #7 in April, 1961.

Our second report, GAP report No. 28, THE USE OF PSYCHIATRISTS IN GOVERNMENT IN RELATION TO INTERNATIONAL PROBLEMS, *is somewhat less general. It focuses specifically on what insights and services the psychiatrist has to offer in government and reviews the experiences of some psychiatrists who served in various capacities in the governmental agencies with international responsibilities. It is essentially enumerative and descriptive, and contains little content in the nature of psychiatric knowledge.*

Our third report, GAP report No. 41, WORKING ABROAD: A DISCUSSION OF PSYCHOLOGICAL ATTITUDES AND ADAPTATION IN NEW SITUATIONS, *is more specific and contains much more psychiatric material. The reception and use of this report, which was far greater than that of the other two, make us feel that psychiatrists—and our committee—can more effectively contribute to the field of international relations by identifying and reporting on those specific areas of international relations about which psychiatrists have intimate knowledge and information.*

We are presently working on a report in the specific area of cross-cultural communication. We are trying to define and delimit the areas in which the psychiatrist has information and understanding in

a) *the process of communication and*

b) *methods of facilitating communication between people, cross-culturally or transnationally.*

We feel that before we as psychiatrists can contribute significantly to this field, we must become more familiar with the insights developed by our colleagues in the other behavioral sciences. Accordingly, we have invited behavioral scientists representing psychiatry, cultural anthropology, and sociology to participate in this symposium. The symposium should give guidance to our committee so that it can begin to develop the psychiatric insights and information which will be of some use to people who are interested in fostering better, more effective, cross-cultural, and transnational communication.

Dr. Bryant Wedge, a member of our committee who has long had an interest in transnational communication, will begin the symposium. He will draw on material from his experience as a psychiatrist in Hawaii, where he worked with people of many cultures, and from his travels as an Eisenhower Exchange Fellow to Russia, the United Arab Republic and many countries in Europe.

TOWARD A SCIENCE OF TRANSNATIONAL COMMUNICATION

Bryant Wedge

For the purposes of this symposium, I shall offer three propositions:

1. The discipline of psychiatry is concerned with the practical science of communication between persons.
2. Communication across national boundaries presents special problems which call for a systematic approach suitable for wide use.
3. Psychiatry can and should contribute to the development of an applied science of transnational communication.

The Psychiatric Approach to Communication

Psychiatrists try seriously and systematically to understand and communicate with a variety of individuals who are not in complete contact with the ordinary world—from withdrawn schizophrenics to adolescents, who so frequently reside in social worlds of their own. Psychiatrists try to work with persons of various social classes and various national origins. Every psychiatric interview aims at understanding and communicating with other persons, and may be looked upon as an experiment in transcultural communication, for no two persons represent precisely the same cultural experience. I believe that it should be possible to abstract from this wealth of experience models and techniques which can be usefully applied to problems of communication between nations.

The psychiatrist views a communicative relationship as a two-way process. He is interested in arriving at an estimate of the meaning and purposes behind the forms of discourse and in making his own interpretations and purposes understood. To the psychiatrist, successful communication requires taking account of and respecting the other person's particular way of doing business, and moreover, considering his own styles and biases. Finally, the psychiatrist has developed techniques to apply these viewpoints systematically to further the processes and aims of communication. It should be added that he does so without sacrificing his own proper role and position in the relationship. I submit that this represents a desirable model for transnational communication: to learn what is in the other person's mind and to convey one's own views in understandable form, while maintaining a proper definition of one's own role.

I think the things I have just said are basic to the psychiatric view of communication, but this approach is rare outside the interview sciences. In fact, the notion that one must consider the other fellow's communicative world is so deeply accepted in psychiatry that it is difficult for psychiatrists to realize the gulfs in communication which exist just because this is not taken into account.

This is not to say that psychiatry has all the answers to communication problems. It is obvious that knowledge from the consulting room cannot be transposed directly to the requirements of international interchange. I am suggesting that the basic attitudes and knowledge and techniques of the psychiatric interview can be adapted to these requirements. Psychiatry, as an applied science which approaches the problems of communication systematically, has the means, ready at hand, to contribute to the development of a science for transnational communication. Such contributions would not only fill a need, but, if they can be developed in communicable form, would be greatly welcomed by those who are involved in the practical management of affairs across national boundaries.

Problems of Transcultural Communication

When N.S. Khrushchev visited the United States he was photographed grinning and shaking his clasped hands above his head. In the Soviet convention, this gesture represents the expression of friendship between brotherly peoples. American papers, however, captioned the photograph as representing a gesture "similar to a victorious prize fighter's." Apparently a considerable error had occurred between the expressive intention and the receptive interpretation of this very simple communicative interaction. Mr. Khrushchev was a little angry at the American press before his visit was over. Compounded thousands of times, on many levels, such misunderstanding may have very considerable consequences, in an age of global interdependence and massive international contact.

The members of a national society share highly organized patterns of communication. These patterns differ between national societies; the differences provide ground for mischance and failure in communication between nations and between individual members of different nations. International contact always involves a degree of transcultural communication; that is, the process which takes place whenever the words, acts, or attitudes of a member of one society are recognized and responded to by members of another society. My colleagues on the panel will illustrate some of these problems, so that I need not go into that.

Problems which arise in transcultural communication can be suggested by listing some of the factors involved in communicacative processes:

Semantics

The meanings attributed to and evoked by symbols, words and gestures differ, sometimes considerably, in terms of the social framework within which they are expressed or interpreted. In America, for example, "freedom" implies the ability to change one's ways, to become what one wishes; in Holland, "vrigdom" suggests the right to continue one's status, civil or religious, without interference, but not the right to change.

Styles of Communication

Each society evolves its own mode or style of expressions or discourse which forms a model for communication. It is said, for example, that Americans "discuss," the English "converse," the Arabs "bargain."

Concepts

Communication within a given society rests upon a series of hidden assumptions which provide an operative conceptual framework, a kind of commonly accepted measuring stick. Because these concepts are more often implicit than overtly stated, and because they are deeply ingrained, it is frequently assumed that similar measuring sticks are used by one's fellow man.

Feeling Tones

The range and kind of feeling involved in communicative interchange is strongly patterned by cultural experience. Since this "language of feeling" varies with culture, the feelings associated with all communicative activity are liable to transcultural misinterpretation. I have seen American men shudder with distaste at the warm embrace of greeting between men in other countries.

Values and Attitudes

Each people holds dear a particular set of concepts, institutions and symbols, closely related to accepted social patterns or ways of life. Such values determine the attitudes which are taken toward ideals and events so that the same occurrence may provoke a positive and accepting attitude in one cultural context, a negative and rejecting attitude in another. The English people value physical privacy; for example, in Russia, insistence on privacy is regarded as antisocial.

Last year I had the privilege of traveling quite widely for the purpose of "advancing the cause of better understanding between nations" under the sponsorship of the Eisenhower Exchange Fellowships. The course of my activities brought me into contact with a number of officials of various governments and also gave me an opportunity to learn something of the problems of the United States official abroad. My experiences during this period made me acutely aware of the difficulties created by gaps in communication across cultural barriers. I met very few officials who were "natural communicators," able somehow to establish and maintain working contact with their counterparts. I met others who were painfully aware of the problems of understanding and being understood and only a few who were completely blind to these issues. The facts are that there are all too few natural communicators, that attitudes toward social communication are generally formed in circumstances of cultural limitation, and that education and training only rarely focus on the communication process. Therefore, it seems likely that achieving reliable means of transnational communication must depend upon developing a teachable science applicable to this problem.

General Approaches to Communication

To my mind, there are three general approaches to communication between differential cultural systems.

(a) The most common is the ethnocentric position: each side expresses itself and interprets the communications of others in its own terms. This contains the dangers and disadvantages of misunderstanding and miscalculation by each participant which may lead to chain-reactions of error.

(b) A more precise approach involves recognizing cultural differences and taking these into account in communicative acts. This may involve high levels of expertise in "understanding the natives." On the more sophisticated level of cultural relativism, it may include attempts to recognize and take into account one's own cultural biases as well. Communication based on this pattern has the advantage of leading to much more precise acts of expressions and interpretation. It has the weakness of requiring a thorough grasp of concepts of culture and a high degree of specific knowledge concerning the societies involved in interchanges. Truly bi-cultural individuals are rare—there certainly aren't enough of them to fill these needs.

(c) Another approach to transcultural communication involves attention to the dynamic processes of communication itself. This approach has the disadvantage of lack of specificity—details of complex dynamic processes cannot be precisely predicted or predetermined—but it has the advantage of containing the potential for self-correction.

In recent years a number of models of dynamic processes of communication have been developed. Experimental and social psychologists—and advertisers for that matter—have been concerned with questions of persuasion, attitude change and opinion and are developing experimental means for testing hypotheses concerning these matters. Communications engineers and, in a very parallel way, neuro-physiologists, have found common ground in theories of communication and information with the use of such concepts as feed-back, signal-noise ratios, and self-steering mechanisms. A number of mathematical models have been constructed, using such bases as von Neuman's *Theory of Games* and Wiener's *Cybernetics*. Of all the approaches to communication problems, however, that which is encompassed in the psychiatric interview would appear to approximate most closely a systematic approach to processes of communication between persons.

A Little Experiment

I cannot offer a model for an applied science of transnational communication, but I would like to report on an experimental attempt in communication with Russian university students. I visited universities in several Soviet regions, but I shall speak only of meetings with Russian students, as those of other Soviet nationalities use different communicative patterns and techniques. The Soviet Union is not quite so monolithic as appears from the outside. However, Russian culture is so strong and Russian society so uniform that my experience in social communication was almost identical in cities several thousand miles from one another.

Establishing Communication

Establishing a communicative relationship requires definition of role, of purpose, and of attitude. In transcultural situations particularly, it is necessary to formulate these definitions in ways which make sense to one's counterpart. In the case of Russian students some experimentation was required to find circumstances and definitions conducive to fruitful interchange. Very quickly I observed that sharp limitations were put on conversations by the presence of officials or an interpreter; students watched the interpreter for cues and direction instead of relating directly to me. I arranged to meet students independently. At once another phenomenon became apparent: these students were quite uncomfortable when approached by a foreigner when they were alone or even in small groups. They would be polite enough, but obviously uneasy and restless. Often they would call friends to join us, or a group would spontaneously gather in support of the beleaguered ones. If a group did not materialize, the students would quickly excuse themselves on some pressing business. On the other hand, once a sufficient group had gathered, usually when it had grown to more than six or eight persons, all traces of uneasiness would disappear, discussion would become freer, and interchanges warmer and more spontaneous. I tested this phenomen many times and came to accept the condition that satisfactory conversations with normal Russian university students required meeting them in groups. The larger the group, and—the closer, too, physically—the freer the discussion became.

Once a group had formed there arose the question of finding a social role and of stating the business at hand. The idea that I, as an individual, should be pursuing a personal interest in student life proved to be both unbelievable and distressing to my young acquaintances who simply could not stomach such "individualism," a rather bad term in Russia. They were much more comfortable thinking that my business was somehow official, so I accepted the term which was thrust on me, and which was close enough to the truth, and became "an American delegation." Of course, to say that I was a psychiatrist made even less sense, for psychiatry in the Soviet Union concerns itself almost solely with gross mental illness, with little interest in personality. Consequently, I accepted the second term which was offered me and admitted that I was "an American delegation concerned with university education," whereupon my interest in student life was at once comprehensible and acceptable. One further step remained in establishing the relationship: this was to demonstrate a knowledgeable and friendly interest in students and their lives. Some inquiry about examinations or study load generally served to show my interest in student life and elicited an enlightening flow of information. In this way, by processes of observation and adjustment of response, by keeping in mind how I might be perceived as well as what I was seeing, a communicative relationship was established.

Exploration and Clarification

Next came a phase of *exploration* or scouting areas of common interest. This proceeds simultaneously with processes of *clarification.* These are essentially processes of getting to know viewpoints, opinions, and attitudes in increasing detail. Exploratory communication was encouraged by seriously and attentively listening to my new acquaintances with a willingness, at least temporarily, to accept their terms. If transnational communication is to be a mutual process, serious and thoughtful response to inquiry was also necessary. The familiar acts of constantly attending to the flow of interchange and maintaining awareness of one's own actions, so that their impact on the process can be observed, are basic to exploratory communication. One knows that communication processes are proceeding successfully by the broadening and deepening of subjects of discussion in a natural progression and by the appearance of possibilities for clarifying questions which arise.

Physical and Emotional Responses

As it happened, the cues to difficulties in communication were particularly evident with Russian students. I have mentioned that a condition of discussion was meeting these students in groups; an extension of this was the tendency of the group to physically incorporate me, and the more I allowed this the freer the discussion became. This physical incorporation was quite literal. It would be manifested by a degree of leaning, touching, and closeness—irrespective of sex—that is quite unfamiliar in our culture. The groups tended to settle in some quite small room. I had the feeling that they felt "the closer, the better," and incidentally, I began to understand something of the Russian tolerance for living so closely packed together. So long as we were in harmony this close contact would continue, but whenever I made a "blooper" or transgressed some code of decency in my remarks the group would literally physically withdraw, often with a hushed silence and sometimes with fairly evident vasomotor responses of blushing or blanching. It interested me that such withdrawals occurred almost solely in relation to some discussion of the Soviet State—particularly if any comparisons with other countries were involved—and never in relation to any detail of personal or social life.

When such a cue to faulty communication became apparent, our discussions invariably became more stereotyped and superficial until I was able to trace back and correct whatever action on my part had led to the difficulty, or when I acknowledged the impropriety of a subject by quickly turning to another. For example, when I remarked on the rather obvious presence of a good many military people on the streets of Stalingrad, I learned, by the hush and withdrawal of my counterparts, that this was not a subject to be discussed, at least with foreigners. Recovering from such difficulties was achieved by a tacit agreement not to pursue this question, changing the subject to more neutral areas. In short, respect for the limitations imposed by the social milieu is necessary to maintain communication.

Any response which recognized proper social styles and forms of communication served to facilitate a flow of discussion. Phrases of a kind that regularly appear in student phrase books, such as "I am happy to convey the greetings of the students of Yale University and American universities to students of the University of Tashkent," reciprocated a certain formal necessity for these young people who regularly regard themselves as personal representatives of the State. Allowing engulfment by the group certainly helped, as did an exchange of cigarettes or the acceptance of a cup of tea; but of all gestures the most effective was recognition of the progress of their country.

It was inevitable that discussion would raise many questions which required clarification by close inquiry and by increasing definition and counter-definition. Such efforts took the form of presenting a piece of information as well as it is understood and offering such formulation for correction. Russian students were very interested in the question of belief in God among Americans, and I was equally interested in their own attitudes in this matter. It took some fairly careful efforts at definition to establish the meaning of individual conscience to Americans, to separate the problem of belief from the Soviet notion of religion as an "anti-progressive force." Clarification did not mean agreement, but simply a recognition of differences of view—differences which did not prevent each of us from understanding the position and even the motives of the other.

Termination of each period of interchange required a summary or restatement of views in light of the discussion, in order to keep communicative channels open. We generally agreed that it was good for people to know each other and we frequently acknowledged that there were real and understandable differences between our ways of life. Naturally my student friends asked me to convey their greetings to fellow students in America. This rounding off both clarified the whole discussion and left open the possibility for further acquaintance, as I think both sides wished.

Formal leave-taking from a Russian group is recurrently charming. One is always seen to the door or to the street by the entire group, often joined by the entire dormitory and clapped or waved out of sight. Such gracious gestures to guests seem to call for the same kind of gesture which Mr. Khrushchev offered in his American speeches, the gesture of clasped hands of friendship.

Psychiatric Contributions

Psychiatry can contribute to an applied science of transnational communication by research, training, and consultation. I will review some of these possibilities, acknowledging that the individual psychiatric discipline has a social responsibility to assist in the development of a systematic approach to this vital problem.

(a) *Research* on problems of transnational communication has both theoretical and applied aspects; it is necessary to develop general theories as a basis for understanding the practical processes. This implies the careful statement of hypotheses or approaches to given phenomena and the testing of these hypotheses by actual experience. I suggest as an overall hypothesis that the approach to communication embodied in clinical psychiatry can be adapted to the purpose of transnational communication.

This general hypothesis requires a good deal of specification and testing in the field. Fortunately, there is a good deal of opportunity for research of this kind in the course of present-day psychiatric activity. Psychiatrists repeatedly meet with individuals and groups in transcultural context, and so are able to observe and experiment with communication processes. What is required is that careful attention be paid to the communication process itself and that this be explicitly described. Some models of interview processes have been developed in detail; it remains to apply these to the special circumstances of transnational discourse.

Furthermore, many psychiatrists have opportunity to participate in transnational discussions of various kinds, as consultants and observers and as travelers. It might prove very valuable to record and describe problems and experiences of communication in these circumstances in terms of interactions and techniques involved. This is what I have tried to do briefly in describing my discussions with Russian students. Chances of this kind occur even without much travel, as in Margolin's discussions with Ute Indians, or in contacts with subcultural communities within our boundaries.

(b) The *teaching* of approaches to communication based on psychiatric experience presents considerable problems. For some years the Washington School of Psychiatry has offered courses with a broad psychiatric orientation, which have interested persons concerned with problems of transnational communication on official levels. Other psychiatrists and even larger numbers of social scientists have acted as consultants to branches of the State Department and to private and public organizations concerned with the conduct of affairs across national boundaries. Psychiatrists are being consulted more in the selection of personnel for overseas duty, yet it cannot be said that the penetration of dynamic views of communication is widespread or very deep in circles practically concerned with these problems.

I believe the responsibility for this disparity lies in large part with the communications professions themselves. Officials sometimes complain that they have been unable to get practical help from these disciplines when they have asked for it. They say that their consultants are apt to be incomprehensible, a bitter comment for the communications professions to swallow. Certainly it is difficult to formulate concepts concerning communicative processes in human interaction, but I suspect that we have a tendency to be too ambitious. We try to teach a whole frame of reference and scientific language rather than to address our efforts to the problems of the practical worker on his own ground. If this is so, it will be necessary to evolve methods of teaching which are suitable to these needs, a nice problem in communication itself. Fortunately, the use of the psychiatric process possesses a "how-to-do-it" approach, and fortunately in a multi-sided society there are always plenty of opportunities for direct approach by students.

I believe the conditions for teaching contributions are eminently present: there is a decided need; there is a wish to learn, at least among some practical workers; and there is a body of applicable knowledge and experience. Consistent efforts are needed to develop formulations and teaching approaches adapted to these problems.

(c) The *consultant's role* is already familiar to the psychiatric profession. Various applications of this role have been suggested, such as the role of clarifier which Dr. Frank Fremont-Smith has suggested for international meetings. Psychiatrists have been asked for assistance in understanding the behavior of individual persons, particularly leaders involved in international negotiations. As consciousness of communicative problems grows, I believe that further roles will develop for consultants and that, increasingly, specialists in human communication will be asked to assist in understanding specific impasses as they arise. Fortunately, the independent consultant enjoys great advantages of objectivity and noninvolvement in details and possesses technical skills which provide powerful possibilities for clarification in such situations. This role, consciously developed, may prove of considerable value to the cause of transnational interchange.

Dr. Torre: *The next speaker on our panel is a member of a very unusual husband and wife team, both possessing degrees in the joint specialties of sociology and anthropology. Dr. Ruth Useem received her doctorate in cultural anthropology and sociology at the University of Wisconsin in 1947, and is presently a research consultant in the Department of Sociology and Anthropology at Michigan State University. She and her husband have conducted two rather extensive and detailed research efforts in India. The first was in 1953, when Ruth and John Useem went to India to interview Indians educated in Amerca and in the United Kingdom to discover how they had used their cross-cultural experience and education in reintegrating into the economy of India. This resulted in the publication of their book,* THE WESTERN EDUCATED MAN IN INDIA.

The second project, which was recently completed, she will now report to you in some detail, focusing on the communicative aspects of Americans in various official and unofficial capacities who try to interact, interrelate and communicate with Indians. Both studies in India were sponsored by the Edward W. Hazen Foundation. She and her husband have also undertaken research through a National Institute of Mental Health grant on "The Stresses and Resources of Middle Management Men," published in the book by E. Gartley Jaceo called PATIENTS, PHYSICIANS AND ILLNESS.

INTERPERSONAL RELATIONSHIPS BETWEEN INDIANS AND AMERICANS IN INDIA

Ruth Useem

It would be presumptuous of me to say what psychiatrists have to contribute, so I am going to take as my approach the setting within which interpersonal relationships between Americans and foreigners take place.

Recent changes in the nature of cross-cultural relations have been so swift and intensive that events often seem to outpace our understanding. In my own field of sociology, the study of cross-cultural relations has been based largely on America's peculiar national history. During previous decades Americans met strangers from other societies primarily in the role of immigrants from Europe, forced migrants from Africa, and subordinated American Indians. Foreigners typically entered American society as part of a low-status minority group, were expected to replace parental traditions with the customs of the dominant group, to assimilate the American way of life, and to become identified with the community and nation as loyal citizens. Out of this period developed our concepts of assimilation, accommodation, acculturation, marginal persons, minority groups, etc.

Now increasing numbers of Americans are moving into alien societies where they count locally as foreigners. Typically, the Americans move in at a high status—in fact a higher status than they usually enjoy at home. Americans are supposed to adjust and adapt to local cultures and societies, but are expected to maintain strong attachments to American society and to be representatives of America abroad. The sociological constructs and concepts accumulated from past experience offer us few theoretical guidelines for handling these types of cross-cultural relations.

The present international movement of Americans and other nationals also differs significantly from the movement of colonial administrators who entered alien cultures in positions of power and authority. We have had instances of Americans as administrative governors of Japan and Germany, but since that period Americans have been entering alien societies not as administrators with authority over foreign peoples but, hopefully, as influencers. The receiving nations have more to say as to what foreigners enter their midst than was true under colonialism or military occupation, and the host societies have more control over what the foreigners can do after they arrive. Consequently, more so than under colonialism, it is truly a two-way process in which both sides have a part in the determination of the relationship.

What I would like to report on is part of a larger study of Americans in cross-cultural relations, the field research for which was done in India in 1958. We were trying to discover some of the social patterns which occur when members of American society live and work in another society, but today I will concentrate on interpersonal relationships between Americans and Indians.

There are about 2000 American households or approximately 5800 American men, women and children resident in India. (There are many thousands more tourists but these were not included in our study.) From this universe we interviewed in depth a sample of 190 "heads of households" of whom 82 per cent were men and 18 per cent were professional women. In addition, the wives and some of the teenage children of the married men of the sample were interviewed separately and in depth.

Americans are in India for a number of different purposes and under a variety of sponsorships. The sample was stratified so as to include some from all of the following backgrounds: 1. the three branches of U. S. government—foreign service, U. S. Information Service and technical assistance ("Point Four" or ICA); 2. Americans connected with international agencies such as WHO, ILO, United Nations Technical Assistance; 3. businessmen—Americans who are managers and technicians for American firms in India, who do contract work for the Government of India or who are employed directly by Indian firms; 4. missionaries, both Catholic and Protestant, who are engaged in nonevangelical activities such as education, welfare, medicine, agriculture; 5. voluntary associations and foundations which sponsor technical advisors, lecturers and specialists; 6. students—both graduate and undergraduate; and 7. a miscellaneous category which includes free-lance writers, newspaper reporters, American women married to Indians, residents of Hindu centers, etc.

India is a subcontinent with a variety of cultures, with 14 different languages and hundreds of dialects, with social patterns going back thousands of years and with modern, urban, industrial development. Interviews were conducted with Americans living in all the major regions in India and in 27 different communities.

Obviously 5800 Americans cannot interact on a personal plane with close to 400 million Indians. What sections of India, then, are available to and sought out by Americans? Americans are neither the first nor the only foreigners in India, for India has had a long history of contact with foreigners. Out of these contacts, patterns have been worked out for the incorporation or the isolation of foreigners which contribute to the type of personal interaction which can and does take place between Americans and Indians.

Variables Influencing Interaction

1. There is first of all the community variable. In New Delhi, the nation's capital, the dominant theme is structured diplomatic relations between Indians and foreigners. In this center the patterns are not greatly different from those in Washington, London, or any other national capital. On the other hand, in Calcutta, which was a major center of British business, there is institutionalized separation of Indians and foreigners. The latter have their own clubs, living areas and social life; the main contacts between local inhabitants and foreigners occur in the work roles. Bombay, in contrast, has developed over the years interpersonal interaction between foreigners and upper-class, Westernized, English-speaking Indians. Well-established missionary endeavors, such as hospitals and schools, have regularized interaction between foreign workers and local Indians.

Most Americans who go to India have their first contacts with local residents through these already structured relationships. There are some Americans who go into communities or sections of communities which have never had a foreigner or an American there before and hence have no regularized patterns for interrelating foreigners and Indians. Examples would be a Fulbright professor who is the first foreigner to teach at a particular university or a technical assistance person working on the introduction of new seeds in an isolated village.

2. A second variable contributing to the type of interpersonal interaction which takes place between Indians and foreigners is the number of foreign groups within an Indian community. The larger the number of foreigners resident in any one community, the more likely is each foreign group to confine its interaction with Indians to those initiated by its own members; and around each of the foreign groups will be a number of Indians who interact only with that set of foreigners. There is little overlap in these circumstances between the Indians who interact with, say, the Americans or the British or the Russians. On the other hand, in those communities which have but a sprinkling of nationals from several Western nations, being a "Western foreigner" becomes a bond uniting all Western foreigners and forging a common channel into approximately the same group of Indians.

3. The larger the number of Americans within a particular community, the more likely is the American contingent to break down into a series of subsections, each having its own channels into India. Thus in New Delhi and Bombay, one group of Indians will commonly associate with the technical assistance group, another with the United States Information Service, another with businessmen, etc., with little overlapping between the subsections. In contrast, in a community such as Trivandrum where there is but one USIS person, one Fulbright, and a couple of missionaries, there is greater sharing of contacts among the members of the American community.

Whether or not the patterned channels are open to the individual American depends in part on the role he assumes when he arrives in India. Thus, a single representative of an American business firm in New Delhi, or a student in Bombay, or a missionary in Calcutta may be as much isolated from the regularized channels into India as the American who goes alone into a community where there are no other foreigners, because there exist no patterned relationships for this type of person in this particular community.

At the risk of overgeneralizing, the characteristics of the Indians whom Americans meet in the regularized channels are: upper class and upper middle class, English-speaking, Westernized in style of life, educated (although not necessarily Western-educated), nonorthodox Hindus, Parsees and Sikhs. Social interaction takes place in Westernized kinds of settings—homes, social clubs (comparable to the American country club), or modern-style hotels. Activities include dinners, cocktail parties, receptions, golf, tennis, bridge. Interaction is carried on in English; Western-style food and drink are served; and the gatherings are relatively large—eight to 75 people.

Inclusion in these groups gives the American a sense of belonging and a feeling that he is getting to know Indians. The patterned contacts reduce anxiety and strangeness and give the American an environment in which he can have personalized contacts with local people without seriously breaking local cultural norms. In the institutionalized interpersonal relationships, the Indians tend to be more permanent members than the Americans, among whom there is greater turnover.

Ready-made contacts do not demand unique talents on the part of individuals, and persons with modest talents can maximize their sense of belonging and effectiveness by utilizing these channels. The greatest demand on the individual is that he be sensitive to the particular established folkways of the group. If the common recreation pattern is golf, then he plays golf; if cocktail parties are the expected mode of entertaining, he gives and goes to such gatherings; if certain topics are eschewed in conversation, he does not bring them up. Each community or subgrouping tends to have its own established folkways and as one moves from New Delhi to Madras or from the business community to the diplomatic community, one observes these slight variations.

Ordinarily the American new to India is introduced to these groups under the auspices of other Americans or foreigners. However, if the American is the only replacement for a single American in an isolated post, it is the Indian group who surrounded the former holder who now initiate the first contact and introduce the American to the on-going American-Indian relationship.

General Reactions to Membership in Patterned Groupings

1. For some Americans, these relationships are consistent with their purposes or ends for being in India, or at least con-

sistent with part of their purposes. Most businessmen, for example, see no reason to break out of them, for they tend to reinforce their position in India. The Indians they meet under these circumstances constitute that segment of India most important for furthering their purposes for being in India. Similarly, it would be fatal if members of the diplomatic corps ignored the structured diplomatic set.

Another group of Americans, while feeling that these ready-made contacts are satisfying and comfortable, go on to build them up and expand them, including a few more here and there. Also these groups become the place where an individual can first meet and test out an Indian and then move on to establish a deeper personal relationship outside the group.

2. A second reaction to these patterned channels is acceptance at first but with a growing feeling of being constrained by them. Usually by the time an American feels uneasy or dissatisfied and begins to view the Indians he meets under these circumstances as "hangers-on" or not "real" Indians, he is so encapsulated and involved that it is difficult to disentangle himself. Early acceptance of the pathway has precipitated a set of obligations to and expectations from others which are not easily abrogated. Occasionally "home leave" is used as a period to break out of the pattern, but this works best if accompanied by a change in community.

3. A third reaction is to eschew the ready-made groups as much as possible and make contacts with the local population on one's own. This reaction, with some modifications, is comparable to the situation faced by those who have no readily available groups—either by reason of being the first American in a community or because there are no other Americans under similar sponsorship in the community.

Variables Affecting Interpersonal Relationships Outside of Regularized Channels

The Indians who are available to and ready to accept Americans form three main types:

a. The first type are Westernized, English-speaking, educated, upper middle class and upper class Indians who have not previously had an American in their midst. In addition to the top echelons of the local community, this type includes Parsees, sophisticated recent refugees from Pakistan, and Indians from other regions of India—all of whom are "strangers" themselves, inasmuch as they do not have ties with the dominant Hindu communities of an area and may not even speak the local language. Americans who make their way into these groups find they have tapped Indian segments not greatly different in social characteristics from the ones available to them in the regularized channels. However, considerable satisfaction is taken by the American in having made these contacts on his own, in being the first member of an exclusive Indian sports club, or in being the first American to participate in a little theater group putting on Western plays. Often these contacts can be institutionalized and passed on to other Americans.

b. The second type include Indians who have something to gain personally by contacting Americans. Like many countries of the non-Western world, India is a nation of millions living a marginal existence, with thousands of unemployed among the educated—a nation whose economy provides few consumer goods and limited opportunities for the individual to improve his lot in life. In India, the "have-nots" have well-developed techniques for extracting from the "haves" some bits for themselves; Indians in positions of authority and wealth have, in turn, well-developed counter-techniques for dealing with this persistent and constant harassment.

Americans in India have a relatively high status and are thought by the "have-nots" to be rich and powerful, to have influence, contacts, jobs to offer, and import privileges of highly desired goods (cars, liquor, manufactured items, etc.). Many Indians view the Americans as another group that can be tapped (Americans call it "laying siege"), to maximize if ever so slightly their own lot in life. This varies from the most obvious open begging on the street, through tradesmen who want to sell brass articles and Kashmir rugs, to persons, less open and more roundabout, who cultivate Americans in hopes of getting a nephew a scholarship in America, of getting a job with an American organization, of having the inside track for getting a book published, of being invited to parties where liquor is served, or of enlisting the aid of the American Women's Club in raising money for a local charity.

Most Americans when they first arrive in India do not have

the techniques for handling any of these situations. They soon learn to protect themselves from the open beggary and obvious "sieges." But they are least adept and suffer most frustrations where the Indian's purpose is most hidden, where they have missed the cues and find, as they put it, that "friendship has been presumed upon," that they have been "taken," or "used."

This might be summarized by saying that those Indians who have the most to gain from Americans are the most readily available, but they are not the ones the American wants to know, or in terms of his purpose for being in India, has to know.

c. The third group is composed of those Indians with whom interaction is necessary to fulfill the American's purpose for being in India and at the same time fulfill India's purpose for having the American there. Interpersonal relationships between Americans and these Indians are, to our way of thinking, the most crucial and often the most difficult to establish and maintain. They are the "go-betweens," mediators, or "men in the middle" relationships. The participants are not just *individuals* from different societies relating themselves *personally* to each other but *representatives* from different societies relating *their societies* (or at least segments of them) to each other by way of their interpersonal relationships. This is not to say that personal benefits cannot or do not accrue to the individuals. It does say that unless the relationship serves more than unique personal ends, it is a failure no matter how personally satisfying it may be to the individual American or Indian.

Let us give an example of what we mean. The Government of India has requested a foreign expert to advise on the introduction of better seed corn; the U. S. Technical Cooperation Mission has sent a man with knowledge in the field. The degree to which knowledge can be transferred will depend to a considerable extent upon the interpersonal relationships that can be established between Indians and the American expert—and yet there may be no prior channels of communication for effecting this transfer. To work out these interpersonal relationships takes time, considerable skirmishing, and testing of each by the other in order to establish, as they say in India, their *bona fides*. Ordinarily, more effort is put into this process by the American, for although the Indians may know who the American is, the latter may not know who the Indians are to whom he must relate in order to fulfill his purpose for being in India—and some Americans finish out their tours never knowing. The presence of a foreign expert may be a real threat to the Indian in-groups, which, like all in-groups, develop techniques for protecting themselves against the threat of outsiders.

The Social Characteristics of Americans

We shall make some generalizations that are open to qualifications in certain circumstances but which hold true in the main. It should be remembered that the qualities we are about to discuss are qualities as viewed in the Indian setting.

a. Those most anxious to break the patterned channels into Indian society and to strike out on their own, and those for whom there are no channels available, are most often those with the least experience in cross-cultural relationships. They are not only in India for the first time but also in overseas service for the first time. We have termed these the "plungers" for they are least selective in their initial contacts. The breathless new arrival who reaches out for everything Indian, who accepts all overtures extended by Indians, who has preconceived notions as to the dimensions of his role in India and does not want to be told by resident Americans what he should do, who says "I prefer to make my own mistakes," who is quick to criticize other Americans for their behavior—this man is a repetitive phenomenon viewed with varying degrees of tolerance by "old hands" in the American community who remark, "Give him time, he will learn the hard way the reasons for our approach to India and Indians or else he will be here a short time and be gone." Many of the "old timers" are right, for the Indians who are quick to seek out an American are the ones who have something to gain personally by contacting him.

b. The longer a person is in India or in overseas service, the more selective he is in his contacts and relationships with locals—he learns to be a "toe dabbler" before being immersed. If there are other Americans in his community, the more likely is he to follow the established channels; if there are not ready-made channels, he follows unchanneled pathways with more caution and less early commitment. The seasoned person in cross-cultural relations knows that the most readily available locals outside the channeled pathways are not necessarily the ones most important for his purposes for being in India and he tries to avoid encapsulation by them.

Those who are more specific in their purposes for being in India have narrower contacts than those who are less targeted. Or putting it another way, the role, and not just the individual occupant of the role, defines the segments of India into which the American can move. Cultivating interpersonal relationships outside of regularized channels is not open to all Americans. To clarify this, one might contrast the role of the Ambassador and that of a roving scholar. The latter role allows the person to interact with Indians in a number of different environments, to talk with people from various walks of life, to meet people on third-class trains and in first-class hotels, to enter the homes of Maharajahs and the huts of villagers. For the Ambassador such informal movement is impossible. Between these two polar types are varying degrees of role definition which delimit in varying degrees the segments of India within which the individual American can establish interpersonal relationships. The less-targeted person is more likely to suffer from aimlessness and estrangement but he can, and often does, penetrate areas of Indian life not open to other Americans with more specific purposes.

The American's Acceptability to Indians in the "Mediator" Role

Although our emphasis has been upon the establishment of new contact into India and not the ready-made variety, some of the following discussion also applies to the latter.

a. The higher the status of the American individual within his own organization, the more acceptable he is. This is in part because authority is more centralized in India than it is in the United States. Not only is the status of the individual within his own organization a key to acceptability but also the reputation which the organization itself has in India. This reputation may fluctuate both in time and in space. An example of this would be the missionary who becomes less acceptable after an anti-missionary pronouncement of the Central Government; furthermore, he may be *persona non grata* to the Central Government but enjoy high prestige and acceptability in his local community.

b. Older persons are more acceptable to Indians than younger persons. This is understandable in a society which emphasizes respect for its older and more experienced members.

c. Single professional women are acceptable to a wider range of Indians than are either single or married men. (This is quite in contrast to what is found in Japan.) Professional contacts are open to them because of their professional status, and Indian women are more available to them because of their sex.

d. Skin color is a double-edged thing in terms of acceptance. The American Negro is suspect if it is thought he or she is incompetent and was sent as a propaganda gimmick; but darkness of skin may enable both sides to feel easier in highly interpersonal relationships. On the other hand, fair skin, in a society which puts emphasis upon it, may actually be an advantage.

e. In contrast to what one might expect, the American's having children is more likely to impede than to extend wide penetration into India. This is not because Indians reject children—for they do not. It is rather because the more children a family has and the older they are, the more time and concern husband and wife must spend in easing their children's adjustment, advancing their education, establishing Western modes of living for the protection of their health and keeping viable the American way of life. And the less time they have for pursuing in depth Indian relationships.

f. Health and vitality are crucial considerations. To get beyond the institutionalized channels and establish relationships with other than the Westernized segments of India propels one into standards of cleanliness below that acceptable to Americans; into forced feeding of foods indigestible by American stomachs; into the searing heat of India in non-airconditioned homes and hotels; and into unsanitary and disease-producing situations. Even within the Westernized segments Americans must take precautions. A rugged constitution and indifference to one's bodily comfort are "musts" if one is to go very far beyond the upper middle class style of living. Many find their spirits willing but their bodies not. As one missionary put it, "Living in this large, Westernized home may mean that we do not live as close to the people as we might, but we certainly are going to live longer."

g. Whether or not it is necessary to learn a local language

depends upon one's purpose for being in India. The majority of missionaries do learn and use a local language in their work but other Americans can get along in India knowing only English. But knowing English is not enough—more Americans have had difficulties and frustrations because they were inarticulate in English than have ever suffered from not knowing a local language. We did find that it was more important for the wife to know local languages in terms of her interaction with servants and vendors than for the primary employee to speak a local language inasmuch as most of his interaction is with English-speaking Indians.

h. After we have said all of this there still remains the personality component. We said earlier that patterned relationships do not require great talents other than modest sensitivity to variations of local folkways. To break through and establish workable relationships, particularly of the "mediator" variety, requires considerable resourcefulness, tenacity, and ability to maintain a sense of perspective despite threatening and frustrating circumstances. It requires willingness to be self-conscious about one's daily behavior and sensitivity to cultural differences.

Conclusion

I think it is in the area of personality structure where psychiatrists do have considerable information that they could be of great help to Americans overseas. No American and, for that matter, no Indian can maintain the pace required to establish and maintain interpersonal relationships across cultures without some escape valves. We found that for the married men, it is most often their wives who become their emotional wastebaskets. For some it is escape back to the familiar—"all-American parties," where Americans can let down their hair with each other in a safe environment, a "home leave," reading American publications, maintaining an American-style home abroad. Some very few Americans can relax with selected Indians, but these are extremely rare exceptions—so rare that their occurrence is always noteworthy. These unusual instances are less likely to occur between professionals of the two societies and more likely to be established between an American wife and an Indian woman. The latter can relate themselves on a common human level and neither threatens the other in an occupational role.

As one would suspect, there are more notable innovations in the mediator relationships and more abysmal failures. These relationships take a long time to establish, need constant cultivation and are highly fragile. By their very nature, every American-Indian interpersonal relationship has inherent in it a breaking point—because of the ultimate loyalty of the participants to structures which can and often are in opposition to each other; because of basic commitment to a cultural way of life in which neither the Indian nor the American can go any further in his acceptance of the values of the other; and, of course, because of political loyalties to two different countries.

I should like to end on this point. Except for expatriates, Americans who reside overseas establish interpersonal relationships with local people not just for their personal satisfaction and fulfillment, but primarily as bridges between two societies through which can flow knowledge, technical know-how, and greater understanding. Bridges are useless unless there are roads on both sides leading to the bridges. Consequently, an important aspect of cross-cultural interpersonal relationships is maintenance of contacts with other members of both societies. Americans need as much help in relating themselves to the members of their own society when abroad and when back at home as they do in relating themselves to members of another society.

Dr. Torre: *The next speaker, Dr. William Caudill, received his doctorate in Social Anthropology at the University of Chicago in 1950. He has had longstanding ties with psychiatry, and has had training as a non-medical candidate in psychoanalysis at the Boston Psychoanalytic Institute. His contact with psychiatry began in 1946 in Chi-*

cago, where he worked for four years with Dr. Charlotte Babcock on a study of Japanese-Americans. From 1950 to 1953, he was with the Department of Psychiatry, Yale University, where he taught psychiatric residents and did research in a small psychiatric hospital. This work was published as a book entitled THE PSYCHIATRIC HOSPITAL AS A SMALL SOCIETY, *Since 1953 he has been a member of the faculty of the Department of Social Relations, Harvard University. In July 1960, he plans to join the staff of the National Institute of Mental Health in Bethesda, Md. Today he will describe some observations on the communication process he made while carrying out research in Japanese mental hospitals. He spent 18 months in Japan in 1954-55, and another 15 months in Japan in 1958-59.*

SOME PROBLEMS IN TRANSNATIONAL COMMUNICATION (Japan - United States)

William Caudill

I have not made a study of the topic of transnational communication, but through my anthropological research during 1958-59 in three small psychiatric hospitals in Japan I have participated in the process of such communication, and perhaps my exerience may be of some use. I have been stimulated in this direction by the consultant role that I have been taking during the last two days of GAP committee meetings.

If, in my words here, I seem to duplicate some of the points made by Drs. Wedge and Useem, it is because such points were important in my own experience. For example, I certainly participated, at first, in what Dr. Useem describes as patterned channels of communication—those established places and persons in the local culture that were set up to be of service to, and make their own use of, foreigners coming to the country for myriad purposes as tourists, businessmen, diplomats, educators, and so on. What I want to say here I hope will, to a greater or lesser extent, be applicable to Americans (and people of other nationalities) in all of these groups who go to a foreign country to live for a period of time.

I went to Japan first, as Dr. Torre has said, in 1954 after several years of work in psychiatric hospitals in New Haven and Boston, and, before that, four years of work with Japanese-Americans in Chicago as part of a team of social scientists and psychiatrists studying the acculturation and personality adjustment of these people. In my two trips to Japan I feel I went through four stages in the transnational communication process and I should like to begin by outlining these.

Stages in Communication

The *first stage* consisted both of initial enthusiasm for the culture, and somewhat later, estrangement from it. This early period of uninformed interest and enthusiasm was coupled with the belief that I was communicating, until something would happen to indicate that quite obviously I was not. This would be followed by a most unpleasant feeling of estrangement accompanied by a mild but very real depression, and with thoughts such as, "These people do not understand what I am trying to say," or, "I don't understand what they are saying." After several bouts of this kind, I came to realize that I had been somewhat too prideful, that I really knew virtually nothing about this language (even though I had studied it for over a year before going to Japan) or about the meaning of interpersonal relations in Japanese culture.

I do not think that my initial reactions were atypical. A foreign culture is a highly convenient vehicle onto which to project, or to use to deny, one's own fairly "normal" conflicts. Common early reactions are overacceptance or overrejection of the foreign culture.

Somewhat more complicated is the denial of problems in one's *own* culture (concerning, say, the existence of social classes, the position of women, and so on) and then seeing just these problems in the foreign culture. For example, in Japan, it is not uncommon to find the American housewife who has decided to pay her Japanese servant a "decent wage" and to "treat her as a person." This very frequently ends in the servant taking leave with rather feeble explanations—feeble because she cannot communicate her real reasons for leaving across the language barrier. Even if this barrier did not exist, the servant would not openly voice her real reasons—even to a Japanese employer—because it is not good form to do so in Japanese interpersonal relations. Her unstated reasons are, however, probably of the order that she does not want to be treated as a "person"—American style, but rather wants to be treated as a servant—Japanese style. Involved in the latter is the assistance of her employer in finding a husband for her should she desire to get married, the giving of gifts at the appropriate times to her and to her family, and her identification with the hopefully rising status of the employer's family in the community. But the American housewife is not likely to know or to understand these matters, and when the servant leaves unexpectedly the housewife is left with feelings of frustration, outrage, or depression, and with such discomforting thoughts as, "Something went wrong," or, "I can't communicate with these people." This sort of reaction, in a somewhat more technical context, is not an unusual one for anthropologists to have during the first few months of a period of field work. Frequent responses to this condition are withdrawal, getting drunk, or deciding to become active—to plan "to do something." This latter response is particularly characteristic for Americans, who, if they are living in Tokyo, will decide to take a trip to Kyoto, or to go to Hong Kong, or plunge into a course in flower arranging, and so forth.

The *second stage* that I felt I went through was one I find it hard to label neatly, but I am calling it here a period of attenuated childhood and dependence as regards certain aspects of the reality with which one is faced. Supposing that the process of the first stage is broken into by some event, one is then faced with the reality of communication difficulties, and with a somewhat sobering view of one's own knowledge of the inner and outer world to be contended with—perhaps not so much in one's sphere of technical competence (providing you could communicate your area of technical competence), but certainly in many areas of general living. If one pays attention to these sobering thoughts, there starts at this point a fairly long period of "growing up in the culture." This is accompanied by the feeling that one "is as a child" and "is being treated as a child." This can at times be very comforting, given the indulgence of children in Japan, and, at other times, at least for me, infuriating. In any case, I think perhaps Americans are especially threatened by the need for such dependency for a period of time, whereas this sort of dependency is the stuff of life for Japanese. If the American is embarrassed, or angry, or brusquely shakes off such helpful overtures, the Japanese person is likely to withdraw into *enryo* (a passive reserve) and once again, to use Hearn's statement in 1904 (which might be more indicative of his state of mind than perhaps of reality) the American is faced with "walls of everlasting ice."

The *third stage* is what I call the technical task phase. About this time, assuming one has managed to survive successfully the preceding stages, one turns sensibly to one's technical work. It is only for so long that I, for one, can enjoy exclusively such general initial experiences as sitting on *tatami*, and of learning to name and eat the various parts of raw tuna, which are graded by the fat content in the flesh (I happen to like the part with the least fat best). So, with an American-educated research assistant, who some five years later was to become my wife, I started on one of my tasks—learning about Japanese psychiatric hospitals.

Observations on Japanese Attendants with Patients

During my first year of field work in 1954 in these hospitals I saw a type of "action" communication—I am making a distinction here between communication through actions and through words—in the use of a subprofessional type of nursing personnel known as *tsukisoi*. These are women who act as attendants, housekeepers and companions for the patients. In the private psychiatric hospital, each patient has his own *tsukisoi* who is with the patient 24 hours a day, 7 days a week, month in and month out. The *tsukisoi* sleeps on a separate bed beside the patient at night. If he awakens, she talks with him, soothes him, and in the morning arises before her patient in order to give him breakfast, and so on. During my first field work I "saw" this type of interaction, but I did not know much about the meaning of it. I could "hear" about it to some extent, but only through translation at this point rather than through my own ears.

In this way, for example, I heard a *tsukisoi* say to her patient after returning from a trip to her home, "I saw the ripening persimmons on the tree." The patient replied to this, "It would be so nice if I could eat the ripe persimmons." I asked the *tsukisoi* what she thought the patient meant, and she said, "I thought he was pointing to my immatureness." So I did not know quite what to do with that. The exchange between the *tsukisoi* and the patient sounded a bit like an exchange of poems between lovers in the *Tales of Genji*. It seemed to me the patient was indicating his desire to eat his *tsukisoi*, to incorporate her, and it was very evident from the contents of his diary at this time that he was much concerned with primitive oral wishes. But this was not something that I knew when

I first "saw" and "heard" the interaction between the *tsukisoi* and her patient. And, in general, my understanding of this relationship was very partial and fragmentary.

About this time I left Japan, having gained a rather simple, descriptive understanding of Japanese psychiatry, such as how many hospitals there were, how many patients, and so on, and, more personally, having made warm contacts with a group of psychiatrists. I also left with people still praising me for my efforts to speak in halting Japanese, a praise which indicated to me that I was still in the childhood stage in general living, although I had made a start toward achieving competence in a technical role. When Japanese stop praising you, then your language ability is improving. This may be true in any culture, but I feel it is accentuated in Japan.

Three years later, by the spring of 1958, I had studied more Japanese in the interim, and upon returning to Japan I picked up once again the technical task of coming to understand and to describe Japanese psychiatric hospitals and the treatment of patients. This time the technical task was easier to enter into directly, and the city of Tokyo, rather than seeming exotic, was disappointingly familiar. Moreover, this time, in order to keep from going through the whole process again, I used a confidential consultant, Dr. Takeo Doi. Dr. Doi had been trained in the United States, and we were interested in some of the same questions. We met together each Friday evening so that I could talk over my work and feelings during the preceding days and he could give me the benefit of his knowledge and reactions. By this time my technical understanding of communications through both actions and words had increased.

Observations on Doctor-Patient Relationship

I was impressed by the ease with which patients talked about their problems in Japan. By this I do not mean that patients talked easily about very deeply felt or very private matters. But they did talk freely about the nature and content of their symptoms, the incidents that led to their hospitalization, their personal background and family history, and so on. This was particularly evident in a series of case conferences which occurred over a period of six months at one of the hospitals. At these conferences quite sick patients would be brought in and would talk with the examining doctor for an hour or even an hour-and-a-half in the presence of six or seven other doctors. American patients are, of course, brought into case conferences, but it is usually not for such a long period of time, and it is seldom that they seem to feel as much at "ease" as did the patients in the Japanese hospital.

Nature of the Relationship

I believe that one thing that was happening in the case conferences was that the patient was taking the "role" of patient very easily in relation to the doctor. Patients at these conferences would very often literally say to the doctor, "I am completely in your hands" ("*Watashi o omakase shite imasu*"). When the patient says this, he is saying that he wants to be taken care of, and is asking to be allowed to take a passive and dependent position with reference to the doctor. The doctor accepts and fosters this wish; indeed, he is not consciously aware of the wish or of his acceptance in the psychological sense implied here because such interaction is so much a part of Japanese culture.

When this sort of interaction happens, the doctor and patient begin to relate to each other in a way for which it is difficult to find a satisfactory English word. I began by calling it a "colleague relation," because it frequently seemed that the doctor and patient were discussing the patient's illness as if it were a thing apart, and the doctor and patient were in a colleague relationship in trying to defeat the "illness." Shortly, however, I became dissatisfied with this term. The relation is an apparently intimate one, but it has a subtle quality of play-acting on the part of both participants that prevents it from being called a truly personal relation. It is similar in a way to the relation between doctor and patient that existed in the United States when a family would have an "old family doctor." Also it is similar to the friendly but not truly personal relations that Americans used to develop (more than nowadays) with the proprietors of the local meat market, grocery store, or drug store. However, the emotional qualities of the Japanese relation seem to go far beyond the nature of the neighborly relations characteristic of an earlier time in the United States.

In my discussions with Dr. Doi of this "intimate but not truly personal" relation, Doi suggested several terms in Japanese that seemed to fit the qualities of the relation more accurately. One of these terms is *nareai*, which can be translated as "collusion." However, the word *nareai* does not necessarily have the fraudulent connotations that the word collusion does in English. The word *nareai* in Japanese indicates mainly the exclusive relationship between the participants in the sense that only they can enjoy a certain family-like atmosphere while excluding others. And this *nareai* relationship can pass without censure in Japanese culture, although it can very well be put to bad use. This sort of flavor is not very usual in professional relations—as in those between doctor and patient—in the United States. When it happens, particularly in a hospital, it is usually described in English as being "too involved with the patient."

A second term which suggests some of the overtones of the relation is *tokekomu,* which might be translated as "to melt into" or "to fuse with." It could be said that whether one is able or not to "tokekomu" with others is a measure of one's social abilities in Japanese culture.

The "intimate but not truly personal" relation I have been describing could be illustrated in many ways within the hospital. For example, after the discharge of the patient it may lead to the doctor and patient drinking together to celebrate the patient's recovery. In some situations, for example, the psychoanalytic one, it has not infrequently happened that during or after therapy the suggestion has been made to the patient that he might want to attend professional psychoanalytic discussions. In general, such behavior seems to be an admission of the patient to a rather privileged relation with the doctor after his discharge. This goes considerably beyond the continuation of the doctor-patient relationship after discharge in the United States.

The particular relationship I have described exists not only between patients and staff but also between the various staff groups. For example, it was quite obvious during the fall and spring trips which members from almost all role groups in the hospital took together. The picture of a group of senior doctors, junior doctors, nurses, office workers, kitchen and maintenance workers going off together for a day's outing or a weekend at an inn is not an unusual one in Japan. But it is not one I have seen very frequently in hospital settings in the United States.

Behavior Outside the Hospital

At this point in my work, then, I felt (as I hope is indicated in what I have said by way of example) that I could understand something of the meaning of communications in actions and words in the Japanese hospital, and I began to wonder how this behavior was related to what went on outside of the hospital in more general life. Thus my attention was drawn back again to events in the wider culture.

Mutual Dependence

It seemed to me that one way of linking interaction in the hospital to that in everyday life was to examine the relative emphasis placed on independence or dependence in behavior in Japan when compared with the United States. Perhaps for Japan, the phrase "mutual dependence" is a better one than simply "dependency" since in the family, for example, the parents are almost as dependent (particularly psychologically, although also in many other ways) on their children as the children are on the parents. I wish to be quite clear about my meaning here. All people in both cultures have, of course, the need to be independent and the need to be dependent, the need to assert oneself as a unique person and the need to be taken care of or to take care of others. However, a person in the United States, particularly a man, is likely when faced with a problem to choose to emphasize his independence whereas a Japanese man would more often express his dependence.

Patterns of mutual dependence can be seen in many areas of Japanese culture and throughout the life span—from childhood to old age. In adulthood, for example, the Japanese person tends to stay with the same company, university, or hospital for the major part of his productive career. Moreover, in his relations with his supervisors he asks for and receives their advice on many matters which would be considered personal in the United States—problems in the family, marriage partners, financial difficulties and so forth. In contrast, the person in the United States is free to, and expects to, move from one job to another fairly often. The commitment in Japan to one channel of action—and hence the dependence on superiors in that channel—starts often in childhood with the fierce competition to be accepted by the correct kindergarten as a road to the correct primary school. This school leads to the appropriate university and later to a favorable job. Again, this is in some contrast to the United States where, at least prior to college, children may, and frequently do, change from one school to another.

Mother-Child Closeness

Moving further back to the pre-school years, the patterns of sleeping and bathing during childhood are quite different in the two cultures. In Japan, the child sleeps in the same covers with his parents (usually his mother) for a long time (anywhere from two to five years), and also receives the personal care and stimulation that is involved in bathing together with his mother or grandmother for many years. In the United States, a middle class child tends to be given a separate bed, and often a separate room, fairly soon after birth, and he is bathed by his mother rather than the two of them taking a bath together. The difference in emphasis between the two cultures in these regards is one of "closeness," or perhaps in how such closeness is expressed. In Japan the relation between mother and child is for a long time almost a symbiotic one where words are not necessary since emotions are communicated in actions. In the United States there is less communication through direct action. There is also more emphasis on the independence of the child, and more use of words between mother and child to try to express feelings that are left unsatisfied.

In psychoanalytic terminology a distinction is sometimes made between "talking out" one's problems as a more acceptable solution than "acting out" one's problems. Neither of these terms applies very well to the relation of the Japanese mother and her child, nor to the normal relations of adult Japanese persons. Dr. Joseph Michaels of the Beth Israel Hospital in Boston, upon hearing the presentation of some of these materials, suggested the term "living out" for the relation of the Japanese mother and child. This seems an appropriate term as it avoids the negative implications of "acting out," and yet allows one to call attention to the large amount of physical contact that goes on for many years between mother and child.

Final Stage in Communication

With the partial shift of my interest out of the hospital and into the family and community, it seemed to me that I began to move into a *fourth stage* in my efforts to understand and to communicate in Japanese life. I would call this a movement from a predominantly rational-technical emphasis in communication to a more general process that included some ability to have emotional understanding of life in the culture.

Throughout the four stages in adjustment that I have sketched, has run the theme of a gradually increasing ability to deal more successfully with communications in actions and words on both rational-technical and emotional levels. Since I hope the spelling out of these stages has some applicability to other persons living in a foreign culture and not merely to myself, I would like in closing to spend a few minutes on this general theme of problems in communication in national (or intra-cultural) as well as in transnational (or cross-cultural) situations.

The Communication Process

Communication, as we know, is a difficult business at best within one's own culture. It is conducted largely through use of the symbols which, in combination, make up the system of the particular language being employed. Such symbols are more or less shared as to their meaning by the communicating persons. Benjamin Whorf's often-cited example of the "empty" gasoline drum that blows up in your face on putting a match to it is a good illustration of the imprecision of such symbols at the level of everyday usage. In addition to language symbols, communication can, of course, take place non-verbally through actions, pictures, and so on, but let us stick with questions of language here.

Spoken or written language symbols are used in everyday speech and in technical vocabularies which attempt to provide greater precision. The technical vocabularies help immensely in transnational communication. For example, the following situation, although hypothetical, is concocted from my own painful participation in, and observance of, many similar, all-too-real situations.

Let us say that Mr. Jones, an American manufacturer of electric motors, comes to Tokyo accompanied by his wife. After some trouble, via intermediaries, Mr. Jones locates Mr. Tanaka who also manufactures electric motors, and who, in the past, spent several months on business in the United States. Mr. Tanaka drags Mrs. Tanaka, who would not usually go out with her husband in Japan, down to the lobby of the Imperial Hotel for a meeting with Mr. and Mrs. Jones. Mr. Tanaka asks Jones "how he likes Japan," and after that is over, Jones asks Tanaka "how he liked the United States." This exchange is very painful and frustrating for both sides, particularly if done through interpreters, as is highly probable. Neither party has the slightest knowledge of the meaningful details of the other's general culture or way of life. And it is with the greatest of relief that Jones and Tanaka turn to the technical discussion of electric motors, as perhaps sensibly they should in this situation.

Emotional Meanings of Words

Now such words, especially from everyday language, that Jones and Tanaka employed to tell each other how they liked Japan and the United States, have, in addition to their explicit meaning, an underlying emotional meaning. This underlying meaning involves what anthropologists call a body of "shared understandings" among men—that is, culture. This is Redfield's definition, and it is a moot point whether a national state as opposed to small folk society of relatively homogeneous people can have a body of "shared understandings."

Examples, of course, of "shared understandings" or the lack of them are familiar to all of us. Friday night in this hotel a waitress and I were chatting about my having just come from Boston, and about her having grown up in Boston. At the end she said to me, "Do you have all you want, dear?" Now, I did not grow up in Boston, but I know what she means by this "dear," and yet my emotional associations with this word I think go in a somewhat different direction from where I imagine hers do.

A second example also comes in a way from my personal experience as it is hard to find such examples in the literature. I have a liking for the word "fuzzy," a feeling I know from past experience that some other people share, because this word is associated in my mind with teddy bears, squirrels, and my mother's fur coat. I wonder what pattern of emotional associations a Japanese man would have with this word since it was learned late in his life? Or, if we turn the question around, the Japanese word which is used when referring to one's own mother is *haha,* while the more honorific word used to refer to someone else's mother is *okasan.* If one wants to refer rather roughly and familiarly to one's own mother, one may use the word *ofukuro*. This word, without the prefix "o" which is honorific, means a "bag" or a "sack." If a Japanese patient working with an English-speaking analyst were to refer to his mother as an "honorable bag" I expect the pattern of the analyst's emotional associations with this would go off in directions other than those of the patient's. The term has invidious connotations in English that it does not have in Japanese.

My general point here is that for certain kinds of transnational communication to be effective, it is more important for the parties involved to know about the emotional feelings associated with everyday events and objects in each other's culture than for them to be deeply steeped in more formal knowledge as regards history, economics, and so forth. For example, in order to understand emotions in Japan, it is probably more important to know the feelings aroused by the smell of fresh *tatami* mats in the house than it is to know about the history of the Tokugawa period.

An "Expectable Map"

In an even more general way, what I want to call attention to here is the expectation that is built up, at both conscious and unconscious levels, in the mind of a person as he grows up in a culture, concerning (to paraphrase Hartmann's concept and apply it somewhat differently) an "average expectable set of interpersonal relations." Such an "expectable map" of interpersonal relations plays a large part in transnational communication. When the American psychiatrist visiting in Tokyo says to his young friend who is a Japanese psychiatrist, "Why don't you apply for a fellowship to study in the United States, and I'll help you," the American has in mind one set of expectations that includes the presumption that an individual can act relatively autonomously in attempting to translate his desires into reality. The young Japanese psychiatrist has in mind a different map of expectations which includes the mutual dependency of people on each other within a tight network of superior and subordinate relations. Because of this the American psychiatrist may be annoyed that his query calls forth embarrassment and evasion.

I think we are just at the beginning of our exploration of the interrelations between the rational-technical and the emotional meanings of words and actions in the communication process, and how these are influenced by the development from childhood through adulthood of culturally patterned maps of average expectable relations.

Since, however, we obviously must keep trying to communicate transnationally across cultural boundaries, I hope that the outline I have given of the four stages I felt I went through in adjusting to life and work in another culture has at least some suggestive usefulness.

Dr. Torre: *The next speaker is Dr. Bertram Schaffner of our committee. Most of you know that he has had rather extensive experience in cross-cultural communication, that he worked with Dr. Margaret Mead at Columbia University in the project "Research in Contemporary Cultures" on the subject, "Pre-Soviet Russian Culture." He also worked in Germany with the Information Control Division of Military Government, and in 1948 published a book,* FATHER LAND, *which deals with authoritarianism in German family life. He has been a consultant in mental health to the Government of the U. S. Virgin Islands and to other Caribbean organizations. He has led and participated in numerous international conferences, and is very skillful at facilitating communication.*

SUMMARY

Bertram Schaffner

Dr. Torre asked me to summarize today's meeting, to point out the psychological-psychiatric implications of what the speakers have said, and to indicate the plan of our approach to this problem of cross-cultural communication. Our committee has really just begun to delineate some of the basic questions and to correlate the material that the speakers have given us.

We are getting under way by asking what insights psychiatrists can contribute toward solving the problems of cross-cultural communication. We wish to learn whether there are any insights we can offer that are different from those which other professionals or experienced lay people might offer.

Dr. Wedge started off with the suggestion that perhaps the doctor-patient relationship in itself could serve as a useful model. The committee members raised the question whether that relationship in itself is useful, or rather must we utilize today's improved understanding of human nature, intrapersonal dynamics, and interpersonal interactions, particularly during cross-cultural as opposed to intracultural communication.

The committee also indicated a need to be much more specific about the type of cross-cultural communication taking place. For example, the conversation with Russian students Dr. Wedge described might be regarded by some as an example of one-way or informational communication. However, Dr. Wedge mentioned that the students also asked him questions, that they were doing something to get to know him and to clarify issues. Nevertheless, there is such one-way communication, as for example with a student or a tourist in a cross-cultural setting.

Classification of Kinds of Communication

Naturally we are more interested in two-way communications, of which there are several types, the structured and the ritualized as Dr. Useem brought out, as well as the informal and unstructured, which sometimes occur separately and sometimes appear together.

Communications may also be divided into those which are designed to be very short-term, say three days, and those which last longer, e.g. for three months, or three years. There are communications which go on in one's own language or in a language foreign to the speaker, with or without an interpreter. When an interpreter is present another problem has been added, anxiety as to whether one is being interpreted correctly or not, and whether one has understood the other person correctly. There is also the question of intent of the communication, and the difficulties that could arise if one member in the discussion is not as interested as the other in resolving difficulties or problems in communication.

Today's speakers have also emphasized the importance of success or failure in communication. The interpersonal communication problems about which the psychiatrist might have something to say cannot always be understood without fuller knowledge of the sociological setting, as Dr. Useem pointed out, or of the cultural setting, as Dr. Caudill emphasized.

Different conditions obtain with different intents of the particular purposes of the communication. Is it for instruction in technical matters or is it for consultation? Is it for innovation to bring about changes? Is it to be a professional exchange leading either to the sharing or the concealment of knowledge? Is it a communication with the purpose of resolving tensions or of increasing tensions? The latter could also come under the classification of communication, even though our current approach to the subject usually implies a major interest in increasing or improving communication. We must also determine whether the communication is in the nature of a diplomatic exchange or a business negotiation in which personal elements are kept to a minimum, or whether the communication is, for example, in the nature of espionage. We could further specify communication problems, according to whether one is dealing with persons from one's own profession, economic level, social group, religion, culture, and so on.

Communications can also be classified as to where they take

place. Our discussion this morning has centered chiefly around Americans who are abroad. We might also ask about problems when communication takes place at home, for example, when an American in his own country receives people from different cultures. Are the problems different when one is an isolated American abroad facing a group of non-Americans, or when one is on home soil in the security of one's own group and dealing with a foreign national who has the insecurities of being a stranger?

Dr. Caudill explained yesterday the difficulties that the Japanese would experience even to conceive of doing a cultural or anthropological study of Americans because of their conception of themselves and their conception of Americans.

There is another area that needs further study: the emotions and reactions of Americans during communication in cross-cultural settings. There has been great emphasis today on the need for adequate time to learn the process of cross-cultural communication. Knowledge of ourselves and knowledge of another culture are not all we need; time and experience make a big difference.

Anxieties of Americans Abroad

In cross-cultural situations, especially abroad, many Americans seem to suffer from considerable anxiety about personal health and safety. Frequently American citizens experience anxiety as to whether they are liked or accepted as persons in their own right regardless of class status or official function. Some Americans are prone to confusion over foreign values in the areas of kindness or morality, confusion about what Dr. Useem calls "somatic manners," and degrees of honesty. There are special problems for Americans over whether or not to act in terms of one's own previous self-identity, or to adopt a new code of behavior. This sometimes leads to confusion of identity or challenges to the sense of integrity, where compromises are required.

As Dr. Useem brought out, there are particular problems for Americans committed to the idea of individual initiative, when required to live under imposed group conformity. This usually raises threats to the sense of independence and self-determination. In Japan, as Dr. Caudill brought out, there would be particular temptations to some Americans to accept greater dependence but with complicated effects upon the self-esteem. I mention these as matters which can lead to anxiety and thereby lead to impaired functioning in interpersonal communication, to difficulty in sensing situations or sensing other persons properly.

For Americans in particular there may be a growing sense of incompetence or inadequacy, due to unpreparedness for dealing with problems of class, caste, religion, race, or, as was brought out this morning, extreme poverty. Sometimes this may produce powerfully negative feelings toward one's own background, even a sense of estrangement from one's own group, together with a feeling of the impossibility of ever belonging to the foreign group that is admired. The American abroad is often brought face-to-face for the first time with his own blind spots and rigidities, and then the difficulty of deciding what to do about them in the cross-cultural setting. For many it is a difficult problem to have to accept a childlike period of learning for the second time, to learn the basic facts of life about a new people.

Lastly, there can be a threat to the sense of achievement, success, or usefulness that is especially important to Americans. This may be compounded in cross-cultural communication settings, since the individual now deals not only with his own personal achievement, success, and usefulness, but he has in addition a role as representative of his country. There is an additional dimension in which he might fail, an additional dimension with which he must cope, in the cross-cultural situation.

Questions Yet Unformulated

There are some essential questions that we have not formulated as yet; for example, to what degree or in what circumstances must one really have knowledge about the other culture? Can knowledge of the other culture sometimes act as a hindrance or even a burden in cross-cultural communication?

The committee is also asking about individual differences in capacity for communication and what to do about them, and how to use psychiatric insights to prepare people for cross-cultural communication. Finally, we will come to the most important question of all: what actually takes place during the process of communication between two people from different cultures?

5

WORKING ABROAD: A DISCUSSION OF PSYCHOLOGICAL ATTITUDES AND ADAPTATION IN NEW SITUATIONS*

FOREWORD

This report has been written partly for the use of psychiatrists and other related professional groups, and also for administrators and personnel officers responsible for the selection, training and effectiveness of personnel abroad.

The report consists of an investigation of the special psychological problems of persons working in foreign lands, together with recommendations as to how these problems may be met. Although this study is based chiefly on the experiences of U. S. citizens abroad, its observations may be equally applicable to citizens of other nations working or studying in foreign countries.

I. SIGNIFICANCE OF THE PROBLEM

A. Numbers and Distribution

This report was undertaken because of the tremendous increase within the last twenty years of the numbers of United States citizens working abroad, because of the importance of their work to the welfare of this country and to the world, and because of the special adjustments in living which have to be made by persons who work in foreign, intercultural settings.

In 1938, there were only 1,218 Americans in the Foreign Service of the United States and another 1,079 working abroad for all other federal agencies. By May, 1956, there were 34,052 Amer-

---

*Formulated by the Committee on International Relations, and first published as Report #41, in December, 1958.

ACKNOWLEDGMENTS: The members of the Committee on International Relations wish to express their deep indebtedness and appreciation to the following consultants who gave invaluable assistance during the preparation of this report: Miss Betty Barton, Dr. Brock Chisholm, Dr. Thomas Detre, Prof. Cora Dubois, Mr. Haskell Ekaireb, Mr. Glen H. Fisher, Mr. Edward T. Hall, Jr., Mrs. Curtice Hitchcock, Dr. Otto Klineberg, Dr. John Lewis, Mrs. Robert J. Lifton, Mr. James M. Mitchell, Dr. John R. Rees, Miss Katharine Taylor.

icans working abroad for U. S. Government agencies other than military—about fifteen times the 1938 total.

This rapid growth has not been due solely to the expansion of federal establishments overseas. Our government has increasingly followed the practice, especially since World War II, of contracting for the services of so-called "voluntary" (private, nongovernmental) agencies to perform specific tasks abroad on its behalf, e.g. agencies specializing in relief and rehabilitation, construction, engineering or economic consultation, child-care or education. It now has contracts with some 75 American colleges and universities to help staff and develop educational institutions abroad.

American personnel also bulks large in the secretariats, research and technical assistance programs of the United Nations and its specialized agencies (World Health Organization, UNESCO, FAO, World Bank, etc.). Over 2,000 Americans are now employed regularly by these organizations, and many others work for them on temporary assignments.

There are also scores of civilian groups—business, banking, labor, educational, religious and philanthropic — which carry on programs similar to those of the national or international public agencies. Some of the industrial companies have undertaken ambitious programs of technical assistance and training, economic and community development, both to improve their local staffs and to create favorable environments for their industrial operations. Labor organizations have established extensive representation overseas. There has been a new surge of practical service projects in agriculture, education, child-care, health and community development on the part of almost all the religious denominations, as well as by various foundations.

In all, "there were more than 100,000 American civilians working abroad on a full-time basis for international organizations in 1956, approximately divided as follows:

United States Government and Government Contracts	37,000
Religious Missionary Organizations	28,000
American Business Enterprises	24,000
Students	10,000
Teachers and Scholars	1,500
International Organizations and Agencies	3,000
Voluntary Agencies and Philanthropic Foundations	1,000

In addition there were probably another 30,000 United States citizens who went abroad on short-term private or government business. To these figures might be added the unknown number of Americans who work directly for a foreign government or foreign business or who are self-employed in foreign countries. For the purpose of emphasizing the problem of education and training for civilians in service overseas, the one million American troops stationed outside the continental limits of the United States have not even been listed. And *none of the figures includes the wives or dependents* of personnel at work abroad."*

It is most important that Americans overseas carry out their jobs successfully. The premise underlying these many assignments is that the United States has committed itself to a policy of international responsibilities, designed not only to promote the welfare of the United States or United States concerns (as in former days) but to promote education, economic growth, political advancement and social progress, which it hopes will be conducive to world peace through international cooperation. Probably these assignments abroad will increase in numbers and scope in the years to come, and much larger numbers of Americans will be preparing themselves for and making their careers in foreign settings.

The mental health of the individual working abroad appears to be of even more critical importance than it is at home, because of its effect upon the vital program the man is responsible for carrying out. In many countries around the world, our contacts with their citizens are not limited to the few traditional ones, i.e. contacts with higher officers in governmental positions, for which there is protocol. Contacts have been extended to many persons at all levels — civil servants, technicians and educators, village headmen, farmers, doctors, nurses and social workers, businessmen, and labor leaders — who now meet on many human levels and not only as officials. Customarily these contacts have the purpose of bringing about profound changes in established technical and social patterns, through the exchange of information and concepts. These results depend upon the ability of both parties to establish mutual trust and satisfactory interpersonal relationships — often a delicate and difficult matter.

Therefore the mental health of the U. S. citizen working abroad has special significance. His individual state of well-being and the

* See Bibliography, Reference 22

quality of his social relationships are most important. He must have a capacity for successful communication and collaboration with persons from widely differing cultures, as well as a capacity to maintain his own emotional well-being for prolonged periods in conditions quite alien to him.

B. Motives and Expectations

A large proportion of U. S. citizens who take jobs abroad, either in governmental, industrial or "voluntary agency" positions are apparently well-adjusted, well-oriented persons. Whatever their motives for leaving home, these do not seem to interfere with their effectiveness abroad; they seek such jobs or are asked to take them because they have specific educational preparation for the work, genuine convictions about the need for the work, positive interest in it and in the persons with whom they are going to work and live. Such persons are usually able to work effectively with the people of other countries, to carry out their assignments well, and to deal with the various impacts and conditions of their work abroad. Because of their attitudes toward people, toward themselves and toward their work, they usually take the foreign conditions and cultural differences in their stride.

There are other Americans working abroad, fortunately few in number, who fail in greater or lesser degree to adjust to life and work there. The more serious failures are relatively few. The absence of readily available facilities for dealing with them may make the few failures more noticeable, as well as also making it far more difficult to give such individuals the help or treatment which they need. There is a small number whose difficulties may result in psychosomatic illness, alcoholism, "nervous breakdown" or suicide. The primary concern in this report is not with this small group, but with the larger group of persons who though frequently very competent in their special fields of work cannot function well in the special situations which arise when they live outside their accustomed environment. It is among this group that one may find the commoner symptoms that are evidence of poor adjustment — such as desire to leave the job before completion, frequent requests for transfer, widespread dissatisfaction or indifference, high incidence of quarreling, frank disregard of regulations, increased sickness or accident rate, work of poor quality, absenteeism and alcoholism.

The foreign situation in itself causes some of the difficulties, although certainly not all. There are often conflicts with values, ideas and customs of the peoples or the co-workers in foreign countries. There often are gross inequalities of privilege and opportunities. Personal relationships with one's own fellow countrymen abroad may be more limited or difficult than similar relationships at home. There are stresses in certain climatic and geographical locations, and in certain cultures, particularly, the greater their differences from Western cultures. The special stress, however, is often to be found in the particular personal or social position in which the U.S. citizen finds himself, or in his reaction to the specific frustrations in his work.

These difficulties are not necessarily an inherent part of the situation; when they are present, training which provides understanding and ways of dealing with the situation, may considerably ease them. Organizations themselves can sometimes bring about changes in the work situation – changes which may be able to lessen an individual's difficulties in living or working abroad.

The psychological challenge of living and working with nationals of other lands is a universal one, and certainly not limited to U.S. citizens. When any person lives within his own country, he does not ordinarily need to be consciously aware of his own culture and of its profound differences from others. He may even believe that "all human beings are fundamentally alike and therefore it should be easy to get along with one another." However, nearly every human being learns his own cultural patterns without much conscious thought about them. When he travels abroad, he is likely to assume naively that his own ways of living are "the natural ones" and would be taken for granted by anyone he meets. He may not even have thought enough about his own culture to be able to describe or explain it, or to compare it usefully with other cultures. He will probably not be prepared to see another culture as a natural variation among the many systems that different groups of people establish as their own accepted way of life.

Fortunately there is more general recognition now that the causes of difficulty in adjustment to overseas living may lie *within the individual himself*. Emotional difficulties may have troubled him to a certain degree at home, but abroad they may become accentuated and also harder to cope with. Often, unrealistic expectations prior to going abroad lead to excessive disappointments, and consequent disturbances in mental health. The presence of personal problems is often hard to detect; whether an individual will have more or less difficulty abroad is not easy to predict, especially since conditions that are trying to one person may not be to another — indeed may be sources of satisfaction.

The emphasis in this report will not be upon the usual factors considered for promoting and maintaining mental health in the home situation. Instead it will concentrate upon the special problems affecting the mental health of U. S. citizens when they work and live abroad. It will deal with the possibilities of prevention (e.g., through personnel selection, predeparture education for life abroad, and special orientation in understanding and communicating with the people among whom the U. S. citizen will work), and the possibilities of assistance to the individual, assistance to the group, and education of those in positions of responsible leadership, in the foreign situation.

II. SATISFACTION AND STRESS IN WORKING OVERSEAS

The psychological rewards for the individual who decides to take an overseas assignment are many. At first sight, the work may represent mainly an opportunity for personal advancement, escape or variety. But no matter what the immediate motivation, the chance to live and work outside one's own country over a period of time often satisfies a deep human need to have personal experience of the world beyond one's horizon.

There is of course the satisfaction of the particular work accomplished. Then there are additional satisfactions for the man with specific interest in foreign affairs, cultural studies, political science, economics, or language studies. There is a reward for the person interested in world-wide cooperation in specific areas of business or science. There can be special pleasure for those who love to teach or to be taught. There are others who derive their satisfaction from patriotic motivations, as well as those who particularly seek rewards in the form of honor, status or prestige. Some derive much-needed financial security in the form of higher salaries and pensions, as well as others who go abroad at considerable personal self-sacrifice for a specific humanitarian reason. The motivations are many and varied; the rewards may be great or small, depending upon the individual himself and upon circumstances he cannot foresee or control.

In general it may be said, however, since the majority of persons (except those in governmental or military service) go abroad of their own free choice to live and work, that the rewards of working overseas are obvious and real to those who choose to go. Nevertheless, even for them, there are psychological stresses, which are not either apparent or anticipated.

A. Environmental Changes and "Culture Shock".

When an individual moves from his home to *any* new and unfamiliar place, it involves certain basic changes in his habits, relationships and sources of satisfaction, and produces a different pattern of stresses from the ones to which he had become accustomed. When the change is the still larger one of moving to a different country and culture, the adaptation required assumes even greater significance. Inherent in such a move, of course, is the opportunity to leave behind, if only temporarily, one set of relationships and life-patterns, and to enrich one's life by establishing new ones, with new satisfactions. Nevertheless, even the well-integrated person sent overseas is likely, especially at first, to have a sense of geographical dislocation or isolation, a feeling of "being out of things"; he often finds an intensified need for communication with home, a sense of frustration over the inevitable slowness of establishing the feeling, of "belonging" locally, and a feeling of boredom brought about by the monotony and limitations of social life.

"The overseas employee and his family are required to adjust to the foreign situation with its frequently more difficult climate, poor sanitation, lack of formal entertainment, inadequate housing, circumscribed social activity; they are expected to work effectively with people who have a different temperament, language, religion, culture . . . different ways of doing things, different values . . . different concepts of time, etc. The most difficult jobs are those which require the employee to work extensively or exclusively with the indigenous people with minimal supervision or support."*

Primarily, the success or failure of the adjustment to the overseas situation depends upon the individual's personality, temperament and capacity for adaptation. (This is not meant to exclude group and social factors which will be considered later.) Generally it has been found to hold true that if a man has been able to live and function happily and effectively at home, he is likely to be successful in his transition to overseas life. When there are unsettled psychological or emotional difficulties, these are usually transferred to the new situation. Occasionally, the new environment may be favorable for the individual and his particular emotional difficulty, but far more frequently the difficulty becomes aggravated. This likelihood emphasizes the importance and value of careful screening with special reference to the nature of his work and the country to which he will be sent.

---

* See Bibliography, Reference 4

Surveys show that those who have worked well and happily abroad generally have the following qualities: flexibility, personal stability, social maturity and "social inventiveness". They either have fewer prejudices or a greater awareness of them and the ability to tolerate the objects of their prejudice.

An important psychological factor relating to emotional stress abroad is the degree of reality in the individual's expectations. Some persons' anticipations are quite unrealistic, even grandiose. For instance, some people with adolescent phantasies take overseas jobs hoping to "save the world." They have irrational concepts of "self", of others, and of the amount of time required for changes in attitudes and habits. For the person whose expectations of himself or of his job are excessive, the frustrations may be so great that he will find it hard to concentrate on the work to be done, or to see his role in it in proper perspective.

If an individual is unable to relate his new experiences to his old ones, to see the foreign situation in terms of his own country's past development, to see the needs of another country through its own eyes, or to reach desired objectives through new or still-to-be-discovered methods, he may become disappointed, frustrated and discouraged. Such feelings are then often expressed in the form of bitter criticism and hostility toward the foreign country, and are not recognized as the result of his excessive optimism, or his lack of realistic understanding of the problems, or of himself.

B. The Role of the Family

Marital situations may also cause either special psychological distress or satisfaction overseas. Ordinarily the man who goes abroad with his family finds that he is thrown into a more intense relationship with them than he had at home. For some Americans, this greater proximity results in greater intimacy and understanding than had been the case at home. For others, basic difficulties within a family relationship become accentuated in the closer living with fewer opportunities for diverse activities or substitute outlets.

Many men who go overseas find a continuity in their work, which makes a bond between their life at home and the life abroad; some even feel a greater sense of usefulness overseas than at home. Certainly many men find their new job very challenging and their time fully occupied. But some wives, particularly those who may have given up jobs or careers in order to accompany the family, experience a greater change of living habits than their husbands. Most wives find housekeeping radically different abroad with entirely new problems to cope with, e.g., having either much more or much less free time than they had at home, or completely new relationships with servants. Problems of schooling, shopping, transportation, can defeat even the most devoted and resourceful wife. And there are such matters as face-saving and "squeeze" – i.e. being obliged to pay higher prices due to lack of knowledge of local language and resources and being dependent on certain local persons – which she must be prepared to meet. Often when she calls on her husband for help, he may not know what to do any more than she does and he may take refuge in his own work and his more pressing problems.

For these reasons, agencies which send employees abroad tend nowadays to consider the prospective applicant *and* his family as a *unit,* and try to determine not only the man's but the *wife's* and the *family's* readiness for life and work overseas. In the words of one Foreign Service officer, "The adjustment and training for overseas for wives is as important as the adjustment and training of the men. I have seen men overseas, doing well at their jobs, become unhappy and dissatisfied because their wives became dissatisfied."

Still another source of psychological reward or distress for the individual may arise from the living arrangements and customs of the group with whom the American employee is to associate. While technical assistance and voluntary agency personnel often live separately because of the nature of their work, the majority of Americans working abroad tend to live within American groups. When, for example, the employing organization provides organized housing, many Americans overseas derive considerable security from being able to live in circumstances of physical comfort and safety not too different from those at home, in a small community of fellow-Americans to which they can "really belong". Often, however, such "colonies" or "compounds" interfere with any real contact with the native population, and may involve social ostracism of individuals who have the interest or desire to make such contact. The U. S. citizen who derives sufficient satisfaction from his work, his family relationships, and the limited community, may feel quite content. On the other hand, the individual who was inclined to go abroad in the first place because of his interest in or curiosity about other cultures, or out of a sense of adventure, may find himself seriously limited and frustrated.

In considering the psychological rewards and stresses for anyone going overseas to work, one should not make the mistake of emphasizing only rewards and stresses as the determining factors in the ultimate state of mental health for any individual. They are probably only of somewhat greater significance overseas than at home. In the overseas situation, the primary factors in an individual's mental health are his already existent *personality*, his degree of satisfaction or adaptation in his family, his work, his social contacts, his *recreational* situation, and the particular dynamic balance between them.

C. Varying Patterns in Overseas Services

Adaptation to the overseas situation may be conveniently divided into early adjustments to the general foreign way of life and later adjustment to the specific features of a given job and a particular country. The early short-term adaptation problems are probably universal, and the speed with which they are met depends largely upon the individual's ability to assess his new environment quickly and accurately, his possession of the necessary social aptitude for such a situation, and the degree and kind of training for the assignment that he brings with him. The later long-term adjustment depends more upon the length of time of the assignment, the individual's goals and motives for accepting the overseas work, the place it occupies in his life-plan, the degree of or significance to him of changes which take place, and the successful or unsuccessful outcome of his work. In this respect, differences in types of overseas service present varying challenges. For example, in brief overseas assignments the individual's way is often made smooth for him and his adaptation problems may be minimal, while in the career service or in assignments lasting a number of years, the adaptations required may be major and continuing. For the career service man, in general, the adaptation problems tend to diminish with each succeeding assignment.

However, a man's desire to remain in overseas service does

not necessarily stay constant. It may waver or decrease, due to many factors. While good selection of personnel may be counted upon to meet a part of the problem of maintenance of interest, it is more and more realized now that the attitudes of the administrator and the policies of the organization have a very strong bearing on the long-range mental health of the overseas employee. Recent conferences and research studies consistently emphasize the vital effects of satisfactions and dissatisfactions within the work situation.

That these satisfactions or dissatisfactions are primarily psychological and social in nature, and not necessarily financial, is given recognition in the phrases "psychic income" and "psychic deficit" which have recently come to be used in administrative circles. For example, a recent United Nations report* listed four points under the heading of "psychic income": a sense of belonging, the opportunity to do constructive work, the recognition of good work, and a reasonable sense of security.

In order to give the reader an idea of the different kinds of conditions and factors affecting "psychic income" abroad, several different types of overseas work will now be briefly described. This review is not intended to be complete, but rather to point out some common characteristics of overseas services.

1. The Career Employee

For a long time, the career officer in the U. S. Foreign Service had what was regarded as the best conditions of any U. S. citizen employed abroad. Social status as a diplomat was high; there was economic security even though the salary was not especially large. There was a sense of genuine belonging to a diplomatic corps, which had integrity and the loyalty of its members. To a large degree, there was a sense of personal identification with the diplomatic mission and its importance.

Personal satisfaction within the Foreign Service naturally varies according to the type of assignment and also according to a man's position within the diplomatic hierarchy. The chief of mission may understandably derive greater pleasure, from his intimate knowledge of affairs and from his status, than the file clerk. In most missions, the subordinates are largely dependent upon the chief or

---

* See Bibliography, Reference 16

his senior staff for their satisfactions in the work situation. Consequently, the personality and habits of the chief become critically important.

For example, the chief of mission in one of the Asian countries, himself a gifted diplomat who received recognition both from the State Department and ambassadors of other countries, carried out diplomatic negotiations himself but also saw to it that his entire staff could participate with him. He set up regular conferences with them, shared the information he received, and invited them to take part in making decisions. His staff acquired an intimate understanding of policies and felt that they had roles of responsibility in the mission's accomplishments. In his mission, there were requests for extensions of assignment rather than resignations or requests for transfer, which are reliable indices of the state of satisfaction within an organization. By way of contrast, the staff working under another chief of mission, who was equally successful in diplomatic negotiations but remarkably poor in relation to his staff, showed a number of personal and professional difficulties; these were directly traceable to the unfavorable attitudes of the mission chief.

A frequent factor leading to special emotional hardship is the rigid structure of communications within the State Department. People in foreign posts usually lack opportunities for informal channels of communication. They are often irked by long delays in replies to official requests, and by occasional failure to obtain recognition or approval from Washington for local programs which they wish to undertake on their own initiative and which they consider vital. A system currently in use, in which inspectors come to the post from the United States, and then send written reports back to Washington, has been a source of friction. This type of friction has been offset to some extent by the practice of having inspectors discuss their reports with the mission staff before leaving the post. Such discussions with the staff, and joint working out of the problems, have proven to be of great help. In some cases, the staff has been able to correct reports in which the inspector has unintentionally misconstrued a situation. In others, the inspector has worked out with the staff new procedures to improve the situation. In such cases, fear of the contents of the report is reduced, and the problems reported are solved before the report reaches Washington.

Sudden changes in government policy work special hardships on men who have become personally committed or publicly identified with previous policy. For example, some U. S. consuls in Germany had helped prospective emigrants make plans for leaving, and then had to reverse their own previous instructions when U. S. immigration laws suddenly changed. In other situations, conflict over having to enforce laws at variance with one's own personal feelings, can create great strain in some individuals.

Security investigations had a profound effect upon some members of the Foreign Service. It is hard to work under the shadow of suspicion, or while feeling constantly vulnerable due to changes in administration policy. The withdrawal of support from the very authority that had been counted upon, was in many cases a serious blow to the mental health of the individual.

2. *The Technical Assistance Expert*

The technical expert has many sources of pride and pleasure in his work. He usually has a specific project and knows that his particular field of competence is needed for the completion of a definite program. He works "in the field" and has the satisfactions that come from direct contact with people and program, in contrast to the relatively removed and routine work of the administrators. He is more likely to see the fruits of his labor, and he receives more direct recognition, usually both from his colleagues and local populations. Though his protocol position in the mission is lower than that of a diplomat, and his fringe benefits (housing privileges, pensions and the like) are fewer, he enjoys great prestige.

On the other hand, since he is often employed to meet temporary needs or to help in specific programs, his assignments are usually for only one or two years. He has neither the security of job continuity nor of job advancement. This temporary aspect of the work prevents some technical experts from experiencing the satisfaction which can come from seeing one's project through to the end. It may place other experts in the position of having to continue another man's project without adequate background information.

The contact with the local population may be extremely frustrating and irritating as well as satisfying. Often the technical expert must work with a local counterpart whose skills and knowledge are considerably different from his own. Usually, programs which a man might carry out at home in a short time, take far longer than he expects abroad. For this reason and others, the technical expert has little opportunity to develop his set task creatively. In terms of his social relations, he is rarely in one area long enough to make a real place for himself in the community. Despite the fact that he is welcome, he remains essentially a newcomer or an outsider.

3. *Civilians Working for Voluntary Agencies**

The staffs of the voluntary agencies are largely composed of civilians from different professional disciplines (social work, education, medicine, etc.). They also usually include nationals of the foreign country whose participation in the work is part of their training process. U. S. civilians in voluntary agencies do not come as officials or representatives of any government, although they sometimes get partial government financial support for their programs. Often they are invited abroad by a non-governmental group in the foreign country. Even when carrying out a program under government contract, they do not receive all the privileges given to government employees.

Civilians with voluntary agencies have a greater degree of independence than most other U. S. workers overseas. They can often determine their own programs and can be most flexible in their procedures. They associate freely with the local population, and because of the nature of their work they usually do not live on the higher standards provided at most governmental and industrial installations. Although they are usually provided by the U. S. Government with adequate medical facilities and certain supplies, their standard of living is closer to that of the local group with whom they are working. This is not ordinarily a cause for any emotional problems, since the staffs of voluntary agencies usually take overseas assignments with the motives of service and usefulness and the understanding that they will work together with the people of the country. Their purpose, in general, is to understand the local problems in terms of the local culture and personalities,

* The term "voluntary agency" is usually given to private, non-governmental, and often non-profit organizations whose work is primarily educational. It includes religious and relief organizations as well.

to help develop local initiative and leaders who will ultimately work out solutions to local problems in ways that are feasible and acceptable to their own populations.

One can see that a well-integrated and successful civilian working in a voluntary agency might obtain deep satisfactions from his work and life abroad. The desired relationship, however, with the local population is not easy to attain, and is highly complicated at best. Though the individual U. S. civilian may be eager to function as an equal, non-directing partner, the local group may still view him in terms of its own national stereotype. Also, a man's very capacity to identify with the local population can create a gulf between him and his own compatriot group.

Not infrequently the local group opposes and frustrates the voluntary agency worker, whom they have themselves invited, for unexplained reasons which it may take months to ferret out. Sometimes the difficulty is resolved; if not, the worker may have to be recalled and another sent in his place. The sense of isolation and frustration can be very great. Nevertheless, on the whole the voluntary agency worker because of his special attitude of service, his training to work with people, and his convictions about values, tends to be capable of coping with his emotional problems.

Industrial employees fall into two categories, as do the government employees. Some of the long-established, large overseas industrial operations are staffed by career employees who spend their lives abroad in the overseas posts of their company. The psychological aspects of the work of these employees are similar to those in the U. S. Foreign Service and international civil service.

A much larger group of Americans in industry abroad are on a temporary basis. Their motivations, goals and expectations are quite different. Many of them expect to live in a state of physical and social deprivation and do so for the money which is offered. The personnel policies of industry frequently require the man to leave his family in the U. S. for the duration of his overseas assignment. Although a higher salary will recruit personnel willing to undergo this kind of arrangement, such personnel living in a state of deprivation reflect this in their human relations with the local people and adversely affect the morale of the American community where they are stationed.

While there are other large categories of U. S. citizens working overseas, such as employees of the U. S. Government both in and outside of the Department of Defense, employees of the U. N. and its agencies, and exchange students, it is unnecessary to deal with each group separately, since the conditions and stresses more or less resemble and overlap the descriptions already sketched.

III. PROBLEMS OF PERSONAL RELATIONSHIPS ABROAD

It is now axiomatic that good working and social relationships are important to a satisfactory frame of mind — to good mental health. Developing a sound working relationship with members of the local population is a basic part of the overseas worker's job. Social relationships abroad are necessarily complicated, not only because of the barrier of the foreign language and the deep gulfs between cultures and unexpected changes in social status. The degree of difficulty which any individual encounters abroad can vary with the degree to which he lives among his own compatriots or among foreign nationals. The Western European cultures probably seem most familiar to the U. S. citizen; the Slavonic, African and Asian cultures are increasingly strange and difficult to feel at home in.

Lastly, the individual's mental health is likely to depend to a considerable extent upon the type of relationships he desires or finally achieves: whether he has a need to be wholly accepted by the foreign culture and to become part of it; whether he rejects it or is rejected by it; whether he is able to develop and sustain the unique relationship imposed by the overseas work situation. Much will depend on whether, as an outsider, he can succeed in establishing good relationships with the local population, without developing serious feelings of isolation or experiencing threats to his own sense of identity.

A. Natural Difficulties

The U. S. citizen brings with him his American cultural attitudes and ideals, e. g., belief in a relatively classless society, willingness to meet all kinds of people at their own level, a generally pragmatic way of thinking, an emphasis upon individual initiative, "team-work", and so on. Sometimes these attitudes are helpful in his social relationships; sometimes they are not. United States attitudes concerning the desirability of change, concepts of time, national and racial stereotypes have often caused friction. Certainly those individuals who have acquired a degree of awareness of their own cultural background and habits, some information about the culture in which they are going to live, together with an appreciation of the meanings of cultural differences, seem to fare much better than those who did not get such preparation.

The foreign nationals who receive the U. S. citizen overseas suffer, of course, from similar limitations. They have equally strong and usually unconscious convictions about their own way of life, and equally preconceived images about foreigners in general and about Americans in particular. Such popularly held images or stereotypes about one another tend to increase the natural confusion when the U. S. citizen and the foreign national meet. Unnecessary resentments may develop merely from this confusion, as well as from specific misconceptions. When a foreign tongue is added to other cultural differences, communication can become even more difficult.

Only one example among many will be given here of the interaction between U. S. citizens and different cultures, since it illustrates the general principle of such interactions: an American arriving in Japan, eager to proffer friendliness in his accustomed way, may be puzzled by a general attitude of reserve in response to his outgoing heartiness. He may be pleased with Japanese politeness but not know what to make of smiling which comes at moments when he would not expect it. When he is most eager to speak directly of a point, he may be irked by what he regards as indirectness or evasion. On the other hand, the Japanese who meets the U. S. citizen for the first time may have been expecting him to behave in an overbearing or militaristic way corresponding to the anticipated stereotype. He may find himself pleasantly surprised that the American is friendly and treats him as his equal; yet by Japanese standards he may consider the American oddly garrulous and insensitive. Not infrequently, each person generalizes from his contact with perhaps the one individual from the other culture that he has chanced to meet. He may conclude that "all Americans are friendly but insensitive" or that "all Japanese are polite but evasive". To learn the meaning of his culture to the man who lives in it, to learn about its expectations, its values and its consistencies, and in turn to explain one's own culture to that man, is necessarily a slow process. But it is well worth the time and effort, though not one for which everyone is equally gifted or prepared.

B. Distortions and Prejudices

The reactions of U. S. citizens to the encounter with foreign persons, referred to as "culture shock", vary enormously. A few Americans feel so uncomfortably isolated that they go to the extreme of trying to merge with the foreign culture, dressing and living in all ways like the local population, giving up as far as possible their own previous identity. Sometimes this is not due to a sense of isolation in the foreign land, but results from an emotional conflict within the individual about belonging to his own family or his own social group at home. Such a flight into the foreign culture may also take place as a result of naive over-enthusiasm.

In contrast to this reaction, there is a second group of U. S. citizens with an equally unhealthy attitude: they reject the local population and culture, and may even become actively hostile toward it. Their distrust or disdain is often due to prejudice carried over from early life at home, and not — as they often suppose — due to an objective evaluation of the culture or people among whom they find themselves. Often it is prejudice against certain religions or colors, sometimes simply a bias against anything foreign. It can seriously undermine peoples' emotional well-being, as well as do damage to their country's relations with the host nation.

Another group of U. S. citizens earnestly tries to learn a little of the local language, to understand, respect and participate in local customs, and yet possesses a comfortable sense of differences, and has good human relationships despite the differences.

It is among the first and second groups that the larger number of mental health disturbances may occur. The individuals whose unresolved family problems and prejudice lead them to over-identification with or rejection of the local population, might better have been discovered and eliminated in selection procedures, or given psychological assistance prior to going overseas. Others who feel rejected by the local population and in turn reject it, or who never are able to establish any kind of rewarding relationship with it, should either be eliminated before going overseas or else should be given special assistance or counselling in the field abroad. This is not only for their own welfare, but because of the pronounced effects such people usually have on those around them.

It seems apparent that the ways in which the important work is done overseas and the quality of personal relationships developed by the people doing it, are bound to affect public relations between the United States and the host country. Ordinarily, patient exploration on both sides and mutual forebearance are required for good cross-cultural social relations. Gradually the image each has of the other may become realistic instead of pre-formed and biased; gradually the personal experience may outweigh the stereotyped preconception, and mutually satisfying friendships may emerge.

IV. FACTORS IN ADAPTATION TO OVERSEAS SERVICE

The following are excerpts from letters of a technical consultant from the United States who was recently sent to assist an Asian country in the development of its public health program. These excerpts may provide a useful background for a discussion of personal qualities necessary to the mastery of stress and a satisfactory adjustment abroad:

> May 7th: As I look out the office window here and see the oleanders and honeysuckles in bloom, I think about the difference in temperature at home. It's 90° now, but they say it will soon be really hot here. We are still not settled in a house; I was glad we got a furnished apartment while house-hunting. I find myself getting very anxious at times, which I attribute possibly to failing to meet unreasonable expectations of myself. Things do move more slowly than at home and everything is tremendously complicated. There are the difficulties of language and concepts, of course, but also the physical difficulties of transportation and communication; I also find the idea of scheduling is something strange to the ——————s. I have planned with the Minister for a conference between his staff and ours; hopefully we will be able to agree on common objectives and learn how to break some of the program bottlenecks.
>
> May 23: We are not used to living in such an atmosphere of distrust, and it is frustrating to wait all day and have people not show up. There is a problem of keys too. Everyone locks everything up; we often find someone else, or the guard, has the key. There are only two keys to the gate; once after I had left, the guard locked the gate with his, and my wife could not get out. You have to watch the car carefully too. To take all precautions advisable to protect your property, slows mobility considerably. . . . It is common practice to have three scales of prices, one for the ———s, one for the ———*, and one for the Americans.
>
> The practice has become so institutionalized, that the ————s will not accept the regular price from Americans; if they are per-

* Another Western nation.

suaded to do so, they feel cheated. The practice is equally intolerable to the Americans, who even though they can afford it, feel that they are being made "the sucker", which is an affront to the ego. It sometimes results in hostility to the natives, who engage in sly practices in return. . . . There should be training in how to introduce technical changes, in terms of the human relations element involved. Everything we suggest is in some way an implied criticism, hence learning to deal with relationships in introducing change is of critical importance. I still don't know how I am doing. One change I've made is to deal directly with the Minister on all matters; heretofore our staff had been seeing any one they thought might be sympathetic, as a result by-passing the Minister, who remained ignorant of our operations. I have been gradually mastering the intricacies; but while learning pathways of getting things done here, I felt trapped since I couldn't fulfill the high expectations I had. Recognizing this, I was able to struggle on and gradually move forward. Hopefully, something will take hold in the program. I do wish the Minister would come to me with matters that he would like help with. But I doubt that one can expect it for a long time. In the meantime, I keep dropping suggestions which he can think over and take up if he likes; otherwise they will wait.

July 20: Periodically I get a compulsion to inactivity, a kind of withdrawal of energy from anything that requires initiative. The misunderstanding and mistakes that arise in our work are very real events, not just theoretical. So are the doubts and suspicions on both sides of the cultural division lines. I try to evaluate all the factors involved in each frustrated effort, and ask myself questions to confirm or refute my impressions. It's awfully difficult to understand what the ———s think about our proposals; it's very difficult to get the simplest data on their operations. It's like walking around in a strange museum at night; you bump into something, get an impression, and then start feeling to determine what it is. You feel it is marble, make out some features, think it may be a statue, but on feeling further you discover it is on a very wide base. Is it a sarcophagus, or what? You discover any number of objects, and can't tell what they are or what they are used for. You find someone to explain, but what he says does not seem to make sense. You suspect he is telling you what he thinks you would like to hear. It is a wonder, with all of the reasons why nothing can happen, that nevertheless they do happen. Out of a welter of confusion, a new water supply system *is* established, candidates appear for training (a week after being advised that no candidates could be found). It's very difficult! Occasionally we get a small indication of interest in something; then we work hard on that until I sense that it has gone far enough.

> Sept. 13: I became interested in malaria last week because we are going to assist in the eradication program. At the moment I feel well informed about it. Something has happened in my relations with the Minister. He has suddenly become most co-operative, insisting on immediate action on my suggestions, where before there was procrastination or even no response, which I ignored but inwardly felt as a signal that every detail was going to be a long drawn-out process with little to show for the effort. Now his speed is almost as much worry to me, because he gives orders to his staff based on my recommendations without giving much thought as to how they are going to be carried out. But overall, I feel much more optimistic than I did a few months ago. I am beginning to like ——— as a place to live; the little annoyances and inconveniences don't bother me as much as before, as I take them into account in my activities. I have just been doing some reading I have wanted to do. This life appeals to me very much.

From the feelings expressed in these letters, it becomes apparent immediately that a deep interest in and dedication to one's work plays an important role in a person's sense of well-being overseas. This is of course also true for U. S. citizens at home, but is more intensified abroad. It is not merely "work for work's sake", nor work to gain fame or money, but a direct sense of satisfaction and pleasure from performing the work assigned. None of the accessory pleasures can compensate for basic dissatisfaction in one's work, but as illustrated above, satisfaction in work may compensate to a large degree for some of the inevitable irritations.

A second factor of major importance is the quality of response to the challenge of the new and the unknown. An attitude of healthy curiosity, of willingness to try to learn and understand, of patience when answers are not forthcoming or are very difficult to obtain, and lack of fear in facing the answers, is obviously valuable. Flexibility and adaptability to the unknown and unforeseeable are very much needed. Even so, frustration and discouragement are almost inevitably to be met, and the man who can bear them well is clearly better equipped for his overseas assignment.

A third factor might be called "social imagination"—the capacity not only to see oneself in proper perspective, but also to sense the situation of the other person as he himself might see it.

It is worthwhile in all human relationships, but especially so in the overseas situation, to be able to estimate the degree of readiness of the nationals with whom one works, and to visualize the next step that they will be ready to take and accept.

A sense of isolation can have a most harmful effect on an individual's sense of well-being overseas. It is not always easy to find a person with whom to share and compare one's experiences and questions, or from whom one can obtain necessary explanations. The stability of many a man has been maintained through the companionship of a wife, a friend, or an experienced counsellor. For a number of Americans working abroad, their well-being has depended to a considerable extent on the closeness and communication they have been able to establish with another member of the staff or team, with one of the local population with whom they have been working, or with the links to home through correspondence.

For numerous Americans, the inevitable criticism leveled at them, either personally or as a group, or failure to achieve cooperation or acceptance and understanding of their program and efforts, may become a source of difficulty. With still others, the disparity between their own government and that of the host government, may form major psychological hurdles. Some suffer from the fact that they live on a higher scale than others in the population, some may feel too much personal responsibility for undesirable social conditions that they encounter.

V. DISCUSSIONS AND RECOMMENDATIONS

Assuming that the number of U. S. citizens working abroad will continue to grow larger in years to come, it is a matter of practical importance to review existing administrative procedures with special regard to their implications for mental health, and to formulate new or additional policies and procedures in the light of further experience. For purposes of discussion, the usual administrative areas may be roughly grouped into three main categories: (A) selection, (B) orientation and training, and (C) mental health measures overseas.

A. Selection

The process of selection of applicants for specific work situations is generally based on three findings. The first is an evaluation of a man's technical or professional qualifications; the second is an evaluation of his physical health; the third is an evaluation of his personal qualifications. An evaluation of the spouse should be included whenever possible, since the successful adjustment of the family as a whole is so important.

Unlike selection at home, where there may be many more candidates available than there are jobs to fill, there are frequently only a very few people to choose among for overseas positions. This is especially true when the overseas position requires highly specialized skill and training together with working knowledge of a foreign language. A number of organizations report that they spend most of their time finding even one person with the necessary technical competence, and consequently have little or no opportunity for selection on the basis of personality. But fortunately, in the majority of overseas jobs, it is possible to exercise some selectivity; then the psychological evaluation of the individual can be given more significance. In general, technical specifications for overseas jobs have in the past been given more importance than personal qualifications, and more was expected from the overseas employee with reference to his craft than with reference to his personal relationships. Recent experience suggests that sending the right kind of person is so vitally important, that it is worthwhile to lower the technical requirements on occasions, even better at times not to fill the job at all, than to send someone well-trained who is likely to fail on a personal basis or who may cause embarrassment in his public relations.

Methods of selecting men along lines of technical and professional competence for work abroad do not differ essentially from selection in the domestic situations. Only the most progressive selection methods used in the U. S. seem adequate for the foreign situation. These procedures should certainly include the careful appraisal of the training and experience of the candidate, finding men with previous experience in work abroad, special efforts to determine their reactions to re-location, and interviews by more than one psychologically trained interviewer.

The second consideration in selection is a man's physical health. Both routine and special duties must often be carried out under strange, trying and shifting conditions. The physicians examining candidates for the Foreign Service have been instructed to reject persons who do not enjoy "*more* than average health".* The health of a man's family of course also calls for the most careful attention. Adjustment to new conditions usually entails physical strain and medical facilities are limited in many parts of the world. Worry over health matters can assume greater proportions overseas. Chronic ill health, even though minor, has been known to give rise to increased psychological strains abroad, which in turn may affect an individual's general health adversely. Persons with histories of psychosomatic illnesses have been repeatedly found to do poorly in difficult foreign climates. It has been the experience of a number of agencies and industries that persons given medical waivers and allowed to proceed overseas to work, have shown poor efficiency in their work, have had to return to the United States for medical reasons more often than other employees. In addition, they have returned to the United States for non-medical reasons prior to completion of service more often than other employees. The cost to the agency which has to send a man or his family home is very high, not to mention the cost in worry to the administrators and the man himself.

---

* INSTRUCTIONS FOR EXAMINING PHYSICIANS, April 15, 1949, Department of State, Foreign Service.

The third consideration, and the most important, is the psychological evaluation for work abroad, which has to differ considerably from selection for work at home.* When men have failed overseas, it has rarely been found to be due to deficiency in their professional work. It is nearly always due to a personal difficulty, such as lack of ability to adapt to local conditions or inability to deal with the complicated interpersonal relationships in the foreign situation. Consequently, greater demands have been made upon the psychological selection process for the foreign situation, and these are not easy to fulfill.

First of all, it is harder to define the specific psychological conditions and personal requirements in an overseas job than in a comparable one at home, although a more careful analysis of the job to be filled is helpful. It is still difficult to make predictions with accuracy about individuals' abilities to maintain good mental health overseas. There are many imponderables. Sometimes the existence of strong, sound enthusiasm for the overseas assignment has been found to be a reliable indicator of probable success. Certainly one would want to learn about a man's previous record of exposure to situations involving national and racial differences and prejudice, and to know about his capacity to cope with it with a minimum of strain or friction. Obviously, overt cases of mental illness would be rejected for overseas duty. However, the non-acute and the mild or subtle emotional and mental disturbances can be extremely difficult to detect, even for the trained observer, unless the candidates cooperate in revealing them, or unless a long period of observation and acquaintance with the candidate is possible. Such periods have usually not been possible in most practical situations. Degrees of dependence, degrees of states of fearfulness, sense of helplessness, sense of despair, are not easy to measure in brief interviews. Consequently, although it is gradually becoming possible to make more reliable predictions concerning probable success or failure abroad, a great deal more research is needed in this regard. It is still far from easy to evaluate human

* It should be noted that employment adjustment problems are by no means uniform even within the United States itself. "Problems at certain places in the United States may bear a resemblance to many of those in the overseas situation. . . . There might reasonably be found some parallels . . . to the environment and working conditions in (Indian) reservation work. . . ." P. 45, RESEARCH PROJECT ON SELECTION METHODS FOR OVERSEAS EMPLOYEES, Ref. 14.

beings in terms of their future reactions. There is much to indicate that a person who has successfully done a technical or professional job at home will not *necessarily* be able to do a similar good job at the same work in a *different* cultural situation.

Frequently people are asked to do something they have not done before, either to perform similar jobs under entirely different interpersonal and social conditions, or to act as *consultant* when previously they have been primarily carrying out the work themselves. To help others to do a job by themselves is quite a different psychological role from doing the job oneself. This is a change which is hard for many otherwise competent people to tolerate. It requires being able to communicate one's technical knowledge to others in an acceptable way, and is likely to be found in those who have a bent for teaching and talent for leadership in group situations. It may give certain consultants less satisfaction than they receive when they do the entire job alone; frequently, the consultant has less opportunity to develop his individual job than do the local personnel with whom he is working.

In many instances, in working with a local counterpart, he has to learn to adjust to his counterpart's strengths and weaknesses as well as his own. Sometimes consultants cover up their own inadequacies by placing the blame for failure on the counterpart, and by such a scapegoat method they prolong the job in the field for a longer time than a job would last at home; this is highly undesirable. Special problems are therefore presented in trying to predict a person's potential skill as a consultant.

Another way to regard selection, and perhaps one with the greatest promise, is to use selection as a way of determining not only existing qualities in a man, but to attempt to measure his *potentialities for growth* in the new job and situation. This re-emphasizes the point that it is important and beneficial in the long run to choose men and women with psychological flexibility and adaptability even though they have less technical skill than would be immediately needed. It is desirable that they not be too rigid and that their work history demonstrates an ability to face difficulties successfully. Certainly, a previous history of successful coping with separation from home and accustomed environment, and a history of good working relations with colleagues would be good indications, since under overseas conditions, the official working team has to operate under far closer, and therefore, often far more trying conditions of competition and rivalry.

The principal methods of carrying out selection have been the personal interview (including the panel interview), questionnaires, letters of reference, records of previous experience and adjustment both in work and personal life, and trial and error. More lately, selection methods have included psychological testing, assessments, observations and evaluation of an individual *during* his training or probationary period, i.e. after he has been employed but while he is still in the United States. Some industrial companies use their appraisal of a prospective overseas employee during this training or probationary period as a final stage in their selection process.

Psychological tests can give valuable information concerning flexibility and rigidity of charcter, social adaptability, tolerance for frustration and other kinds of endurance, inner resources, levels of aspiration and the quality of drive toward achievement, and strength of motivation. Tests in combination with personal interviews, have been found to be more helpful than tests alone.

There are a number of ways to increase the reliability and validity of predictions as to success or failure in an overseas job. The background appraisal includes a review of as many facts as possible about the person's psychological maturity. It is better when it includes the opinions of subordinates and peers as well as supervisors. The employment interview, or preferably several interviews, should be conducted by competent persons who have been carefully trained to use the insights of psychiatry, and who periodically add to their training through follow-up studies of the selections they have previously made. Such interviewers can then better integrate the material found in the background appraisal and in the psychological tests, with considerations of the individual and his particular place and type of assignment. In addition, it helps a great deal if the interviewer is personally familiar with the setting and conditions in the country for which he is selecting a prospective employee.

The candidate can be a useful partner in the selection process. Most Americans, if given full information about the nature of the job and the living conditions, can assist in assessing their capacity to cope with the situation. Since most of the candidates are successful in their present jobs, they will probably refuse to take the proffered job if they feel it is beyond their capabilities.

Sometimes a naive or overzealous recruiter in order to obtain a candidate for a post which is difficult to fill, will glamorize and distort the description of the assignment. Although this may result in finding some one to fill the job, the possibility of this person failing is much greater. A candidate recruited through subterfuge is denied the opportunity of accurately assessing his own ability to handle the job and adjusting to the local conditions. He is usually quite resentful and dissatisfied when he discovers that he has been given false and misleading information.

B. Orientation and Training

1. *Orientation*

Nearly every organization, governmental or non-governmental, that sends personnel abroad to work, attempts to provide some sort of "briefing" before departure. This in itself indicates the widespread recognition of the need for pre-departure orientation. The word "briefing" reveals how regrettably little attention and time are usually given to this phase of going to work abroad—a phase with critical importance for a new overseas worker's eventual adaptations.

In most briefing, the emphasis is usually primarily placed upon necessary factual information (travel requirements, vaccinations, housing, baggage, money, and the like.) Usually descriptions of the country and the people in the new country are given, and a sketch of the organization or agency and its overseas purpose. Until the present time, the difficult human relations involved in work abroad have been neglected. Either it has been assumed that most human beings will be able to communicate and relate to their new neighbors without assistance, or else the difficulties inherent in the new relationships were underestimated. Perhaps the need for satisfactory interpersonal relationships as part of good international political, social and economic relationships, was not sufficiently understood. More likely, ignorance of the process of teaching people how to adapt to new cultures caused most briefing instructors to avoid this area of orientation and training. In any case, the absence of consideration of human relations in orientation constitutes a grave weakness in any such program.

It is unfortunate that, in preparing personnel for work abroad, orientation programs are not making more use of modern psychiatric knowledge concerning the nature of anxiety, the ways of recognizing it in oneself and in others, the ways in which it disables people, and the ways of coping with it or reducing it.

Painful or faulty communication between people abroad is due to more than the language barrier. Interpersonal difficulties, both at home and abroad, are often due to attitudes either caused by or characterized by increased anxiety which, even when unconscious, is nevertheless real and potent. The overseas employee, while in training, could receive some understanding of the nature of anxiety and how it can affect his relations and communications with others, which he could profitably apply in difficult situations abroad.

Factual information is one effective means of reducing a man's or a family's anxiety and insecurity in the new situation; therefore adequate knowledge of the host country's history, religion, economics, political and traditional culture is of basic importance. Equally important, is a man's knowledge, his expectations of himself, of the expectations that others will have of him, together with his probable ways of reacting. But the imparting of such knowledge ought not to be attempted only through lectures or reading of books and pamphlets. It would be most desirable to supplement these by giving the man an opportunity to ask questions relating to his specific areas of inadequacy and self-doubt, to get answers from people who have already worked abroad and have had foreign experience — preferably in the very area to which the new employee is going. It would be most helpful to hear how others fared and how they eventually mastered their own situation overseas.

Such opportunities before departure to learn about the personal side of the new experiences, have rarely been given. In one country the following list of pointers was prepared as a means of stimulating prospective employees to examine their attitudes, guide themselves in the overseas situation, and thereby have a more meaningful and profitable encounter with the host population:

1. Expect some hardship at first, because of the shock of coming into the new culture. You will be under some strain, and so will the people who are receiving you.

2. Learn about the people by letting them tell you about them-

selves. Although you have read something about them, you know less than you think you do. Don't be afraid to ask them questions; they will appreciate your interest. Expect that they will ask you lots of questions too. It may be uncomfortable to answer some of them.

3. Be prepared to appreciate and admire what they already are and do, as well as being prepared to give something worthwhile to them. Participate in unfamiliar customs, if you can. It is natural to be prejudiced against some of them, just as it is natural for them to be prejudiced against some of your customs. You may find your prejudices decreasing, and theirs too.

4. Expect criticism. It will come from them, just as you will find yourself being critical after a while. But take it, think about it; it may be worth something to you.

5. Try to discover how they see you, in what social position, how they expect you to behave, what it will mean to them if you do not. Try to decide how you can strike a balance for yourself between what you are used to doing and what they will expect from you. Try to find a person in the community who can help you solve conflicts of this kind; there usually is at least one. Try to put into words what puzzles you about the new community, and share your concerns with him. He may be of great help.

6. Examine your own motives towards these people. How strong is your desire to 'change' them? How would you feel if an outsider came in with the avowed purpose of 'changing' you? What bad results might you fear if 'change' were successfully brought about? Under what conditions might you accept an outsider's help? What conditions or limitations would you want to set for him? How would you want him to work along with you? You personally and your work will get on much better as long as you try to see things from the local population's point of view as well as your own.*

In line with the emphasis given throughout this report on the desirability of regarding the overseas employee, his wife and his family as a *unit*, rather than the employee alone, it is important to give complete orientation whenever possible to the man's wife, and to their children if they are able to participate. Furthermore, it is desirable that ample time, much longer than usual, be given for the absorption and digestion of this information. In the case of the technical expert who is ordinarily sent overseas for a few

* See reference 24.

weeks or months only, there is little time for such extensive orientation. When persons go abroad for long periods, however, orientation before departure might well begin four to six months in advance, with greater stress on all matters pertaining to personal adaptation and interpersonal relations.

2. *A Foreign Service Training Center?*

The need for different kinds of methods and for new knowledge has made many people hope for the establishment of some kind of over-all foreign service training center. Such a center could provide a setting for training, consultation and research. It is not the purpose of this report to define or solve the complicated problems involved in establishing and administering such a center. The obvious need for such an institution may emerge clearly from a description of what a hypothetical center could offer.

Much of the work now being done abroad, is studied by a variety of different organizations. Separate research projects are carried on under the auspices of various governmental agencies, universities, and colleges, industries, foundations, religious and other private organizations. At present there is no systematic center for integrating and coordinating the results; for research, evaluation and consultation; for conducting concerted pilot training programs and follow-up studies, for systematic supervision and correlation between preparations at home and success or failure abroad. Such a contemplated center would not, of course, duplicate or replace any existing facilities, but would provide links between them and means of coordination, which do not yet exist in this field. Preferably such a center should be accessible to all governmental, industrial, public and private personnel, including foreign personnel working in the United States. It could serve as a clearinghouse, enabling all the individuals working in this field to profit from each other's experiences, instead of, as has often happened, doing overlapping jobs and duplicating studies without knowledge of each other. It could reinforce studies being made at universities, and in turn serve as a feed-back to them, enabling them to strengthen their curricula.

By means of its coordinating functions, it could make possible more consistent policies for training and preparing personnel for going overseas, and for their management and for such remedial measures as are undertaken. It could begin to accumulate information from many different parts of the world, and make this available in a systematic way to new organizations and new persons going overseas. It could also serve as a directory of expert consultants; every agency knows from bitter experience how difficult and time-consuming it is to try to locate the special person needed for a particular situation. A staff of consultants, able to travel when they are needed, might be available for special services such as evaluation, supervision, consultation and research in overseas installations. Such a center might conceivably function not only in the service of U. S. citizens going to work abroad, but also in the service of foreigners coming to study or work or teach in the United States. It might provide them with guidance and assistance, and also make use of their services in teaching U. S. nationals better methods in international situations. It would naturally be necessary to have interprofessional cooperation, making use of today's psychiatric insights.

Such a center could perform a special service by introducing into the entire range of overseas activities, concepts bearing upon individual and social psychology. It could teach the principles of mental health, both theoretical and applied, and cover such matters of agency policy as selection, pre-departure orientation, life overseas, and the employee's return home. Indeed it could make an ideal place for the widespread introduction of mental health considerations, and also for further research into the nature and causes of poor human functioning abroad, which in turn could be useful to persons responsible for selection.

Further research could be carried out on a continuing basis about life, work, missions abroad, social problems and the solutions they require, and especially into new ways of helping people who will be going abroad develop their capacities. Such an institute or center might also help to establish a tradition of "international-mindedness"— a valuable attitude acquired in many United Nations agencies, and of long-standing in some Old World countries — but still new for many younger ones.

3. *Mental Health Measures Overseas*

In the adaptation of U. S. workers overseas, two chief factors call for consideration: first, the environment and the strains it produces; second, the personality of the individual with its inherent stresses and susceptibility to stress. Emotional difficulties with consequent loss of productivity and satisfaction result primarily from the interaction of these two factors. Remedial measures may therefore be divided for practical purposes into (a) management of environmental factors, (b) assistance to the individual in his efforts to function in his milieu, or (c) removal from the situation.

The environmental stresses previously enumerated in some detail may be summarized as separation from familiar people and routines of living, and confrontation by strange and unknown people, customs, ideals and material facilities. Some degree of anxiety and insecurity inevitably occur, with an accompanying increased need for emotional support. Administrative procedures designed to alter the environment and thereby lessen such "separation-anxiety" and "culture-shock", have usually been similar to procedures used at home in industrial and military establishments. In this category are measures like increasing "fringe-benefits", better housing and recreational facilities, more "creature comforts" and luxuries, and so on. Such procedures may diminish stress to some degree.

In the overseas situation, however, there is the complicating factor that the creation of a so-called "Little America"* may increase the psychological distance between U. S. employees and their local contacts. Such distance deprives the U. S. worker and his family of close meaningful relationships which might otherwise be formed. This in turn creates another type of isolation, with diminished satisfaction, resulting in poorer general performance. Anxiety is thus brought about. Furthermore, disparity of living standards can lead to a sense of guilt and embarrassment on the part of some U. S. workers, or resentful withdrawal by the local population; this again results in anxiety and tension. With these considerations in mind the administrator can readily see the limitations in merely improving living standards; he must not expect to solve all adjustment problems in that way. He may, in fact, be able to avoid his own frustration which would naturally follow

* The phrase "Little America" has been used to describe the circumscribed compound type of community, inside which houses and living arrangements are like those in the U.S.A. and not like those of the host country.

if his efforts to improve environmental factors actually caused greater troubles.

There are other administrative procedures which can directly decrease basic anxiety: improved efficiency in mail service, which will maintain the comforting attachment to home; the creation of easy, accepting, intra-organizational communication, thereby establishing new groups of personal relationships on a friendly basis; further development and deepening of the early "briefing" about the new area and its culture. Encouraging curiosity and facilitating learning about the new region can be quite helpful in relieving anxiety about the unknown; besides it may produce the added advantage of increased job efficiency.

Individuals in overseas situations tend to develop two main anxieties of a very specific nature: "separation-anxiety" (anxiety about *separation* from home and the familiar) and anxiety about the unknown. These are usually most acute at the time of arrival in the new area, but may be revived at any later time when work becomes unsatisfactory, when new environmental stress appears, or when valued personal relationships are disrupted. People vary in the degree to which they develop such anxiety and in their ability to function well despite its presence. These variations are usually related to the individual's previous experiences of separation, desertion, death, loss of close relationships, sudden changes to new homes, new surroundings, and new people. Some people have had little trouble in the past in shifting to new groups of playmates, leaving home for school, leaving school for jobs, changing to married life, etc.; others have made such separations and relocations with great anxiety and have needed extra emotional support. It is obvious that the needs of individuals and the remedial measures required, will vary in kind and degree.

Sometimes when anxiety is high enough to interfere with a man's functioning, it may be lessened by firm understanding and direction from his superior officer, in much the same way that a youngster's uneasiness can be relieved by a strong supportive parent. Close understanding between administrator and individual, can be extremely effective in relieving anxiety and enhancing job performance. Some individuals without previous experience of uprooting and relocation may sustain a double threat, if they develop separation-anxiety, and are then frightened because they do not know quite what has happened to them and do not realize that this is a natural and a manageable occurrence. A chance to air these feelings and to receive friendly reassurance may be all that is needed for rapid adjustment to the "normal", non-incapacitating degree of feelings of separation.

Some persons attempt to assuage anxieties in other specific ways: some try to obtain special recognition and interest from superiors and colleagues, quite unaware of why they need the preferential position. Behavior of this sort can be bewildering, irritating and troubling, not only to fellow-workers but to the person himself. Investigation often reveals that the source of the behavior is the common situation of rivalry in which children feel they must vie with each other for parental affection and recognition. Loss of security in a foreign area may easily revive this old pattern of long-forgotten, adaptive behavior. It is usually impracticable and unwise to meet the special demands which the individual makes at such times; friendly discussion of the problem may help a great deal, especially when the administrator gives adequate time for adjustment to overseas life and tries to treat all personnel with fairness and impartiality.

Another stimulus to anxiety is the loss of familiar patterns in authority relationships, both as to people and as to relative position in the hierarchy, plus the sudden necessity of facing new people and positions. It is often essential in speeding the process of adjustment, to provide further on-the-job orientation, with administrative clarification of duties, responsibilities and "chain of command". Also valuable is the availability of some higher authority for frank, non-judgmental discussion of personality clashes which occur.

The degree of help required by an individual depends too on the newness or stability of the situation. This is comparable to the military situations where it has been found valuable to provide extra emotional support for troops prior to their entering combat the first time — support which could later be reduced after troops had become seasoned. In other words, neither the workers themselves nor administrative personnel need have cause for concern over the extra personal support needed soon after arrival. After the natural, early burst of separation-anxiety and fear of the unknown have been overcome, the normal emotional patterns take over and extra help is usually no longer needed.

Although the types of anxiety and conflict mentioned above are common, they serve only as samples of the basically emotional nature of mental health problems in overseas adjustment, and do not cover the infinite range of human personality problems which occur both at home and abroad.

When separation anxiety and other emotional problems are so great, that ordinary environmental support and understanding human contacts are insufficient, it becomes necessary to seek other sources of help. Then it is desirable to have a competent psychiatrist clarify the problem for both individual and administrator, and to determine methods of treatment, to decide whether an emergency exists, whether the worker can stay on the job, should be hospitalized or returned home, etc. Unfortunately it is not always possible to have the services of a psychiatrist readily available. Relatively few psychiatrists as yet have had special training and experience with problems of public mental health or intimate experience with foreign service, that are needed abroad. Except in large cities and military installations there are usually few psychiatrists available overseas. Even in the best managed post, psychiatric emergencies arise which require prompt removal to adequate treatment facilities. It is useful to have routines thought through and established before emergencies arise, e.g. the necessary administrative steps, funds to pay for psychiatric consultations, nurses, etc. Simple procedures should be established beforehand; at the time of an actual emergency, the administrative personnel are often too involved emotionally and therefore unable to evaluate the situation properly or make sound plans. This is especially true in the case of a very disturbed psychotic patient, or one with suicidal or homicidal tendencies.

Even when a psychiatrist is available, it does not mean that his services are always asked for. He is rarely consulted on community mental health problems, to which he could make a contribution. Sometimes it is hard for persons in higher positions to bring themselves to seek psychiatric help. Therefore it has many times been found advantageous to have a specialist in internal medicine who has a good grasp of mental health and a background in psychiatry.* On the other hand, in situations where the psychiatrist is frequently consulted, the company or organization may expect too much from him, asking for recommendations and decisions beyond his competence. At times a psychiatrist employed by an organization may be faced with conflicts between his therapeutic and his administrative roles. For example, how much, if any, of what he learns about an individual should he be required to report? Where does his loyalty lie, with the patient or with the organization? The organizational psychiatrist is frequently expected to place the welfare of the community above that of any individual in it; this is not easy to do. Obviously, such situations require a high degree of tactfulness and judgment. In some organizations — e.g. the United Nations Secretariat — the newer policy is to separate the medical and administrative functions, leaving the psychiatrist free to function therapeutically.

How then can the psychiatrist's best contribution be made to the mental health of the overseas employee? Apart from the obvious service that he can render in appropriate treatment situations, (such as hospitals, private practice, and child guidançe clinics in the larger posts), it would appear that psychiatrists can be of special value when they are brought into situations for consultation, bringing to them their own special kind of awareness of human relations and mental health factors, which other responsible persons in the situation are not able to observe or to evaluate. By conferring with various people, trying to understand and interpret interactions and reactions, by helping to bring these factors into the open and facilitating constructive discussion of them, a psychiatrist may make a far more useful contribution than if he were to be placed in an administrative position. Clarification of the real human issues, identifying the processes at work and the questions that need to be asked, and indication of possible ways to resolve difficulties, can be the special contribution of the psychiatrist. It is implicit that the value of a psychiatrist's awareness and questioning may be increased when he works in combination with trained persons from other disciplines, who also observe and question in the light of their own specialties.

A special function for the psychiatrist that unfortunately has

* Reference 17.

not yet been widely used, is the care of the overseas employee who has failed at his job — who has been discharged and has returned to the United States. Such a person usually needs better understanding of the reasons why he failed, and would greatly benefit from therapy. Many such persons require emotional preparation for the return to the United States as well as for the difficulties they will encounter in trying to re-establish themselves.

Very often, especially in smaller or more isolated foreign installations, psychiatric help is unavailable, even on a travelling consultant basis. In such instances, aid of some degree may be obtained from other persons. Physicians, general practitioners and other specialists, especially when psychiatrically oriented, have been able to give much valuable help. Social workers, particularly if they have had experience in psychiatric social work, clinical psychologists, sociologists and cultural anthropologists are sources of useful ideas, suggestions and support. With increasing frequency clergymen with training in pastoral psychology have developed skill in understanding emotional problems. In larger overseas posts where a sense of community responsibility has developed, groups of people working with trained leaders have been able to work out many problems through the group process, with great benefit to the mental health of the participants.

In summary, a certain degree of separation-anxiety and fear of the unknown is a natural, expectable occurrence in persons going into overseas work. It presents an emotional problem which can cause much trouble if not understood or well handled; it can be reduced through appropriate measures and correct evaluation, and through certain environmental changes and psychological support. Invaluable in this area are non-judgmental understanding and ease of communication between all persons concerned. This does not imply coddling, but rather applying correct remedial measures in specific situations. Improvement and maintenance of sound mental health is necessary if the overseas worker is to do efficiently the job for which he was selected because of his special skills.

BIBLIOGRAPHY

1. EDUCATION AND TRAINING OF AMERICANS FOR PUBLIC SERVICE, a project submitted to the Carnegie Corporation of New York, Oct. 23, 1956, by the Maxwell Graduate School of Citizenship and Public Affairs, Syracuse University.

2. INTERNATIONAL ORGANIZATIONS, by Arthur Loveday.

3. "Performance and Adjustment of American Personnel in Overseas Missions", by Dr. Mottram Torre, read at Conference on Americans at Work Abroad, held at Syracuse University, March 7-8, 1957.

4. "Observations of Some Aspects of Performance and Adjustment of MSA and TCA American Personnel in Asia," by Dr. Mottram Torre, 1953, unpublished.

5. "Human Problems of U.S. Enterprise in Latin America", by William F. Whyte and Allan R. Holmberg, a special issue of *Human Organization*, published by the Society for Applied Anthropology, Fall, 1956, Vol. 15, No. 3.

6. AMERICANS AT WORK ABROAD, a conference on the problems of education and training for public service overseas, called by the Maxwell School of Citizenship and Public Affairs, held at Syracuse University, March 6-8, 1957.

7. WHEN PEOPLES SPEAK TO PEOPLES; AN EXPERIMENT IN INTERNATIONAL RELATIONS, by Harold E. Snyder, Director, International Affairs Seminars, Washington, D.C.

8. CULTURAL PATTERNS AND TECHNICAL CHANGE, by Margaret Mead, Published by Mentor Books. 1955.

9. SEARS, ROEBUCK DE MEXICO (First Case Study), United States Business Performance Abroad, National Planning Association, Washington, 1953.

10. WHEN AMERICANS LIVE ABROAD, prepared by Glen H. Fisher for the Foreign Service Institute, Department of State, Washington, 1955.

11. AN INTRODUCTION TO LATIN AMERICAN CULTURE, prepared by Charles Wagley, Columbia University, for the Foreign Service Institute, Department of State, 1953.

12. SO YOU ARE GOING OVERSEAS!, prepared by the Employee Relations Department, Standard Oil Company (New Jersey), 1954.

13. SO YOU'RE COMING TO BOMBAY, SO YOU'RE COMING TO SINGAPORE, and INDONESIA BOUND, pamphlets prepared for new employees of the Standard-Vacuum Oil Company.

14. RESEARCH PROJECT ON SELECTION METHODS FOR OVERSEAS EMPLOYEES, A TEST DEVELOPMENT PROGRAM, published by the U.S. Civil Service Commission Examining and Placement Division, Washington, D.C., August 1953.

15. THE DEVELOPMENT OF EXECUTIVES, by William Oncken, Jr., prepared for Office of Civilian Personnel, Department of the Army, reprinted from Pamphlet No. 8, Society for Personnel Administration, in The Federal Employee, April, 1954.

16. "Report of the Salary Review Committee", United Nations. General Assembly, 11th Session, New York, 1956.

17. CONSTRUCTIVE MENTAL HYGIENE IN THE CARIBBEAN, proceedings of the First Caribbean Conference on Mental Health, held in Aruba, Netherlands Antilles March 14-19, 1957, published by The Prins Bernhard Fund of the Netherlands Antilles, October, 1957.

18. THIRD ANNUAL MENTAL HEALTH WORKING CONFERENCE, Division of Mental Health, Virgin Islands Department of Health, April 1954.

19. FOURTH ANNUAL MENTAL HEALTH CONFERENCE, Division of Mental Health, Virgin Islands Department of Health, April 1955.

20. HEALTH AND HUMAN RELATIONS, Report of a Conference on Health and Human Relations, held at Hiddesen, Germany, August 1951, sponsored by the Josiah Macy, Jr., Foundation, New York City and the World Federation for Mental Health, published by Blakiston.

21. CULTURAL BRIEFING FOR TAIWAN, written by Arthur F. Raper, published by Foreign Operations Administration, Mutual Security Mission to China, Taiwan, 1954.

22. THE ART OF OVERSEAMANSHIP, edited by Harlan Cleveland and Gerard J. Mangone, Syracuse University Press, 1957.

23. "The Relation of Culture-goals to the Mental Health of Students Abroad", by Dallas Pratt, M.D., *International Social Science Bulletin*, Vol. VIII, No. 4.

24. A list devised by Bertram Schaffner, M.D., while Consultant in Mental Health to the Government of the Virgin Islands, 1953-1956.

25. NORTHEAST TO THE ARCTIC (DOD Pam 2-15), official Department of Defense publication for the use of personnel in the military service, 16 December 1957.

PART THREE

Forceful Indoctrination

Editor's Note. In the spring of 1955, Dr. Alan Gregg*, then Vice President of the Rockefeller Foundation, wrote in a letter addressed to the then president of GAP, Dr. Sol W. Ginsburg, "Two or three sources of experience suggest to me that there is a field of mental hygiene that needs attention. Though learning how to get along with people might be a good layman's statement of what people often turn to psychiatrists for, there is also (and perhaps more often than is commonly realized) a need in certain groups to learn how to get along *without* people.

"Military outposts such as those in Alaska and Canada make some studies of the psychiatric and psychological aspects of isolation of considerable importance. All businesses maintaining personnel in either the tropics or in places remote from travellers or easy communication furnish another group. A general manager of one of the big rubber companies told me that of his American rubber estates managers who had to be sent home for health reasons, only 15% were for such tropical diseases as malaria, amoebiasis, dysenteries, intestinal parasites (hookworm, etc.), while 85% were sent home for psychiatric reasons. . . . The misfits in the

*Much loved and widely respected medical statesman, Dr. Gregg was one of the very few persons to be designated as an Honorary Member of GAP.

U.S. Point 4 programs have become almost proverbial in point of wastage and lack of adaptation. Possibly the consular and diplomatic services have some difficulties of this sort, though not as frequently since this service can hardly send representatives to really isolated posts.

"Where the emphasis belongs at first would seem to be (1) to describe the types of strain or inefficiency or disorder that occur most often or most seriously in foreign service, and (2) what kinds of people support loneliness best—male and female—and (3) what types of relationship between the isolates and the home office do (or might) improve the proportion of misfits invalided or otherwise poorly adapted.

"I might add that when I lived abroad, and especially in Brazil, I was much impressed by the contrast between the British and the Americans in point of the ability to stand up in lonely jobs. The British were greatly our superiors. Why?"

In recognition of these problems, GAP decided to hold two symposia in 1956 on the general subject of isolation. One of these was to be primarily concerned with the subject of "brainwashing." Because of his own research experience in this area, Dr. John C. Lilly, who was at the time Chief, Section on Cortical Integration, Research Branch of the National Institute of Mental Health, was asked to assume responsibility for organizing and chairing the two symposia.

In accepting this assignment, Dr. Lilly proposed that the first symposium should consider the following: accounts of experimental work on the mental symptoms resulting from isolation from physical stimuli; isolation from other persons, controlled starvation, and controlled lack of sleep, with special emphasis on such factors as regressive phenomena and heightened suggestibility.

Dr. Lilly proposed that the second session be devoted to the more complex situations involving other persons and purposeful use of the situation by some people to coerce and control others. "It seems to me," he wrote, "that the so-called 'brainwashing' is a very complicated and variegated set of processes, and that the session ought to work up to this subject slowly. As I understand it, in the usual procedure, isolation is only one of the conditions imposed on the prisoner; rewards and punishments, starvation, interrogation, sleeplessness, and physical stress are used in varying degrees and frequency."

It was in this context that GAP sponsored the two symposia in 1956 out of which emerged the two documents that follow.

6

FACTORS USED TO INCREASE THE SUSCEPTIBILITY OF INDIVIDUALS TO FORCEFUL INDOCTRINATION: OBSERVATIONS AND EXPERIMENTS*

Dr. Ginsburg: It is now my pleasure to ask Dr. John Lilly to take over this meeting. I would like at this time to express again our very great indebtedness to him for doing such a splendid job in arranging this program.

Dr. John C. Lilly: In this program we are considering some of the basic background factors in the process of forceful indoctrination. The program for next time will be more directly involved in the psychological processes of so-called forced indoctrination, brain washing or thought reform. However, before such a program can be arranged and carried out, it was felt we should assemble the available, experimental material on some of the factors which tend to weaken personalities and make them more susceptible to such psychological processes.

Originally the program started out to be solely on isolation: we found that isolation is extremely important, especially isolation from one's own culture. However, there are other powerful factors in addition to the isolation itself. There is usually semi-starvation, some pain, usually physical illness and injury. There is restraint in many cases, if not all. There is sleep deprivation.

As is well known from published material[1], the Russians purposely use restraint, solitary confinement, semi-starvation and sleep-lack in order to break individuals' wills. When they are in a hurry, they make it a very acute process using a period of only weeks. On a longer term basis apparently these background factors are not used so extensively, especially if they have a large population to deal with. As Dr. Lifton has observed and reported, schools

*The papers and discussions that follow were presented at the meeting of GAP in April, 1956, and were first published as Symposium #3 in December, 1956.

1. STYPULKOWSKI, Z., *Invitation to Moscow,* Thames and Hudson, London, 1951.

are set up in which they have no need of most of these factors because they are not in a hurry. They have plenty of time and hence can use psychological pressures and a form of social isolation until full indoctrination is achieved.

We will start today with Dr. Jack Vernon from Princeton University, who has done some experiments in physical and social isolation over short periods of time with normal subjects.

Dr. J. A. Vernon: Thank you. The story I bring you today is another in the long list illustrating that there is nothing new under the sun. To be sure the social and physical isolation of humans is an old story. I am sure you are all familiar with the problems of "stir crazy" prisoners. We have all heard of the man who divided his candles into small pieces to serve as rationed food that he might survive his accidental confinement in an abandoned wine cellar. You probably are familiar with the account given by Koffka of a case he called "behavior in the absence of an ego".

This was the story of a mountain climber who fell into a deep crevasse and there lost consciousness. Apparently upon awakening he found himself in a very large gray, nebulous world, and was completely unable to render an ego to the situation until he discovered some discrimination in the environment. So perhaps heterogeneity of environment is a very important aspect of our everyday world.

There certainly has been enough exercise recently in terms of constructing brain models and the theoretical considerations concerning brain function to emphasize the importance of normal everyday sensory input. In a way this is all we are trying to look into, but by the obverse process; what happens when you simply shut down rather markedly on this sensory input?

We have coined a term for this process of sensory shut-down: "sensory deprivation"; a term, you will recognize, which is more convenient than accurate. It is obviously impossible to have complete sensory deprivation for you can never stop all the sensory input and retain a reporting organism. Most of you will recall in a report given at the last meeting by Dr. Lilly[2] that even in a very

2. LILLY, JOHN C., Effects of physical restraint and of reduction of ordinary levels of physical stimuli on intact, healthy persons. Illustrative strategies for research on psychopathology in mental health, Group for the Advancement of Psychiatry, *Symposium No. 2*:13-20, 44, 1956.

severe restriction there always remains kinesthetic input. Thus the term sensory deprivation is used simply to emphasize the fact that there is a very drastic reduction in the amount and the variability of the normal sensory stimulation.

Before the presentation of our data, I would like to emphasize one thing. This is a *preliminary* study, and I am going to talk very loosely about it. Whether or not these data are to be substantiated is yet to be determined. The data of the pilot study were collected from only four subjects.

The physical description of the confinement cell is as follows: It is a floating room which is light proof and sound proof. It is a room within a room, each of which has 16″ concrete walls that are separated by a 5″ air gap. The floor of the floating chamber rests on a concrete base which in turn rests on a 5″ layer of sand contained in a cement saucer. This rests on another 5″ sand bed also contained in a concrete saucer which is supported by a bed of gravel. All of this prevents ambient vibrations from entering the room and hence the room is excellently sound proofed. The room which does not touch the building has roughly an 80 db sound loss through it. In addition to the sound proofing each subject is fitted with sealed ear plugs so as to minimize sounds he may make while in the confinement cell.

The subject receives no light stimulation throughout the period of isolation. The period of confinement was 48 hours which was interrupted for testing, for toilet needs, and for an eating schedule. A safe estimate of the summed interruptions of isolation is 1½ hours out of the total 48 hours.

Each subject was introduced into the chamber with something like the following comment, which we felt was very important: "This is not a study in endurance. This is not an attempt to 'break you down'. We are simply trying to find out what happens to humans under these conditions. If at any time the confinement becomes too difficult, you are free to terminate the experiment, and we insist that you do so rather than trying to be heroic. The ante-chamber to the confinement cell will always be occupied by an experimenter." So far we have had only one subject who could not continue the study.

There is still one final restriction on the confinement subjects. Each is equipped with a pair of cardboard gauntlets which extend from just below the elbows to just beyond the finger tips. In a way this is a bogus confinement gadget, but it serves well the function of reminding the subjects to remain quiet, and also they serve as psychological confiners.

A very similar study to the present work is that conducted by Bexton, Heron, and Scott at McGill. These investigators confined subjects for various periods of time. Their subjects were placed in a semi-sound proof room containing a constant masking sound (a motor hum). The room was lighted but the subjects wore semi-translucent goggles which permitted brightness discriminations but not form discrimination.

It was found in the McGill study that with continued isolation there was a progressive intellectual deterioration which fortunately repaired after release from confinement.

It was this intellectual deterioration which suggested to us that perhaps some form of simple learning may be effected by isolation. We decided to use a simple rote memory task, a list of 12 adjectives to be learned by anticipation. We predicted that if the McGill confinement conditions produced intellectual deterioration then the Princeton confinement conditions should render learning a difficult task. The data were quite contrary to our expectations; not only did the subjects not perform worse with isolation, they improved markedly. The learning data may be illustrated by the following table:

Period	*Trials to Criteria*
Pre-confinement	20
After 24 hours of confinement	15
After 48 hours of confinement	8
24 hours after release from confinement	15
48 hours after release from confinement	22

From the above table it is clear that the improvement was confined to the isolation period and that once out of confinement the learning rate returned to normal.

In the McGill study all subjects reported some sort of hallucinatory behavior. Usually they experienced visual hallucinations, but there were also auditory hallucinations, and at least one case of kinesthetic hallucination; the subject reported a double, semi-overlapping, body image.

Not one of our four subjects reported any hallucinations. We have suggested that perhaps this difference in data is due to the difference in the confinement conditions. Perhaps the constant hum of the masking noise and the ill-defined brightness discrimination provided material from which one could generate hallucinations.

We have all played at the game of inventing songs or rhymes to the sound of railroad wheels, windshield wipers, etc., which suggests that perhaps when we come to deal with amorphous stimuli we endeavor to make them meaningful. Maybe we attempt to generate hallucinations out of such stimuli. It is also our belief that even under the Princeton confinement conditions perhaps hallucinatory behavior would occur with longer confinements.

Another vast difference that occurs between the McGill and Princeton studies lies in the area of the visual processes. Immediately upon release the McGill people reported a loss of saturation of hues and stated that the world had taken on a rather pastel array of colors. They also reported a loss in tridimensionality—the world had become somewhat bidimensional. None of our subjects reported any of the above phenomena. We have observed in some subjects an insensitivity to pain from bright lights upon release from confinement. The normally dark adapted eye of most people will receive a sudden bright light only with pain. And while there is a great deal of individual difference in this matter of "dazzle pain" it is, nevertheless, of interest that some lose their sensitivity to "dazzle pain" after 48 hours of dark adaptation.

We have found that our subjects shortly come to resent us. They adopt many forms of aggression, shortness and ill temper which they display toward the experimenter. However, the moment they are released they seem greatly relieved and no longer hostile. At the point of release we give these people a tape recorder and request that they tell us about their experiences in confinement. They usually have a great deal to tell, most of it worthless and mainly chatter. They go on and on which might suggest that they are compensating for a need to communicate. This need may be reflected in other ways. For example, I am reminded of the subject who made a very obviously abortive attempt to steal a lump of sugar from his food tray. Apparently he wished the experimenter to at least engage him in conversation long enough to say "give it back".

The protocols of our subjects were unusual in one other regard. They contained, so it seemed to us, an inordinate amount of four letter language. At the moment we do not wish to emphasize this and we are not prepared to attach any meaning to it.

Another area of human behavior which we felt should be influenced by sensory deprivation is the matter of suggestibility. We attempted to test suggestibility by the old Hull body sway technique. The data were negative but interesting. The pre- and post-confinement tests were not significantly different but in each case the subjects were more able to resist suggestion to sway after confinement than before — not an anticipated finding.

Well, these are the data of the preliminary study and further studies are now being conducted.

Moderator Lilly: Thank you, Dr. Vernon.

We have time for one or two questions of Dr. Vernon before going on to the next paper. Are there any questions?

Dr. Haun: Dr. Vernon, did you make any study of the absence of ego in darkness? I was fortunate enough to meet in New York a Dr. Chang who spent a good deal of time in Tibet. He speaks of the Yogi darkness. The conditions are slightly different. After spending a week in a cool, dark room these phenomena begin to occur. At the end of it, I am certain after 50 days of it, you would begin to find most satisfactory results. I was certain too but indicated that I did not have the 50 days available. I can give you Dr. Chang's address. You will find there is a great deal of data on the phenomenon. I wonder if the 48 hour period is just not enough time. There may be some crucial cutoff point.

Dr. Vernon: I am sure this is quite true. Probably the crucial cutoff point will vary from individual to individual. You recall the now very famous tank experiments[2] where in two or three hours similar phenomena are reported. I have the feeling that there is something important between 48 and 72 hours. Under our conditions, in fact, we have people now who generate hallucinations during 72 hours confinement but this is in the very sharply restricted situation.

Dr. Wolff: The most telling thing you said had to do with the amount of talk that was observed coming out of the confinement. You suggested that there was a good deal of profanity.

2. LILLY, *op. cit.*

Has that to do with the general content of hostility or some other meaning to this?

Dr. Vernon: I wish I could answer this. I suggest that your answer is the proper one, that probably this is an admixture of relief over getting out—emotionality accompanies that—as well as, residual hostility or aggression that they feel as the result of the confinement.

Dr. Furman: Do you want to tell us about those not remaining over 48 hours?

Dr. Vernon: One man to date has walked out on us, so to speak. We are still in the process of analyzing the man on all the follow-up data that we can get. The interesting thing here is that he quit after 11 hours of confinement and that he was the first man we have ever put in in the morning, which is a situation that Dr. Lilly used. Most of our subjects have gone in at six o'clock in the afternoon so that they have only a short period before they seem to go off and spend about 24 hours in sleep but this individual had just gotten through sleeping and was put into confinement and 11 hours later came out saying that he was afraid he was going blind and he could no longer tolerate staying in there. Apparently he had battled this decision for quite some time. He estimated four hours but his excuse, let us say, for coming out was the fear of going blind. He is the only one.

Dr. Wolff: What about time orientation?

Dr. Vernon: This is where we disappoint them all. When they come out they are just as apt to say, "It is 11 o'clock!". They are very disappointed when we don't ask them about time orientation. They have all apparently gotten hold of the Mammoth Cave studies.

Dr. Newson: I am wondering whether this is really confinement. These subjects can leave any time they want to. What is their motivation for staying in the room? Were they paid? They could obviously stop. I wonder if this does not change the conditions of the experiment very much.

Dr. Vernon: The preliminary data that I have primarily given you today involved four subjects, four *voluntary* subjects. Since this time the present studies have involved subjects who are being paid at the rate of $20 a day, a fee established by the McGill study. You are quite right in saying that there is a motivational shift. These people, by and large, can use the money and I do feel that there is probably a strong motivation for them to stay in there. However, I hasten to add that again we are not trying to break them down or anything like this.

Moderator Lilly: Since Dr. Vernon brought up the tank experiments, I want to add one note to his presentation. Apparently this production of hallucinations which excites interest in this type of experimentation is not yet well understood. As you well know, there are probably very great personal variations among the people involved which is one factor that can be controlled only by running many subjects and finding out where the variability is.

If you contrast the amount of output and the amount of input that is allowed the subjects in these three situations (McGill, Princeton, and Bethesda) you will find that the tank experiments have the lowest absolute stimulation level. The amount of confinement in the psychological sphere is minimal; the subject can leave at any time he wishes. This is not quite the same psychological confinement of Dr. Vernon's experiments. In his experiments there is an additional pressure from the observer for the subject to stick it out. Such pressures are not brought to bear in the tank experiments: the observer and the subject are co-existent; it is a perfectly voluntary situation. In addition, I suspect that if you do not allow energy discharge in the biological sphere, hallucinations will occur earlier; however, in any given person the threshold and the time course varies greatly.

We will now go in to solitary confinement with Dr. Milton Meltzer of Bethesda, who spent one and a half years as psychiatrist at Alcatraz.

Dr. Milton Meltzer: What I have to say this morning is based on my experience and observations as Chief Medical Officer at Alcatraz Federal Penitentiary during 1951 and part of 1952. At that time the institution confined about 230 federal prisoners, one half of whom were serving the equivalent of life sentences. The rest had sentences ranging down to a minimum of five years for auto theft. The inmates had come to this prison from other institutions in which they had proved to be intolerable or incorrigible. There were a few exceptions who were direct commitments because of their extreme notoriety.

The prison was organized to achieve detention and some degree of isolation. Comforts, distractions and rehabilitation programs were secondary. Maximum custody was achieved by a variety of means; isolation, armed supervision, controlled movement of the population, frequent counts during which all activity was suspended, custodial alertness and penological know-how. Discipline was enforced or implemented by combining the difficulty of escape with a reward-punishment orientation predicated on the prisoner's wish to retain his good time and earn a transfer to another institution where comforts and privileges were more abundant.

As chief and only medical officer, I supervised a United States Public Health Service staff of technicians in our daily sick call and hospital service. Psychosomatic reactions were frequent, especially those which seemed to relate to intense oral needs expressed psychophysiologically or symbolically in upper gastrointestinal complaints and cutaneous reactions. There was little hypertension but much tension headache. There was a great craving for barbiturates, narcotics or any drug which could actually or by reputation produce some kind of a "kick", which in that context meant any kind of profound physiologic reaction or alteration of consciousness.

My conclusions and impressions stem exclusively from a non-experimental, clinical observation method. Much of what I learned came about through the scrutiny of my own counter transference reactions and anxieties. I was able to observe the recurrent integrations and reactions which were evoked in the fairly stereotyped situations in prison life and prisoner-authority or prisoner-doctor relationships. Little interviewing was possible since it meant a realistic hazard to the prisoner and to myself.

Let me describe for you now the physical setting of the prison. The housing consisted of a cell house of three tiers of cells in two cell blocks facing each other. Each cell had a bunk, toilet, sink and small writing surface. There was one man in each cell. A disciplinary and segregation section was in a separate wing, had slightly larger cells but was in a single unit so that on looking out of his cell an inmate would see a high wall and out into the bay. Here were the solitary cells, regular cells behind an extra partition so that the open grill work at the end of the cell was closed off from contact with the rest of the section. A peep hole was present for observing the inmate from outside and an electric light was controlled from the outside. In several cells the toilet fixture was absent and there was only a hole in the floor connecting to a floor drain. A blanket and mattress replaced the bunk. Clothing was sometimes removed from the inmate. Diet was the regular prison fare except for the deletion of premium items and an emphasis on bland and monotonous substitutes which were calorically adequate but not particularly appetizing. The inmate knew that he would be visited and talked to at least once on each shift by a member of the medical staff and by a member of the custodial staff. With ingenuity he could holler into the toilet bowl or rap on the steel bulkheads and communicate with others in the unit. Noise would sooner or later bring the guard to see what was going on. If he had medicine to take this was brought to him. Later, he could write letters to his congressman or others, complaining of cruel and unusual punishment and often enough have his letters produce a temporary diversion while matters were investigated. Prisoners were rarely confined for periods beyond a week. It usually came about, almost by tacit agreement, that there would be an intermission for a day or two in the defiance and then he would reprovoke and go back in. An indeterminate stay was rare. The inmate knew that he could get out by capitulating or seeming to capitulate if his sojourn was in the service of forcing a change in his attitude. Often enough his stay was for a specified number of days for some infraction.

In describing the more specific effects of solitary, it must be kept in mind that a highly selective process operated. Only certain inmates found themselves in such a situation. I would estimate that two-thirds of the population rarely if ever were in the "hole". I am not certain as to what factor or factors operated in this selection process but it seems that inmates with acting out tendencies, impulsivity, great preoccupation with power and prestige operations and a more paranoidless depressive makeup were most often confined.

The motor effects ranged from occasional tense pacing, restlessness and sense of inner tension with noise making, yelling, banging and assaultiveness at one extreme, to a kind of regressed, dissociated, withdrawn, hypnoid and reverie-like state at the other. Interest seemed to be withdrawn from the usual objects in the surroundings and one would have a feeling on visiting the inmate of having roused him from a state of retreat into inner fantasy.

It appears that the sense of self, the ego and ego boundary phenomena are profoundly affected by the isolation. The body ego prototype re-emerges with an intense investment in various aches and pains, disabilities and body functions. Hypochondriacal states of a transient type are evident. One is told "when you're in that cell and have a headache, your headache fills up the whole cell".

The various aspects of regression and ego alteration or disturbance greatly perturb the custodial officers and inmates in the sense that a preconception which exists is not being fulfilled. The basic assumption is of the hypothetically normal prisoner who for disciplinary reasons is placed in seclusion with the attendant loss of comforts and distractions implicit in the isolation. He is to perceive this as punishment for his misdeeds and is to decide to alter his ways or control himself so as to avoid such a state of affairs in the future, for which he will be allowed to have the rewards of more comforts and satisfaction rather than less. All of this is, in essence, predicated upon reward-punishment having influence on hostility and unacceptable aggression. When the experience of seclusion gets used for gratification of unconscious fantasy or for the living through of unconscious infantile dependency needs the system tends to break down. The authorities had a tendency to place in solitary only those who could "take it". When others who reacted unrealistically had to be punished there was anxiety and ambiguous administrative handling, often with an effort to involve the psychiatrist so as to get around the issue. This often resulted in highly paradoxical situations. There were some inmates who were inclined to use solitary as a retreat and catalyst for a regressive experience of the mystical union type. This was the fellow who instead of being shoved into solitary, would dive into solitary in the way some people dive into bed at the end of a hard day. This was quite outside of the concept of punishment and yet it had to be achieved via the route of misdeed resulting in seclusion. There was the occasional prisoner who would openly ask to be put in solitary, especially when he felt on the verge of panic. When one observed him and saw what went on one had the sense that he had shrouded himself in some of the steel and concrete of his cell and in a few days he would "have control of himself" and be able to go back out into the population.

The dilemma of the prisoner is a difficult one. He has to achieve some kinds of satisfaction and gratification of his primitive and infantile needs, allowing himself to receive from the authorities and yet maintain his malevolent, disjunctive integration with them.

In some prisoners, this character defense of malevolent integration was relatively absent. This man was the older criminal of a previous generation—the "businessman bandit" type. He suffered more pain, had cardiovascular psychosomatic reactions, tended to have a greater struggle with depressive problems and showed historical evidence of a previous heterosexual capacity of relative durability. He had some contempt for the "young punks and hoodlums" who were making up the greater part of the more recent commitments. The staff tended to feel more sympathetic to his plight and it was easier to feel into his personality. This type was a rare exception in the group.

I would like to focus on an idea which gradually evolved as I reflected on what I saw. It has to do with the primitive psychic state of good-bad objects. The prison experience with solitary as a maximum and day to day relative deprivation and restriction as the minimum tends to cause a regression towards this state of development in people who are doubtlessly somewhat fixated there anyway. Other factors and capacities determine whether this state will be largely in fantasy or largely acted out and lived through.

The history of one prisoner may illuminate some of this. This was a middle-aged inmate who had been incarcerated for several years. Prior to his transfer to Alcatraz he had been suspected of being an informer, and his safety was in jeopardy, since the other inmates had threatened to harm him. At Alcatraz he had resumed the same kind of behavior and for a short while had sought to gain favor by informing tactics. He came to grief in this pursuit when it became apparent that his demands were intolerable, and he placed himself in a segregation cell in what was ordinarily the disciplinary unit. He remained in this unit thereafter. The behavior that was so striking had to do with his precipitating a struggle with the institutional administration over the issue of taking baths. I had noticed for several weeks that he was becoming increasingly tense and that he was making extravagant demands for all kinds of medications. Finally it came to my attention that he was refusing to bathe, claiming that a skin condition prevented this. Actually he had a mild case of ichthyosis, and consultants had provided him with suitable ointments for use after bathing. Nonetheless, he refused to take baths for about a month, and it became clear that the welfare of the other inmates demanded some change in his hygiene. The officials informed him that he had to bathe and that there was no medical reason to prevent bathing. He then insisted that if he were going to be bathed "they would have to come in and get him". Several officers came to escort him from his cell to the shower, and he used this occasion to provoke a fight. He armed himself with a homemade blackjack, a cake of soap in a sock, and when his cell door was opened he seized an officer and started to beat him. The other officers entered to quiet the disturbance, and in the resulting scuffle the inmate managed to hurt several officers, and himself received a laceration of the scalp. There followed a period of about a day during which he attempted to defeat treatment of his minor scalp laceration by tearing off bandages and so on. During this phase of disturbance his behavior was actually psychotic. The next day, however, there was a striking calmness and diminution of tension, and he began an extended course of writing detailed letters to the courts and public officials, describing how he was the victim of willful and malicious assault at the hands of the warden and medical officer and demanding and acting as if he expected to get $100,000 damages.

The episode depicts an instance of maneuvering reality to suit certain needs and of a way of relating to real and illusory persons. This instance serves to delineate some features of the super-ego of the inmate.

There is a wide range of concepts about the psychopathic super-ego. Various students have emphasized the apparent lack of super-ego. Others have emphasized the overdevelopment of super-ego. Another conception describes these people as having an impulse neurosis, in that ordinarily controlled impulses gain free access to behavior. My own impression of the super-ego in one type of criminal psychopath is derived from observation of the kind of relatedness he establishes with other persons. His reprojection of his super-ego figures gives us some idea of the kinds of experiences which brought his conscience into being. Unfortunately, our legal systems, social attitudes, and personal defenses all too often provide confirmatory evidence to the criminal that the projected super-ego figures are real, and he is deprived of the opportunity of having a corrective emotional experience. Efforts to get him to see that he provokes a large part of his difficulties collide with his short-term psychic profit he gets out of feeling persecuted.

The reduction in stimuli and suitable sources of acceptable instinctual gratification evokes a stimulus hunger and deficit which the prisoner tries to handle in various ways. He seeks "kicks", he somaticizes his needs, he symbolizes his needs, especially oral ones towards food, drugs. His capacities to tolerate ambivalence and to synthesize contradictions disappear. His interpersonal dealings reflect the good-bad dichotomy. He is all one way and you are all the other.

I would imagine that the prisoner of war in the hands of the enemy is in a state similar to the criminal in the hands of the prison officials. I had the suspicion that the rescue and reunion fantasy was pretty universal, the direction of resolution, towards fantasy or towards acting out, was influenced by previous experiences in a familial setting. A fairly frequent family history in those who act out was of the child living with an alcoholic, bad, punishing father who hated him, and hurt him without cause, and a masochistic "good" mother who rewarded, indulged and gratified him more out of her need for vicarious satisfaction than from any more realistic concept of him as a separate person.

It seems to me that the movement towards the regressed state of good-bad objects is what makes a man vulnerable to external indoctrination, especially when the experience is inflicted upon him rather than being the reciprocal role played out in reaction to him.

As deprivation of stimulus and gratification pushes him in the direction of regression, the bad parent image becomes more real—the good image rises also to fulfill the gestalt and the man is ready to perform the integration with the good or illusory good one should he present himself. This good-bad configuration is the prototype of hope, but magical, undifferentiated and oriented toward oral and narcissistic needs rather than more highly evolved ones.

Lack of resistance to this process might depend upon the paucity of intermediate resources, previous experience which would fixate the process at an operating interpersonal level with the good or illusory good one.

I saw some prisoners who, when isolated, would slip into regression with fantasy gratification with such fluidity that they couldn't be "touched" or reached for the reward-punishment bargaining. In this way they defeated the intent of the process in so far as identification with or incorporation of the good one is concerned.

In one way or another the core reaction had to do with this good-bad dichotomy. Some struggled against it, some sought it purposely in order to have the fantasy of union with the good one for a while. Some made the incorporation but in terms of the physical structure of the cell and not the persons involved. I think I saw one or two old timers whose prison history was one of violence and turmoil in the beginning who were now tractable and seemed to have changed genuinely by having taken in a part of a previously hated official. They had spent much time in the hole. They wouldn't admit what had changed them and would speak only of getting out or getting to a more comfortable place.

To summarize, the prison experience in general and solitary confinement in particular, threatens the inmate's integration by depriving him of stimuli and various sets of reaction patterns or things in the environment towards which he can orient himself and constantly redefine himself in the service of knowing who he is. As these are withdrawn he tends to regress towards an infantile ego state of split and paired good-bad objects. He may pursue this as an end in itself as a way of helping the regression to occur. He may resist it and strive to slow down the regression or arrest it at some point short of this. In this sense one sees an evolutionary spectrum of primitive integrative reactions which doubtless recapitulates that person's development.

To the degree that the basic state is achieved so is the man vulnerable to forceful indoctrination. As his picture of the bad world and bad person mounts, he shows a readiness towards finding the illusory good one and at this point he is capable of massive incorporation, introjections and identifications. In the prison this tends to be forestalled because of his sense of belonging to the prisoner group. He will tell you that he would like to do it "your way" but he has to live with them and handle their retaliation if he deserts them and you cannot provide him with anything to help him escape from that.

Moderator Lilly: We will go on now to "Sleep Deprivation" by Dr. David Tyler, University of Puerto Rico.

Dr. David Tyler: I am very pleased to be with you today and to have this opportunity to talk about a subject I am very much interested in—"The Effects of Prolonged Wakefulness". However, I have many doubts that I can contribute anything to the understanding of the mechanisms that may be involved in the phenomena called "brain washing" or forceful indoctrination. Frankly, I am not quite certain what is meant by this term. During the past few weeks, in an effort to prepare myself for this occasion, I made a search of the literature on this subject. The results were not rewarding for if there are any factual data on the subject of forceful indoctrination it is unavailable to me in the open literature or has escaped my attention. I did find a number of opinionated reports written by individuals whose qualifications as observers or interpreters of medical, psychological or social phenomena I have not been able to establish. Further, those that I did read contained few first-hand accounts or case reports set down by competent recorders but for the most part dealt with essentially uncritical third or fourth-hand reports of the actions and behaviors of vaguely described individuals.[1] Many of the papers referred to as primary sources of references, novels, motion pictures, newspaper articles or articles in magazines such as *Life*, *Newsweek*, *Colliers* or *Time*. I would not like these remarks of mine to be interpreted to mean that I hold accounts in such magazines as untrustworthy, but merely that such sources are generally not satisfactory as primary references for students seeking factual data, particularly in an area that is so emotionally charged. What facts I did gather from my literature search were the following:

a) There were a number of individuals who reported that when they were prisoners the enemy used rather vigorous tactics to obtain information of military value.[2]

b) In operations "big switch" and "little switch" (terms used to describe the exchange of prisoners in Korea) some difficulty was encountered in organizing and getting together sufficient psy-

1. DR. ROBERT J. LIFTON of the Neuropyschiatry Division of the Walter Reed Army Institute of Research, has kindly given me a copy of his paper "*Chinese Communist Thought Reform*: *'Confession' and 'Reeducation' in Penal Institution*", which is in press. This paper describes the results of his interview with 25 European and American civilians after their expulsion from Red China where they had been imprisoned from 2 to 4 years.
2. WINOKUR, G., *Germ warfare statements*: A synthesis of a method for extortion of false confessions, J. Nerv. and Ment. Dis., *122*:65, 1955.

chiatrists to make a thorough evaluation of returning prisoners.[3] This was very unfortunate.

c) Among the returning prisoners it appears there were a few —a very few—who were not sympathetic with our objectives in Korea or elsewhere. There were also some very self-interested and cowardly men.

d) Among these few there were some (from the description given) who had personalities that might be called psychopathic. But whether the psychopathic personalities were established before Korea or during their imprisonment is not clearly established from the accounts, although one report[2] claims to rule out the possibility of preservice impairment of personality in three cases.

What is very confusing, at least to me, are the stories of confessions at the famous (or infamous) Moscow trials. I know of no rational mechanism that can explain the behavior of these individuals except theater, or exhibitionism, or plain fraud and collusion.

Therefore, with these qualifying remarks I would like to discuss the effects of sleep loss. I say "qualifying"—as I should not like it to be interpreted that by this talk I am setting myself up as an authority on the effects of sleeplessness on brain washing or that I infer that certain psychological changes that occur from the result of sleep loss, such as hallucinations or delusions, have real significance on what or what may not be forcefully indoctrinated on an individual when he is subjected to such a stressful situation —or in the ease in which an individual may be convinced of another viewpoint.

We have been studying the effects of acute deprivation of sleep in human *volunteers.* I stress the word volunteers for I am certain that in this audience there are many who are only too sadly aware of the effect of motivation on performance. We made observations on some such 350 male volunteers who remained continuously awake under close supervision for periods up to 112 hours. I am quite certain if these subjects had not been volunteers the results would have been different.

---

3. LIFTON, R. J., *Home by ship.* Reaction patterns of American prisoners of war repatriated from North Korea, *Amer. J. Psychiat., 110*:732, 1954. SEGAL, H. A., Initial psychiatric findings of recently repatriated prisoners of war, *Amer. J. Psychiat., 111*:358, 1954.
2. WINOKUR, G., *Germ warfare statements*: A synthesis of a method for extortion of false confessions, J. Nerv. and Ment. Dis., *122*:65, 1955.

Under such experimental conditions (because of time limit I won't describe in detail these conditions as this has been fully described elsewhere)[4] certain changes occur. However, it appears that those that do occur are confined chiefly to the functioning of the brain and little, if any, significant biochemical, psychomotor or physiological effects are seen.

Let me give you some typical examples of our findings:

First, the biochemical: Blood sugar, adrenalin-like substances in the blood, red blood cells, hemoglobin, white blood cells, basal metabolism, body temperature, urinary nitrogen, creatinine and even the excretion of 17-ketosteroids remain unaffected by prolonged wakefulness. The excretion of 17-ketosteroids has been reported to increase with fatigue of heavy work,[5] but we found no such change during five days of sleeplessness; in fact the results show a slight but statistically insignificant decrease. This appears to me to indicate that the stress of heavy work does not produce identical effects as the stress of sleeplessness.

Second, the psychomotor: We have used a variety of psychomotor performance tests during these studies. For the most part the results reveal that a man without sleep (even after 100 hours) can perform as well, during such test situations, as a normal rested man—provided the test is not made unduly long, tedious or boresome. If it is, then we find some deterioration in performance due apparently to his inability to maintain attention which is particularly a result of momentary dozing off during the long test.

Third, the physiological: the only significant finding we noted (other than a slight increase in body sway) was in the character of the EEG. Briefly, with increasing periods of wakefulness, there

4. TYLER, D. B., *Psychological changes during experimental sleep deprivation,* Diseases of the Nervous System, *16*:2, 1955.
TYLER, D. B., The effect of amphetamine sulfate and some barbiturates on the fatigue produced by prolonged wakefulness, *Amer. J. Physiol., 150*:253, 1947.
TYLER, D. B., J. Goodman and T. Rothman, The effect of experimental insomnia on the rate of the potential changes in the brain, *Amer. J. Physiol., 149*:185, 1947.
TYLER, D. B., W. Marx and J. Goodman, The effect of prolonged wakefulness on the urinary excretion of 17-ketosteroids, *Proc. Soc. Exp. Biol. and Med., 62*:38, 1946.
GOODHILL, Victor and D. B. Tyler, Experimental insomnia and auditory acuity, *Arch. Octolaryng., 46*:221, 1947.
5. PINCUS, G. and H. J. HOAGLAND, Steroid excretion and the stress of flying, *Aviat. Med., 14*:173, 1943.

is a marked depression in the percent time occupied by the 9 and 10/sec. waves and an increase in the faster activity. This may be considered by some to be similar to the desynchronization of the electrical activity of the brain.

PSYCHOLOGICAL CHANGES

It is the findings in this area that make the study of the effects of prolonged wakefulness particularly interesting. It must be emphasized that for the most part the changes that occur are very mild and vary greatly from individual to individual and from experiment to experiment. They would be of little significance were it not for the fact that there also occurred seven cases that showed more severe reactions—persistent hallucinations and paranoid reactions that, in fact, closely resembled those found in acute schizophrenia. Were it not for these cases the mild transitory wave-like disturbances such as the increased irritability, the tendency to hallucinate, the mildly disturbed thinking, the autistic expressions that occurred in all men in varying degrees, would only be a confirmation of the very common observations of the behavior of otherwise normal men who are extremely sleepy.

For convenience, and for no other reason, we are grouping these psychological changes into three categories: (Probably it would be better if we could forget these categories and simply classify all symptoms as mental aberrations: mild, moderate and severe.)

I. *Psychoneurotic*:

Twenty-two percent of the men quit of their own accord or were dropped out for reasons that they developed colds or other minor ailments. Those that quit on their own developed vague fears: they were afraid the experiment was harming them, some felt they would not sleep properly again. Most of the individuals quit during the first 24 hours. One can be fairly certain that in the age group we used, and more so since they were Marines, all had stayed up at parties, and dances (sometimes with girls) for periods longer than they went without sleep in this study before they quit. Many of those that quit gave evidence of psychosomatic complaints, such as headache, and gastro-intestinal disturbances, but on examination little or no physical basis could be found for the ailments they described. Some were extremely irritable and quit without reporting to the observer.

II. *Schizophrenia-like reactions*:

A. *Illusions, Delusions and Hallucinations*:

Approximately 70 percent of the subjects complained of hallucinations, both auditory and visual types. With the exception of four men, all had insight. They knew they were hearing things or seeing things that did not exist. The most common hallucinations were seeing women or hearing dogs—which should not necessarily surprise one as they are common experiences. Four cases occurred where the subjects insisted that what they thought they heard or what they thought they saw actually was occurring. Since these men persisted in their belief, they were dropped from the experiment and put to sleep. Our experiences prompted us to take no chances in such circumstances.

B. *Disturbances in thinking*:

This was difficult to detect during the test situation as during this period results obtained on a wide variety of examinations indicated normal performance. Among the tests used were: the ability to complete sentences, define and associate words, interpret stories, solve elementary problems in logic and the retention and recall of figures, both forward and reverse. Three cases of repetition were noted. That is, the subjects repeated an answer given to a first question to subsequent but different questions. However, disturbances in the thought processes appeared more frequently outside of the test situation and particularly during the spontaneous conversations of the subjects during the day, at meals or at the periodic rest intervals. Very common was rambling, garrulous speech, with little indication of coherent structure or logical connections among the many ideas that were covered in a few minutes conversation. Some appeared to have some difficulty in answering very ordinary questions concerning everyday occurrences or people. Unreasonable, unrelated or silly laughter was not common. While changes in emotional response were difficult to measure and varied greatly from subject to subject, most observers agreed that the swings from euphoria to depression were more noticeable in subjects who were without sleep.

III. *Paranoid Reactions*:

In three subjects reactions occurred resembling acute schizophrenia of the paranoid type. These individuals exhibited marked delusions of grandeur (one claimed he was on a secret mission for FDR), persecution and aggressiveness (all three started unprovoked fights with the intent to do bodily harm) and hallucinations.

The three cases of paranoid-like reactions and the four subjects who were hallucinating without insight constituted the seven severe reactions that resulted in these experiments. Whether this number would have been higher if the subjects had not been volunteers or if those that quit during the first 24 hours had been made to stay on is a question that we can't answer.

It is of interest that all these psychological changes reported here: the mild, the moderate and the severe, disappeared completely after the equivalent of a night's sleep. This rapid disappearance of mental symptoms resembles the state found in the toxic type of psychosis, particularly those reactions coincident to certain illnesses or overdoses of drugs. This toxic-like character of the reactions resulting from sleeplessness suggests the possibility that some substance accumulates in the brain during prolonged wakefulness which may be the cause of the psychotic-like symptoms that are observed.

Thank you very much.

Moderator Lilly: Thank you, Dr. Tyler. Are there any questions?

Dr. Ostow: I want to ask Dr. Tyler, if he saw depression and apathy?

Dr. Tyler: Yes.

Dr. Ostow: Could they be distinguished from the rest of the syndrome?

Dr. Tyler: We saw it. I cannot tell you how accurately it was measured as this is difficult to observe objectively. Depression and apathy were not noticeable during the test situation (the test situation is the period beginning at eight o'clock at night and lasting two and one-half hours) but during the rest periods when the men were permitted to sit down for five or ten minutes under supervision. We found indications of euphoria with subsequent depression but the euphoria in experiments of this sort is a difficult thing to control and I cannot tell you how valuable our observations are in this area. One gets the impression that there are wider swings in mood in sleepless men.

Question: What was the difference between the two groups, the Marines and the conscientious objectors?

Dr. Tyler: With the conscientious objectors there were no "casualties" to speak about. Nobody dropped out. With the Marines we lost 22 percent of which more than half dropped out on their own accord.

Question: Do you have any comments on the possible usefulness of experiments of sleep deprivation as a possible screening procedure for individuals who might be selected for especially hazardous missions?

Dr. Tyler: We did use it for that. At least it was suggested. I don't know whether it worked. One of the reasons we were able to get the cooperation we got from the Marine Corps was because of the friendliness of one of the generals to that idea. We had no trouble getting any number of volunteers during the war because of this excellent cooperation.

Dr. Osmond: What adrenalin derivatives did you test for?

Dr. Tyler: Just total adrenalin-like substances in the blood. I may add that there is a difference of opinion between two of us. I looked over the data and I didn't think there were any significant differences. On the other hand, Dr. Tietz did think the differences were significant and those who know her will agree she is quite competent to judge matters of this sort.

Dr. Osmond: When was that done?

Dr. Tyler: The adrenalin-like substances, in '44.

Dr. Osmond: When techniques were different?

Dr. Tyler: That is exactly true.

Dr. Osmond: The second one, am I right in supposing that among the psychological tests you used you could find very little difference but in observational work you found there were certain differences?

Dr. Tyler: That is right.

Dr. Osmond: Our own work, using other substances suggests exactly this, that these tests are extremely disappointing. Yet, on the other hand, observation is extremely useful.

Dr. Tyler: May I point out that we were not concerned at first with the psychological changes. These became apparent as we were going along. In fact there were a large number of subjects used on experiments of this type, until one of the medical corpsmen who was permanently assigned to our group said, "You know these men act crazy?"

Dr. Osmond: The last one, what is the longest period of time over which the psychological changes persisted? Did they (the men) go immediately to sleep, require more than one sleep or an extra long sleep?

Dr. Tyler: That is a question we have not been able to answer. First, there is the motivation factor. The men got 72 hours' leave if they completed an experiment and you know what a Marine will do for a 72 hour leave. Some of them went into town right after the experiment was over. These were picked up in the streets of San Diego, sometimes asleep. Others, in fact most, on awakening in the morning would go right off on their leave. So we could not evaluate too well the amount of sleep needed for full recovery. Some reported that they required the same amount of sleep; others said it took a few nights to get over the "hangover".

Dr. Wolff: On the method of maintaining, keeping people awake, is there any comment?

Dr. Tyler: We have to keep them active, almost constantly on the move. We tried one "sedentary" experiment where the men sat around the table. We were forced to stop at about 30 hours because of lack of cooperation. You have to keep men moving to keep them awake for prolonged periods. I admire any efforts to run experiments without constant activity. In some experiments the men went on forced marches, totaling around 60-70 miles in the first 48 hours with full equipment.

Dr. Wolff: Sleep loss mixed with physical activity?

Dr. Tyler: That is true, and with muscular fatigue.

Moderator Lilly: Dr. Weinstein will probably have something to say about these matters also. I wish to call on Dr. Weinstein now to talk about "Confabulation with Brain Injury and Sleep Loss".

Dr. Edwin A. Weinstein: The data to be presented were obtained in studies of certain of the behavioral changes which follow brain injury. Such phenomena as confabulation, denial of illness (anosognosia), disorientation for place and time, reduplication for place, time, person and parts of the body and paraphasia have been shown to be not simply manifestations of specific psychological or physiological defects but rather alterations in symbolic organization or language. It is because such forms of language function as modes of adaptation to stress that the observations may be germane to the understanding of "brainwashing". While this presentation is confined to confabulation, it should be pointed out that the same principles apply to the other phenomena as well.

Confabulation may be defined as the narrating of a false version of a particular experience or event. In 100 consecutive cases of the types of brain injury to be described, confabulation occurred in 28 under conditions of routine hospital observation. It is difficult to give statistics because the method of interviewing, the social milieu as well as the type of brain injury and the nature of the disability all affect the incidence. We interviewed patients on an average of twice a week in a structured fashion, using the ordinary questions of the clinical history. We soon recognized that the hospital milieu involved stressful features apart from the patient's disability itself. In cases of head injury, there is a long waiting period often lasting many months before disposition is made. Many of the staff wonder if the patient is psychotic and his symptoms are not exclusively in the sphere of either neurosurgeon, neurologist or psychiatrist. Frequently confabulation does not develop until the patient has been in the hospital for several months and brain function has actually improved. Also patients are more apt to confabulate in formal interviews than they are in conversation with other patients. In our experience, confabulation appeared only in subjects with fairly rapidly developing brain pathology as in tumors, ruptured aneurysm and lacerating brain injuries. The tumors were deep-seated, involving particularly the diencephalon. EEG records indicated involvement of no discrete cortical area but rather showed diffuse, usually bilateral slow wave activity. It should be pointed out that these conditions of altered brain function, while apparently necessary for the enduring existence of the behavior to be described, also are present in many persons who do not confabulate.

The content of the confabulations dealt mainly with the manner in which the patient had sustained his disability. Patients injured in automobile wrecks told of having been in parachute and airplane accidents, or of having been hurt in a football game or of having been wounded in combat. A soldier who had sustained a brain injury in combat said he had been hit on the head by his wife. A soldier who had been struck in the head by a piece of exploding pipe stated that he had fallen off a truck. A patient who had fallen down a flight of stairs confabulated that he had been in a fight at a country club. A man who had sustained a sub-arachnoid hemorrhage said he had been hit on the head while "waiting for a street car". Several women confabulated that they had come to the hospital to have a baby.

Almost all of these confabulations are quite plausible. Patients who give stories of having been in parachute accidents have actually been paratroopers. The confabulation is generally related in a matter of fact, bland fashion and often escapes detection by those unfamiliar with the facts. The story is often told in a rambling circumstantial way, using many apparently irrelevant details, stereotypes and cliches.

It became evident that the confabulation, although ostensibly an account of some past event, was in some degree the representation of some contemporary problem. This relationship is exemplified in the case of a supply officer who sustained a brain injury when his jeep overturned in Korea and confabulated that he had been struck by an enemy shell. He was left with a weakness of his right hand, an inability to write and a mild dysphasia and dyslexia. After having been hospitalized for several months, he would give the following confabulation when asked about his injury, "I had a big job overseas. I was an intelligence officer. There were two men working with me, and I was sent to check on their security. They were as commy as if they had been painted with a red brush. I had to write out everything so it could be read at the court martial for those men some day. I wrote it out and turned it in to headquarters. I had enough written so any jury in its right senses would give those men 40 years without any question. Those two were riding with me the day the enemy shell came over and killed both of them." In interview after interview this account would be repeated in identical fashion. When asked what the security offense had been, he replied that "they were selling groceries at a fraction of their value to make some money". After the disappearance of the confabulation and with the presentation of the man's problems in more referential fashion, his concern with his intelligence, his ability to read and write and the matter of making a living were expressed with considerable anxiety.

The clearing up of a confabulation indicated either that a problem had been solved or that the patient was expressing it in another pattern of language. Thus while a patient might no longer confabulate as such, he might give the content in the form of a rumor or a "confession", stating in effect what was *not* true. What was significant though was the apparent need to continue to express the confabulatory material in some fashion. There is commonly a stage where the patient gives the true and false version of his accident side by side. Some patients introduce the true content in terms of the accident having happened to some one else, for example that a brother was in an automobile accident. Similarly he may displace the accident to a time in the past before he tells when and how it actually happened.

The introduction of a new confabulation about past events, or a change in the original confabulation, usually parallels the occurrence of some stressful incident. One soldier, receiving news that his wife was divorcing him, charged that an old scar had been caused by her having tried to shoot him in the back. The man who told of apprehending the "spies" stated that he had "threatened to shoot them" after his ward officer had refused him leave to visit his wife. Throughout the period of confabulation the patient, despite his disabilities and problems, is generally quite free of anxiety. Anxiety in the form of a "catastrophic reaction" appears only when confabulation ceases abruptly and is not succeeded by other alterations in language pattern. In addition to those cliches described, humor, slang, profanity, vows and threats may appear at this stage and serve a similar adaptive function. Often there is an initial euphoric state, followed by a paranoid attitude before the patient expresses realistic concern over his problems.

In about half of these cases, there is denial of illness, particularly in regard to the brain injury. In general, explicit denial of illness is not accompanied by much confabulation and the more florid confabulations occur in patients who admit the injury. Confabulation, like denial, does not appear alone though it may outlast other changes in behavior such as paraphasia, disorientation and reduplication. Just as confabulation involves a symbolic representation in terms of an event, paraphasia does so in terms of misnaming objects and the various forms of reduplication and disorientation do so in terms of misidentification of places, persons and dates.

Why do people confabulate and present their problems in such a metaphorical fashion? A study of the background of these patients indicates that only one of them could be considered an habitual liar. The others had been very conventional people with a great deal of conformity to family standards. The histories given by families stressed such qualities as goodness, obedience and devotion. In comparison with patients with other forms of adaptation following similar types of brain injury, it seemed as if the patient had formed a self-concept and felt himself most meaningfully related to people in terms of such qualities. In the confabulation the patient similarly uses those symbolic values which had constituted the most significant aspects of their experience, such as those concerning flying, country clubs, driving a truck, etc. These were the roles from which they derived the most prestige and in the fulfillment of which they had felt themselves most significantly related in their environment.

Confabulation is thus a means whereby the patient overcomes isolation and identifies himself with the most meaningful and powerful aspects of his environment. By this he seems to avoid nothingness and to establish a feeling of existing or "reality". This may seem paradoxical in that the confabulation is actually a distortion of reality but the *feeling* of truth or reality may be more closely related to the degree of identification in a culture than to any more logical cognitive process. Following certain types of brain injury the patient seems to be in a state of social isolation or anomy. Many of the alterations in behavior are to be interpreted not as an escape from "reality" but as an attempt to attain it.

DISCUSSION OF DR. TYLER'S PAPER

We were greatly stimulated by Dr. Tyler's work and ran a similar experiment on 26 subjects at the Walter Reed Army Institute of Research. The subjects were studied in groups of five or six, a man serving as a control one week and being sleep deprived for the following week, during which period the various test procedures were repeated.

We found much less disturbance in behavior than was recorded by Dr. Tyler. What changes did occur were mild and transitory and in any group were reported by only one or two men. Several, after the first 24 hours without sleep, described a disorientation for time of day in which they felt that it should be much later than it actually was. Perceptual distortions were also described. One man, looking at a row of circles during a test, saw them as doughnuts. Others saw distortions of the dimensions of the room. One man had the feeling that he was sitting behind himself. In all of these instances the subject was quite aware of the distortion.

The degree to which the overt signs of sleepiness were manifested was very variable. Some men appeared profoundly drowsy after 24 hours, while others at 90 hours seemed only slightly sleepy. Yawning was only rarely seen. Many of the subjects seemed more anxious and irritable after they had awakened from post-deprivation sleep than they had been during deprivation itself. There were somatic complaints, expressions of concern about the subject's family and whether deprivation might have been harmful. During deprivation on the whole, patients did well on psychological tests. Errors occurred mainly in tasks involving prolonged visual and auditory attention.

The subjects were conscientious objectors, members of a religious sect. They were highly motivated and had a strong group organization. Thus they would help to keep one another awake with emphasis on "beating the record". I mention this to stress the point that one cannot consider the effects of physical stress apart from the social milieu.

Moderator Lilly: We will go on with Dr. Joseph Brozek from the University of Minnesota, who will talk on semistarvation.

Dr. Josef Brozek: This conference is concerned with the effect of various kinds of stresses and deprivations on personality and behavior, with special reference to the process of forceful indoctrination. I wish to make it clear at the outset that our presentation, confined to experimental work on semistarvation carried out in the Laboratory of Physiological Hygiene, can be of only limited value in clarifying the basic psychological processes or in quantifying some of the parameters of what has been termed "brainwashing".

The intensity of the stress, judged from the loss of weight per unit of time, is one parameter about which we would like to know more than we do at present. As things stand now, we are not able to predict with desirable precision what would be the results — psychological or physiological — of losing a quarter of one's weight in, say, six weeks rather than six months.

Our ability to estimate effects of *combined* physical stresses is also very limited. In some situations the interaction between the stress factors may yield surprising results and may *facilitate* rather than impair the chance of adjustment and survival. Let me illustrate this in reference to sweat losses in a combined water (900 cc. per day) and calorie restriction (1,000 Cal. from carbohydrate per day) in the presence of moderately severe physical work (daily total expenditure of about 3,000 Cal.). The sweat rates, determined as the weight loss during a one-hour walk on a motor-driven treadmill, were highly predictable, practically constant during the control period. During the experimental period there was a marked decrease in the sweat rates which were reduced, on the average to about 50 per cent of the control value on the sixth day. Substantial water conservation was achieved also by a reduction in the insensible water loss. Rehydration, with continued caloric restriction, resulted in an increase of the sweat rates but by the 10th day the sweat losses reached only 70 per cent of the control level. The sweat rates increased markedly and promptly as soon as food restriction was lifted. The values returned to the pre-restriction levels within a week. Clearly, food restriction, affecting importantly the sweating, would be beneficial rather than a detrimental factor in situations where water deficiency was present (1).

There are several other limitations concerning specifically the psychological impact of prolonged caloric restriction. Firstly, and perhaps most importantly, we have always used volunteers as subjects. This is crucial to the perception of situations as threatening or non-threatening, to the arousal of conflicts and frustrations, to the very definition of "deprivation".

Secondly, the men were treated firmly but with respect. They

1. H. L. TAYLOR et al., Water exchange in man in the presence of a restricted water intake and a low calorie carbohydrate diet, *Fed. Proc.*, *15*:185, 1956.

were made to feel, as strongly and as clearly as possible, that the study in which they participated was a cooperative enterprise. They had the role of a partner in an important scientific pursuit and they were given to know it.

Thirdly, we were concerned primarily with the physiological—psychophysiological, if you wish — effects of a variety of stresses that we investigated, whether this was total or partial starvation (semistarvation), high environmental temperature, or restriction of the water intake, excessive physical work, experimentally induced malaria or lack of sleep. The principal criterion of "fitness" was the subject's performance. As performance represents a product of capacity and motivation, concerted effort was made to maintain morale high, in spite of the developing signs of physical incapacity. Only under these conditions could actual performance (especially all facets of "psychomotor" performance — strength, speed, coordination, endurance) be interpreted as a measure of performance capacity. We were interested in "somatopsychics" (to reverse the order in which these terms are usually put together), specifically in the impact of dietary restrictions and the resulting somatic alterations in behavior. Other environmental stresses, physical and social, were minimized or eliminated.

A part and parcel of the conscious effort on the part of the experimenters to maintain high morale was the provision of adequate sleeping quarters — not very fancy or airconditioned, but livable, clean, with adequate toilet facilities and plenty of soap and hot water. There were reasonably adequate recreation facilities. Positive newspaper and magazine publicity, visits of individuals ranking high in pacifist circles, and contacts with local churches were all important as morale builders.

One feature of the experiment that made it definitely easier to withstand the stress of semistarvation was the fixed schedule. The duration of the individual periods of the experiment — control, restriction, refeeding — was largely determined in advance and was strictly adhered to. No developments took place that would necessitate shortening of the experimental period. The subjects knew that in no case would they be required to starve for more than six months. The presence of a definite "end point" was a factor to which they clung when the going got tough. The thought "Well — it's only 13 weeks to go" was a definite morale booster. By contrast, the very uncertainty about everything, including the length of stay, would constitute a severe stress in the prison or concentration camp situations.

In the personality area we have used a variety of techniques, from standardized complaint inventories to Rorschach ink-blots and sociometric analysis. The focus was descriptive, rather than dynamic and interpretative. The problems of psychopathogenesis presented themselves in spite of, not because of the goals and design of the experiment.

There are 3 things I should like to do:

1) To present the general features of the study and the average changes in the major physiological and psychological variables;

2) To describe the different types of reaction patterns noted in the subjects during maintenance on the severely reduced food intake; and

3) To discuss a small number of individuals with more frankly psychopathologic responses.

This is, clearly, too heavy a menu for 20 minutes. As a workable alternative, I propose to go very briefly over the psychometric picture, point out the increasing docility of the subjects during semistarvation, and indicate the types of the more severe behavioral deviations in a few subjects who had great difficulty or were unable to adhere to the dietary regimen. The details may be found in the literature (2; cf. also 3 to 7).

Design of the Experiment

PSYCHOMETRIC DATA

Thirty-six young men, free of physical or mental disease, served as volunteer subjects. Following 12 weeks of the control period with an average intake of about 3,500 Cal., the food intake was abruptly

2. ANCEL KEYS, J. Brozek, A. Henschel, O. Mickelsen, and H. L. Taylor, *The Biology of Human Starvation*, Minneapolis, University of Minnesota Press, 1950.
3. JOSEF BROZEK, Semistarvation and nutritional rehabilitation: A qualitative case study, *J. Clin. Nutrition, 1*:107-118, 1953.
4. JOSEF BROZEK, Starvation and nutritional rehabilitation: A quantitative case study, *J. Amer. Dietetic Assoc., 28*:917-926, 1952.
5. NANCY K. KJENAAS and Josef Brozek, Personality in experimental semistarvation: a Rorschach study, *Psychosomatic Medicine, 14*:115-128, 1952.
6. JOSEF BROZEK, Harold Guetzkow, and Marcella Vig Baldwin, A quantitative study of perception and association in experimental semistarvation, *J. Personality, 19*:245-264, 1951.
7. JOSEF BROZEK, Psychology of human starvation and nutritional rehabilitation, *The Scientific Monthly, 70*:270-274, 1950.

decreased to less than half this value, with a 24-week average of 1,570 Cal. In the 32 men about whose adherence to the diet there was no question, body weight dropped from 69.4 kg. to 52.6 kg. (Δ=16.8 kg., 24% of the control value). Time of runs to exhaustion on the treadmill decreased from 242 sec. to 50 sec. (Δ=192 sec., 79% of the control value). Speed of hand and arm movements decreased minimally. There was a larger deterioration in the precision of coordinated movements and a substantial loss in strength. In brief tests of intellective functions no change was noted. In complex prolonged tests of intelligence the changes in the total score were consistent, and, consequently, statistically significant. Biologically, in terms of the importance of the impairment, the changes were negligible.

Self ratings stressed apathy and irritability, moodiness and depression, decreased ambition and mental adequacy. Sex and activity drive decreased while concern with food grew throughout the semistarvation period. In the Minnesota Multiphasic Personality Inventory there was a characteristic elevation on the scales of the "psychoneurotic triad" — Hypochondriasis, Depression, and Hysteria. In rehabilitation, which is of no concern to us in this context, the mean scores returned to the pre-starvation levels.

COMMON REACTION PATTERNS OF SEMISTARVATION

The subjects' changes in outward behavior, their reduced energy output, eating habits, subjective symptoms, emotions and attitudes were described in detail elsewhere (8).

For the purposes of this conference, perhaps the most relevant phenomenon was a distinct trend from a critical appraisal of events during the control period and an emphasis on sharing with the staff in the making of decisions affecting the group, to a definite *docility* as the semistarvation progressed in time and in the magnitude of its impact on the organism. I believe that this was not simply another manifestation of the overall apathy. During the starvation phase, the men were quite willing to trust the judgment of the staff of the Laboratory. In the rehabilitation period this confidence and ready reliance on authority definitely decreased. In fact, the men elected a committee to represent their voice in making decisions on various matters concerning their welfare.

8. JOSEPH C. FRANKLIN, Burtrum C. Schiele, Josef Brozek and Ancel Keys, Observations on human behavior in experimental semistarvation and rehabilitation, *J. Clin. Psych.*, *4*:28-45, 1948.

SEVERE PERSONALITY DISTURBANCES

All subjects exhibited, to a varying degree, symptoms of what was labelled "semistarvation neurosis". In a few men the neuropsychiatric disturbances were more severe. In four of the subjects a character neurosis was manifested in their inability to adhere rigorously and consistently to the dietary regimen. It should be noted that, legally, the subjects were free to quit but the moral and social pressures against such an action were strong. In no case were the subjects able, psychologically, simply to quit. One of the four men developed a reaction pattern bordering on psychosis and had to be briefly hospitalized. When the disturbance was relieved, he was released from the experiment. In one subject a psychogenic accident served as means for solving the intense conflict between the impulse to leave and the desire to carry out the original moral commitment.

Perhaps the very fact that such personality disturbances did develop under conditions of uncomplicated semistarvation is more important for our considerations than the details of symptomatology and etiology (cf. 9). At the same time, I believe that we do not deal here with personality alterations resulting from profound physiological changes. The stress probably simply revealed weaknesses present in the pre-starvation period, just as physical exercise brings out electrocardiographic evidence of coronary insufficiency, not manifest in the electrocardiogram of the resting patient.

To some, such a simile may appear tenuous, even questionable. Nevertheless, it is probably useful to differentiate between the reaction patterns that are common to a group of starving individuals and thus, in a real sense, "normal", and those reactions that deviate substantially from this norm.

SUMMARY AND CONCLUSIONS

Thirty-six men, recruited from Civilian Public Service Camps for conscientious objectors, volunteered for an experiment on semistarvation and nutritional rehabilitation. On the average, the men lost one-fourth of their body weight within six months and exhibited profound changes in body composition and physical fitness. In the overwhelming majority of cases they adhered rigor-

9. BURTRUM C. SCHIELE and Josef Brozek, "Experimental Neurosis" resulting from semistarvation in man, *Psychosomatic Medicine, 10*:31-50, 1948.

ously to the dietary regimen. Depression and apathy, curiously interlaced with irritability, rather than intense frustration constituted the characteristic mood. In contrast to the control period and, in particular, to the period of nutritional rehabilitation, in semistarvation the group was easy to manage. Such a docility would favor submission to forceful indoctrination.

One subject developed personality disturbance bordering on psychosis and was removed after a brief hospitalization, from the experiment. Three other men were unable to adhere consistently to the rigorous dietary regimen. One subject, in spite of a psychogenic accident, completed successfully the experiment.

A situation in which food would be offered on certain occasions and would be withdrawn on other occasions would constitute a more intensive psychological stress than food restriction alone. It would result in severe frustration, and would more readily break a man's moral fiber. By combining such a treatment with other forms of deprivation and insult, one could expect eventually to induce a "breakdown" in the majority of adult human beings.

The ethical and legal judgment concerning the responsibility of an individual for his actions under conditions of prolonged, systematic, severe maltreatment appears to lack, at present, a valid scientific basis. We do not have adequate information concerning the critical levels of the parameters (duration, severity, combination of stresses) of the "softening" process, basic to forceful indoctrination. Specifically, the *amount* of weight loss alone is not an adequate criterion of the magnitude and the biological impact of the stress of semistarvation.

Moderator Lilly: We have time for one or two questions.

Dr. Hamburger: I would like to ask Dr. Brozek if he made any attempt to study the dreams of his experimental subjects and if so, would he comment on particular dreams concerned with food and eating?

Dr. Brozek: I am glad that you brought up this question. The results are confusing. We obtained the evidence in two or three different ways. The men kept diaries and in these diaries they quite frequently spoke of food dreams. They reported such experiences in their interviews. However, in addition to this information, at definite periods during the experiment, at times unannounced to the subjects, we asked them systematically, "What did you dream about?" When we used this systematic sample we did not get the kind of differences that you would expect. These are the facts. How you will interpret them I am not quite sure.

Dr. Osmond: There is one point I am not clear on, Sir. The diet is roughly a thousand calories?

Dr. Brozek: 1600.

Dr. Osmond: Vitamins?

Dr. Brozek: Adequate.

Dr. Osmond: Minerals? Was any work done particularly about vitamins being deliberately reduced?

Dr. Brozek: Yes. We have done extensive work in this field but not in combination with caloric restriction. Actually, with developing thiamine deficiency you do have a loss of appetite and finally vomiting so that you come really to a combination of vitamin and caloric deficiency, but not by design.

Dr. Osmond: Did you do any work on niacin deficiency?

Dr. Brozek: No. On thiamine and riboflavin. Most of the work was concerned with thiamine. There the changes were quite marked and pronounced changes would be obtained within a period of 10 to 14 days.

Moderator Lilly: We will go on now with Dr. Wolff on the effects of noxious stimuli in man.

Dr. Wolff: Among the host of effects of noxious stimulation in man is the experience of the sensation of pain. Pain sensation is not essential to a good adjustment, for man is quite capable of making all the basic and many of the complicated adjustments that his life calls for in the absence of pain sensation. This has been demonstrated by carefully studied individuals who have been without pain sensation since birth, and by those who have had pain sensation surgically eliminated. Secondly, pain is a very poor indicator of the degree of damage that a man has sustained, and the intensity or amount of pain is no indicator at all as to whether he will survive a given tissue damaging experience. All of the afferent impulses involved in pain sensation enter through the dorsal roots and ascend the spinothalamic columns or ventrolateral portions of the cord. As yet no one has been able to elicit or evoke the experience of pain by stimulation of the cerebral cortex.

Pain as a sensation can be studied by methods which permit both qualitative and quantitative generalizations. One method consists of measuring the pain threshold by means of thermal radiation from a 1000 watt electric bulb focused on the blackened skin of the subject to be examined. The intensity of radiation just evoking a report of pain at the end of a 3 second exposure is taken as the pain threshold and is expressed in millicalories/cm^2/second. Using this method for measuring pain threshold in many hundreds of people, it became apparent that, by and large, mankind has a pain threshold which is about the same, say plus or minus 16 per cent, from person to person, and in the same person from time to time. Man, woman or child feels pain with about the same amount of thermal radiation regardless of color, race, or political persuasion.

Also, there are a limited number of discernible steps in pain sensation from a threshold to a point beyond which discriminations of more intensity cannot be made. There are approximately 20 such steps indicating that the neural apparatus involved in pain sensation affords a crude kind of perception apparatus. It has been possible to build a pain scale in terms of the intensity of stimulation and the intensity of experience of pain. The pain unit has been defined as two of these discriminable steps, and called a dol.

On the other hand, let us consider the reaction threshold. Individuals vary enormously in how they react to sensations of pain. Although the pain threshold for a given individual on different occasions will remain quite uniform, his reaction threshold or responses to the experience of threshold pain, let us say, in terms of a sweat reaction of the skin (so called psychogalvanic response) varies from day to day, from hour to hour and from moment to moment according to the meaning of pain at the moment and based on his previous experience. This enormous variation in reaction threshold, in the same individual, and from individual to individual explains the confusion about apparent differences in the amount of pain that can be tolerated.

Wherever pain has been perceived it is likely that there is tissue damage, be it ever so slight and reversible. If the skin temperature is varied by one means or another, the amount of energy required to evoke the sensation of pain on the skin will be that which will raise the skin temperature to about 44°C to 45°C. It has been shown that at this temperature certain protein inactivation or breakdown occurs, perhaps with the liberation of polypeptides or other breakdown products. It is suggested that pain sensation may be evoked by some of these agents, accumulating at a given rate.

When tissue is damaged the pain threshold is lowered. Let us take a person who has had a sunburn: the pain threshold in the erythematous skin is very much reduced and a stimulus intensity which is barely threshold for the average intact individual causes the sunburned person to have a moderately severe pain. With the pain threshold so much lowered and a threshold stimulus able to induce a high intensity of pain, indeed anyone who has had a sunburn realizes what a friendly clap on the shoulder means in the way of pain.

Another device which has been used to measure pain threshold pulls upon a hair in the skin. A hair of the skin is attached to a thread and a rubber band with an indicator running along a scale. When the pull of the hair just begins to hurt one makes a reading on the scale. Again, this pain threshold varies but little from person to person.

The pain threshold was sharply reduced in an area of erythema around an injured site in the flare area described by Lewis as part of the triple response to injury. Also, wherever vasodilatation occurred and especially during the process of vasodilatation, there was a lowered threshold. Such an area with lowered pain threshold may be said to have become more vulnerable to other noxious forces.

A third way of measuring pain threshold in sub-surface structures, consists of a simple spring arrangement for pressing against bony surfaces, such as the forehead or the top of the head or the tibia, and measuring the amount of pressure necessary when the subject first reports pain. This method of measuring deep pain thresholds has been useful in studying vascular headaches, including those of the migraine type. A person, for example, who has a migraine headache has a low threshold as compared to the threshold at headache-free periods. Therefore, the hypothesis can be advanced that a "pain substance" or "headache substance" is present when tissues are damaged, temporarily, as during a migraine state. Such local tenderness, regardless of how induced, is called primary hyperalgesia.

Thus, primary hyperalgesia occurs in damaged or injured tissue and is followed by a lowered pain threshold and increased pain sensibility and probably results from a local elaboration or accumulation of agents which excite terminal nerve endings subserving pain sensation. To be distinguished from primary hyperalgesia, is secondary hyperalgesia, this occurring in undamaged tissue and not associated with a lowered pain threshold. However, there may be increased pain sensibility due to an alteration in the central excitatory state so that impulses that enter the nervous system at the usual threshold are perceived as more painful. Such an augmented central excitatory state may arise from and be continued by a site of noxious stimulation adjacent to or remote from the area of noxious stimulation. Thus, noxious stimulation of a small site which may not be perceived as painful can cause a buildup and spread of a central excitatory state which may affect the pain sensibility (not the pain threshold) of adjacent or distant areas.

This was demonstrated experimentally in an individual who had tissue injured locally in the subsurface structures of his back by the injection of hypertonic salt solution, an injury which was completely reversible. As part of the reaction there developed an area of secondary hyperalgesia of the skin, in which pain threshold as measured by thermal radiation remained unchanged from that of the opposite control side of the back, but in which a stimulus of the same intensity as on the control side now evoked a much more intense pain. Therefore the bombardment of afferent impulses arising from a damaged site may so alter the central state of excitation as to alter perception from widely scattered tissue. On the other hand, a central inhibitory as well as a central excitatory state can be demonstrated. For example, take an individual with a damaged hemisphere. If we stimulate first one leg and then the other with a thermal stimulus it is apparent that it takes a greater intensity of stimulus to induce pain on the affected side than on the intact side. If we stimulate both legs simultaneously, then the stimulus intensity necessary to elicit pain on the affected side is greatly increased. Indeed not only is the pain threshold of the affected side raised by noxious stimulation of the opposite side, but the stimulus intensity necessary for motor response to occur is also increased. There is thus a central inhibitory as well as a central excitatory state relevant to pain sensation.

A step further can be taken by asking the question what is the effect of suggestion upon pain perception and upon reactions to noxious stimulation? There can be noxious stimulation without pain and noxious stimulation with pain; also pain as a sensation is to be distinguished from the adaptive, protective reactions that occur with it. Thus, when the left arm of a laboratory subject was struck with a ferrule, there occurred a lowering of capillary tone, not only in the part thus noxiously stimulated and the site of pain, but also in the other arm as well; gradually the capillary tone returned toward the initial control level. Now, without warning, a "sham blow" was introduced in the direction of the left forearm, and the left capillary tone was lowered as it was when the tissue was actually damaged. Subsequently, when a "sham blow" was expected and understood by the subject to be forthcoming, there was no capillary response.

Another experiment carries us a step further in the exploration of the effects of suggestion. The two arms of a subject were immersed in warm water at 37°C. In one set of experiments there was no suggestion made, and the subject experienced the usual warmth of the water. In the next series of trials, it was suggested that one arm would be anesthetic. It was then suggested that the water (still 37°C) in which the arms were immersed, first one and then the other, would "scald the skin" of the arm not suggested as anesthetic. During the latter experiment the individual suffered pain, showed many outward signs of discomfort with flushing and sweating of the face. The skin of the arm supposedly injured became red, and after the skin was dried the pain threshold was found to be lowered. A noxious thermal stimulation of known intensity was applied in comparable spots on both arms. In the arms in which anesthesia had been suggested there was relatively little damage noted during the subsequent days as a result of the burn as compared to the damage in the arm that had been previously suggested as being scalded when immersed in the water at 37°C. It was thus apparent that the attitude or feeling or the individual's concern or conception of the sensation that he was to feel not only played a part in the intensity of the pain experience but also in the intensity of his tissue reaction and in the vulnerability of this tissue to further assault.

In another series of experiments it was demonstrated that an individual who is highly motivated can withstand a good deal of pain, and indeed, while experiencing such pain can perform well on tasks requiring considerable mental effort. Three subjects were used; one woman, who was experienced with high intensity pain during experiments from time to time for many years, and two men less experienced in such pain. The experiment consisted of putting a tight blood pressure cuff around the upper arm, raising the pressure to 230 mm. of mercury and holding the cuff in place at this pressure for a half hour. During this period the subjects repeatedly opened and closed their fists. Within a few minutes they were experiencing a moderate to a high intensity pain and complained bitterly. At this time mentation tests, consisting of learning procedures (digit symbol), mental arithmetic tests, and block design tests were given. In the woman long experienced in pain relatively little change in mentation was seen even when the experiment was repeated after sleep loss of 24 hours. In the two less experienced men the mentation tests were performed well during the pain. They performed the tests slightly less well when pain was experienced during excessive fatigue and following sleep loss.

Another body of information which I am not going to detail at this time because it is not relevant to this discussion concerns the outcome of an opportunity to interview a number of people who were exposed to the duress of prison circumstances and who were exposed to what was called indoctrination procedures. Pain was one of the factors in their experience but the pain played a more indirect role. The pain along with other experiences was instrumental in altering the attitudes of these individuals when it succeeded in convincing them of their isolation and the hostile attitude of their captors and sometimes other prisoners. Such individuals felt humiliated, degraded, cut off or despised. They ultimately became disorganized by the asocial, unfriendly and unsympathetic attitude of their jailers, which was coupled with their isolation, pain and other bodily discomfort. These individuals then became especially susceptible to the contact of a friendly person who might approach them. The pain then in a sense had become one of the several ways of humiliating and disorganizing the individual so that he became dependent or especially related himself to any other human being who would approach him in a friendly way. This injured subject was then more readily manipulated by the latter who could often make him accept or rationalize views which formerly were unacceptable. By threatening to withdraw his support or by assuming an unfriendly attitude he could usually bring the subject to heel. In other words, the experience of pain was only one of the means of so altering the individual as to make him dependent upon the friendly approach of another human being, whose friendly approach could then be exploited to change attitudes and value systems.

In summary, the human subject can be affected by afferent impulses from noxious stimulation which do not give rise to sensations of pain. There are a host of skeletal, vasomotor, gastrointestinal and neurohumoral changes which occur independently of sensation. Then there is a second category of effects which are linked with pain sensation which has its dimensions, as do other sensations. These dimensions have to do with site, quality, intensity, and temporal aspects, all highly definable. The pain experience is modified by a number of factors; i.e. concurrent other sensations, giving it special quality (distension in the gut or tightness in the head or rhythmic movement in the case of intestinal activity). A vastly more important category has to do with feeling, mood, attitude, bodily behavior, and adaptive reactions to pain sensation in which cultural factors are pertinent. We know all painful stimuli are not avoided. Many people enjoy pepper, snuff, needle baths, and similar experiences. We find that analgesics modify attitudes perhaps more than they do the pain threshold. Also, damaging the brain affects the significance of pain. We also have reason to believe that the painful experience is one that has a highly symbolic significance and is closely linked with feelings of isolation and rejection, especially when imposed by other human beings under hostile circumstances.

These elaborate reactions are implicated in the effects of noxious stimulation in man and involve far more than sensation of pain per se.

7

METHODS OF FORCEFUL INDOCTRINATION: OBSERVATIONS AND INTERVIEWS*

Dr. Ginsburg: I would like now to turn the meeting over to John Lilly.

Dr. John C. Lilly: Last April we began this symposium, and we hope to conclude it today. The first half of this subject[1] last April considered that which is known about certain physical factors in weakening personalities, with special reference to increasing the susceptibility to forced indoctrination. We talked about the lack of sleep, starvation, pain, brain injury, and isolation.

This morning we are considering the psychological processes of thought reform and indoctrination with force, or "brainwashing", or whatever you wish to call these processes. The term "brainwashing" has come apparently to have a meaning created by the national press. In this meaning the term is more or less defined by an indoctrinator in the following quotation; the indoctrinator is talking to his victim: "We make the brain perfect before we blow it up. No one whom we bring to this place ever stands out against us. Everyone is washed clean. There is nothing left in them except sorrow for what they have done and love of the party. It is touching to see how they love the party. They beg to be shot quickly so that they can die while their minds are still clean."[2]

Apparently this is one source for this term "brainwashing" and its definition. George Orwell not only wrote a great novel, *Nineteen Eighty-Four*, but he wrote a disturbing handbook for brainwashers which convinced his readers of the reality of an extreme form of forcible indoctrination. Orwell's victim, Winston Smith, was subjected to social isolation, solitary confinement, starvation, lack of sleep, physical beatings, personal betrayal, personal humilia-

---

***The papers and discussions that follow were presented at the meeting of GAP in November, 1956, and were first published as Symposium #4 in July, 1957.**

1. Factors Used to Increase the Susceptibility of Individuals to Forceful Indoctrination: Observations and Experiments. *Symposium No. 3*, Group for the advancement of Psychiatry, December, 1956 (Chapter 6 in this volume).
2. ORWELL, GEORGE. *Nineteen Eighty-Four*. Harcourt, Brace and Co., New York, N.Y. 1949.

tion, treatments with drugs, torture and direct electrical stimulation to his brain. He was told and shown that he was completely powerless, that any possible rescuers were probably fictitious, that the party could and would control his thoughts, and finally that he would love no one and nothing but the party. Apparently Orwell did such a convincing job on his readers that any types of involuntary indoctrination are thought popularly to correspond to Orwell's single definite process scientifically applied by men trained to a fine point, all of whom are as fanatical as O'Brien was in *Nineteen Eighty-Four*.

I spent this time on this fantasy because today we are asking the speakers and their officially appointed discussant to clarify the differences between the fantastic account of Orwell and the real processes actually used in authentic cases.

Our first speaker is Dr. Robert J. Lifton, a Research Associate at Harvard Medical School in the Department of Psychiatry of the Massachusetts General Hospital who will talk under the title of "Psychiatric Aspects of Chinese Communist Thought Reform".

Dr. Robert J. Lifton: I am very glad that Dr. Lilly pointed up some of the misunderstanding about the term "brainwashing". I am going to mention it right now at the very beginning primarily to dismiss it. For our purposes it no longer means anything specific, particularly in view of the manner in which it has been used in this country.

I think it is very significant that among all of the people I interviewed in Korea and in Hong Kong, no one who had been through the experience ever used the term "brainwashing", unless he had first heard it from a Western source. But in searching for a term, or trying to label this process, one runs into a little difficulty.

I remember one suggestion that came to me which may for some people shed some light on the subject. A friend of ours in Hong Kong, a member of the British Diplomatic Service, felt there was too much concern on the part of Americans about "brainwashing", and he particularly deplored the name. He suggested, "Why not simply call the whole thing a 'mental douche'?" But I am not too sure that this would serve as a very scientific name.

But despite much confusion in terminology, the process of *szu-hsiang kai-tsao* — translated as "ideological remolding", "ideological reform", or "thought reform" — is very much a reality. Where applied to Westerners, to either prisoners of war or to incarcerated civilians, many of its methods have been written about popularly, and have to a certain extent, been subjected to psychiatric and psychological investigation. But the process applied to the Chinese themselves, and particularly to Chinese intellectuals, has been very little studied.

For this reason, and also in keeping with GAP's policy of trying to present a certain amount of unpublished research[1], I am going to talk about the most intensive of the "thought reform" programs for Chinese intellectuals as conducted in special institutions known as "revolutionary colleges". These were set up all over China immediately after the Communist takeover.

I wish first to emphasize that thought reform has been applied, in varying degrees of intensity, not only in the special centers I will describe, but also in universities, labor, business and government groups, even among peasants—and in fact throughout the immense population of China. This is in itself a rather amazing accomplishment.

I had the opportunity to study this process in Hong Kong over a period of 17 months, working with twenty-five Westerners who had been in Chinese prisons[2], and with fifteen Chinese intellectuals who had undergone the type of process I am going to describe.

Although I could occasionally conduct interviews in English, where the subjects had been exposed to a Westernized education (generally in mission-endowed institutions), I usually worked through interpreters. That set up a very complicated three-way communication system, which I won't discuss now. I found that it was very important to work with a subject over a long period of time, and the most meaningful data that I was able to obtain came through working with people for over a year. There is a very simple reason for this. It is a Chinese – and East Asian – cultural trait to say what one thinks the listener wants to hear, as a form of politeness and propriety. So I would first encounter many cliche anti-communist statements; one could only get into the real areas of conflict when there developed a meaningful and trusting relationship, and when the subject could realize that I wanted to know about his true feelings.

---

1. Some of this material has since been published. LIFTON, R. J. Thought Reform of Chinese Intellectuals, a Psychiatric Evaluation. *The Journal of Asian Studies, 16 No. 1.* November. 1956.
2. LIFTON. R. J. "Thought Reform" of Western Civilians in Chinese Communist Prisons. *Psychiat.,* 19:173-195. 1956.
LIFTON, R. J. Chinese Communist "Thought Reform": The Assault Upon Identity and Belief. Presented before the Annual Meeting of the American Psychiatric Association, May, 1956. *To be published.*

THE REVOLUTIONARY COLLEGE

Who attends a revolutionary college? Students are drawn from many divergent sources: former Nationalist officials and affiliates, teachers who had been associated with the old regime, Communist cadres who had demonstrated significant "errors" in their work or thoughts, party members who had spent long periods of time in Nationalist areas, students returning from the West, and finally, arbitrarily selected groups of university instructors or recent graduates. Many in these groups came in response to thinly veiled coercion — the strong "suggestion" that they attend; but others actively sought admission on a voluntary basis, in order to try to fit in with the requirements of the new regime, or at least to find out what was expected of them.

The college itself is tightly organized along Communist principles of "democratic centralism". One center may contain as many as 4,000 students, subdivided into sections of about 1,000 each, then into classes of 100 to 200 each, and finally into six- to ten-man groups. The president of the institution may be a well-known scholar serving as a figurehead; technically below him in rank are a vice-president and the section heads, who are likely to be Communist Party members, and exert the real authority at the center. Under their supervision are the class-heads, each of whom works with three special cadres.

These cadres, usually long-standing and dedicated party workers, play a central role in the thought reform process: they are the connecting link between the faculty and the students, and it is they who perform the day-to-day leg work of the reform process. The three cadres of each class may be designated according to function: the executive cadre, concerned essentially with courses of study; the organizing cadre, most intimately involved with the structure and function of the small group and the attitudes of the individual students who make them up; and the advisory cadre — the only one of the three who may be a woman — offering counsel on personal and ideological "problems" which come up during this arduous experience.

I have divided the "thought reform" process into three stages, referring to the successive psychological climates which are created. These are my subdivisions, but I believe that they are very much in keeping with the Communist view of their own process: first, The Great Togetherness — the stage of Group Identification; second, the

Closing in of the Milieu — the stage of Emotional Conflict; and third, Submission and Rebirth — the Final Confession.

1. *The Great Togetherness—Group Identification*

New students approach the course with a varying mixture of curiosity, enthusiasm, and apprehension. When a group of them arrives, their first impression is likely to be a favorable one. They encounter an atmosphere which is austere, but friendly — an open area of low-slung wooden buildings (frequently converted from military barracks) which serve as living quarters and class rooms — old students and cadres greeting them warmly, showing them around, speaking glowingly of the virtues of the revolutionary college, of the Communist movement, of the new hope for the future. Then, after a warm welcoming speech by the president of the college, they are organized into ten-man study groups. And for a period of from a few days to two weeks they are told to "just get to know each other".

Students are surprised by this free and enthusiastic atmosphere: some among the older ones may remain wary, but most are caught up in a feeling of camaraderie. Within the small groups they vent their widely shared hostility towards the old regime—an important stimulus to the thought reform process. There is a frank exchange of feeling and ideas, past and present, as they discuss their background experiences, and hopes and fears for the future. There is an air of optimism, a feeling of being in the same boat, a high *esprit de corps.*

Let me illustrate this with a few sentences quoted directly from one of my subjects:

> "*Everyone felt a bit strange at first, but we soon realized that we were all in the same position. We all began to talk freely and spontaneously; we introduced ourselves to each other, and talked about our past life and family background. . . . The Revolutionary College seemed to be a place which brought together young people from all over with a great deal in common. We ate, slept, and talked together, all of us eager to make new friends. I had very warm feelings towards the group and towards the school. . . . I felt that I was being treated well in a very free atmosphere. I was happy and thought that I was on my way to a new life.*"

Next, through a series of "thought mobilization" lectures and discussions, the philosophy and rationale of the program are impressed upon the individual student: the "old society" was evil and corrupt; this was so because it was dominated by the "exploiting classes"— the landowners and the bourgeoisie; most intellectuals come from these "exploiting classes" (or from the closely related *petite bourgeoisie*) and therefore retain "evil remnants" of their origins and of the old regime; each must now rid himself of these "ideological poisons" in order to become a "new man" in the "new society". In this way, he is told, the "ideology of all classes" can be brought into harmony with the changing "objective material conditions".[3]

Also quoted invariably is a highly significant speech of Mao Tse-tung, the chairman of the Communist Party in China:

> ". . . *our object in exposing errors and criticizing shortcomings is like that of a doctor in curing a disease. The entire purpose is to save the person, not to cure him to death. If a man has appendicitis, the doctor performs an operation and the man is saved. If a person who commits an error, no matter how great, does not bring his disease to an incurable state by concealing it and persisting in his error, and in addition if he is genuinely and honestly willing to be cured, willing to make corrections, we will welcome him so that his disease may be cured and he can become a good comrade. It is certainly not possible to solve the problem by one flurry of blows for the sake of a moment's satisfaction. We cannot adopt a brash attitude towards diseases of thought and politics, but must have an attitude of saving men by curing their diseases. This is the correct and effective method.*"[4]

This illustrates the tone with which thought reform is presented to the student. What we see as a coercive set of manipulations, they put forth as a *morally uplifting, harmonizing, and therapeutic experience.*

Then the formal courses begin — the first usually entitled the History of the Development of Society (to be later followed by Lenin — the State, Materialistic Dialectics, History of the Chinese Revolution, Theory of the New Democracy, and Field Study — visits to old Communist workshops and industrial centers). The subject matter is introduced by a two- to six-hour lecture delivered by a leading Communist theorist. This is followed by the interminable

3. AI SSU-CH'I. On Problems of Ideological Reform. *Hsueh Hsi,* 3, No. 7. January 1, 1951.
4. BRANDT, C., SCHWARTZ, B., and FAIRBANK, J. K. Correcting Unorthodox Tendencies In Learning, The Party and Literature and Art. *A Documentary History of Chinese Communism,* p. 392. 1952.

hsueh hsi or study sessions within the six- to ten-man group, where the real work of thought reform takes place. Discussion of the lecture material is led by the group leader who has been elected by its members – usually because of his superior knowledge of Marxism. At this point he encourages a spirited exchange of all views, and takes no side when there is a disagreement. The other students realize that the group leader is making daily reports to a cadre or to the class head, but the full significance of these is not yet appreciated; they may be viewed as simply a necessary organizational procedure. Most students retain a feeling of pulling together towards a common goal in a group crusading spirit.

2. *The Closing in of the Milieu—The Period of Emotional Conflict*

About four to six weeks from the beginning of thought reform – at about the time of the completion of the first course – a change begins to develop in the atmosphere. With the submission of the first "thought summary" (these must be prepared after each course) there is a shift in emphasis from the intellectual and ideological to the personal and the emotional. The student begins to find that he, rather than the Communist doctrine, is the object of study. A pattern of criticism, self-criticism, and confession develops – pursued with increasing intensity throughout the remainder of the course.

Now the group leader is no longer "neutral"; acting upon instructions from above, he begins to "lean to one side", to support the "progressive elements"; to apply stronger pressures in the direction of reform. He and the "activists" who begin to emerge, take the lead in setting the tone for the group. The descriptions of the past and present attitudes which the student so freely gave during the first few weeks of the course now come back to haunt him. Not only his ideas, but his underlying motivations are carefully scrutinized. Failure to achieve the correct "materialistic viewpoint", "proletarian standpoint", and "dialectical methodology", is pointed out, and the causes for this deficiency are carefully analyzed.

Criticisms cover every phase of past and present thought and behavior; they not only "nip in the bud" the slightest show of unorthodoxy or nonconformity, but they also point up "false progressives"— students who outwardly express the "correct" views without true depth of feeling. Group members are constantly on the lookout for indications in others of lack of real emotional involvement in the process. Each must demonstrate the genuineness of his reform through continuous personal enthusiasm, and active participation in the criticism of fellow students. In this way he can avoid being rebuked for "failure to combine theory with practice".

Standard criticisms repeatedly driven home include: "individualism"— placing personal interests above those of "the people"— probably the most emphasized of all; "subjectivism"— applying a personal viewpoint to a problem rather than a "scientific" Marxist aproach; "objectivism"— undue detachment, viewing oneself "above class distinction", or "posing as a spectator of the new China"; "sentimentalism"— allowing one's attachment to family or friends to interfere with reform needs, therefore "carrying about an ideological burden" (usually associated with reluctance to denounce family members or friends allegedly associated with the "exploiting classes"). And in addition: "deviationism", "opportunism", "dogmatism", "reflecting exploiting class ideology", "overly technical viewpoints", "bureaucratism", "individual heroism", "revisionism", "departmentalism", "sectarianism", "idealism", and "pro-American outlook".

The student is required to accept these criticisms gratefully when they are offered. But more than this, he is expected to both anticipate and expand upon them through the even more important device of *self-criticism*. He must correctly analyze his own thoughts and actions, and review his past life — family, educational, and social — in order to uncover the source of his difficulties. And the resulting 'insights' are always expressed within the Communist jargon — corrupt "ruling class" and "bourgeois" influences, derived from his specific class origin.

The criticism and self-criticism process is also extended into every aspect of daily life, always with a highly moralistic tone. Under attack here are the "bourgeois" or "ruling class" characteristics of pride, conceit, greed, competitiveness, dishonesty, boastfulness, and rudeness. Relationships with the opposite sex are discussed and evaluated, solely in terms of their effects upon the individual's progress in reform. Where a "backward" girl friend is thought to be impeding his progress, a student may be advised to break off a liaison; but if both are "progressive", or if one is thought to be aiding the other's progress, the relationship will be condoned. Sexual contacts are, on the whole, discouraged, as it is felt that they drain energies from the thought reform process.

The student must, within the small group, *confess* all of the "evils" of his past life. Political and moral considerations here become inextricably merged; especially emphasized are any "reactionary" affiliations with the old regime or with its student organizations. Each student develops a 'running confession', supplemented by material from his self-criticisms and "thought summaries"; its content becomes widely known to students, cadres, and class heads, and it serves as a continuous indicator of his progress in reform.

Most are caught up in the universal confession compulsion which sweeps the environment: students vie to outdo each other in the frankness, completeness, and luridness of their individual confessions; one group challenges another to match its collective confessions; personal confession is the major topic of discussion at small group meetings, large student gatherings, informal talks with cadres, and in articles in wall newspapers. Everywhere one encounters the question: "Have you made your full confession?"

Confession tensions are brought to a head through a mass, prearranged, revival-like gathering where a student with a particularly evil past is given the opportunity to redeem himself. Before hundreds or even thousands, of fellow students, he presents a lurid description of his past sins: political work with the Nationalists, anti-Communist activities, stealing money from his company, violating his neighbor's daughter. He expresses relief at "washing away all of my sins", and gratitude towards the Government for allowing him to "become a new man".

As the months pass, "progressives" and "activists" take increasing leadership, aided by group manipulations by cadres and class heads. Where a group leader is not sufficiently effective, if his reports to the class head are not considered satisfactory, or where there is a general "lagging behind" in a particular group, a reshuffling of groups is engineered from above. The weak group becomes reinforced by the addition of one or two "activists", and the former group leader, in his new group, is reduced to the level of an ordinary student. Although group leaders may still be elected by students, these shifts can insure that this position is always held by one considered "progressive" and "reliable".

At the same time, "backward elements"— students with suspicious backgrounds, whose confessions are not considered thorough enough, who do not demonstrate adequate enthusiasm in reforming themselves and criticizing others, whose attitudes are found wanting — are singled out for further attention. Such a student becomes the target for relentless criticism in his group; and during odd hours he is approached by other students and cadres in attempts to persuade him to mend his ways. Should he fail to respond, friendliness gives way to veiled threats, and he may be called in to receive an official admonition from a class head. As a last resort, he may be subjected to the ultimate humility of a mass "struggle" meeting: in ritualistic form, he is publicly denounced by faculty members, cadres, and fellow students, his deficiencies reiterated and laid bare. It becomes quite clear that his future in Communist China is indeed precarious, and the ceremony serves as a grim warning for other students of questionable standing.

In response to all of these pressures, no student can avoid experiencing some degree of fear, anxiety, and conflict. Each is disturbed over what he may be hiding, worried about how he may come out of this ordeal. Some, recalling either stories they have heard or personal experiences, find revived in their minds images of the extreme measures used by the Communists in dealing with their enemies. All are extremely fearful of the consequences of being considered a "reactionary".

I can again illustrate this through the feelings expressed by another one of my subjects:

> *"Towards the middle of the semester the intensity of my anti-Communist thoughts greatly increased. I developed a terrible fear that these thoughts would come out and be known to all, but I was determined to prevent this. I tried to appear calm but I was in great inner turmoil. I knew that if I kept quiet no one would know the secret which I had not confessed. But people were always talking about secrets. In small group meetings or large confession meetings, everyone would say that it was wrong to keep secrets, that one had to confess everything. Sometimes a cadre or a student would mention secrets during a casual talk, and I would feel very disturbed. Or at large meetings someone would get up and say: 'There are still some students in the University who remain "anti-organization".' I knew that no one else was thinking specifically of me, but I couldn't help feeling very upset. The secret was always something that was trying to escape from me."*

Students who show signs of emotional disturbance are encouraged to seek help by talking over their "thought problem" with the advisory cadre, in order to resolve whatever conflicts exist. Many experience psychosomatic expressions of their problems — fatigue, insomnia, loss of appetite, vague aches and pains, or gastrointestinal symptoms. Should they take their complaints to the college doctor, they are apt to encounter a reform-oriented and psychosomatically sophisticated reply: "There is nothing wrong with your body. It must be your thoughts that are sick. You will feel better when you have solved your problems and completed your reform." And indeed, most students are in a state of painful inner tension; relief is badly needed.

3. *Submission and "Rebirth"—the Final Confession*

The last stage — that of the over-all thought summary or final confession — supplies each student with a means of resolving his conflicts. It is ushered in by a mass meeting at which high Communist officials and faculty members emphasize the importance of the final thought summary as the crystallization of the entire course. Group sessions over the next two or three days are devoted exclusively to discussions of the form this summary is to take. It is to be a life history, beginning two generations back and extending through the reform experience. It must, with candor and thoroughness, describe the historical development of one's thoughts, and the relationships of these to actions. It is also to include a detailed analysis of the personal effects of thought reform.

The summary may be from five to twenty-five thousand Chinese characters, (roughly equivalent numerically to English words) and require about ten days of preparation. Each student then must read his summary to the group, where he is subjected to more prolonged and penetrating criticism. He may be kept under fire for several days of detailed discussion and painful revision, as every group member is considered responsible for the approval of each confession presented, and all may even have to place their signatures upon it.

The confession is the student's final opportunity to bring out anything he has previously held back, as well as to elaborate upon everything he has already said. It always includes a detailed analysis of class origin. And in almost every case, its central feature is the denunciation of the father, both as a symbol of the exploiting classes, and as an individual. The student usually finds the recitation of his father's personal, political, and economic abuses to be the most painful part of his entire thought reform. He may require endless prodding, persuasion, and indirect threats before he is able to take this crucial step. But he has little choice and he almost invariably complies.

The confession ends with an emphasis of personal liabilities which still remain, attitudes in need of further reform, and the solemn resolve to continue attempts at self-improvement and to serve the regime devotedly in the future. When his confession is approved, the student experiences great emotional relief. He has weathered the thought reform ordeal, renounced his past, and established an organic bond between himself and The Government. His confession will accompany him throughout his future career as a permanent part of his personal record. It is his symbolic submission to the regime, and at the same time his expression of individual rebirth into the Chinese Communist community.

COMMENT

Although there is not time for much detail, I would like to say a few words about the types of response to the process and the degree of success it seems to achieve, and then indicate what I believe to be some of the more important psychiatric principles it employs and their possible relevance for psychiatric theory and research.

In commenting on the success or failure of thought reform, I can only make what I believe to be a reasonably well-informed speculation, based upon the experiences and observations of my subjects, as well as opinions of many others who had an opportunity to observe its results first-hand. We may roughly identify three types of responses: first, the resisters who felt suffocated by the process, some of whom fled (and I would emphasize that my subjects were limited to "failures"). Some of them had been much more sympathetic to the regime prior to their thought reform, experiencing a reverse effect. But this group would seem to be a small minority. Second, on the other extreme there are the dramatic "converts"— especially among those in their teens and early twenties — who become zealous adherents of the Communist movement. The third, in-between group would appear to be by far the largest, partially convinced but essentially concerned with adapting themselves to these severe pressures and working out some type of future under the new regime. Their attempts to find a way of life and a form of personal identity become more decisive to them than theoretical ideas and beliefs. Some of the people in the second and third groups seem to feel 'purified' by the process, the emotional equivalent of taking 'bad medicine' which was unpleasant but 'good for me'.

Finally, in listing the important psychological areas involved, I wish to stress that the four which I will mention are among the most relevant for us here, but by no means the only ones.

1. *Milieu Control.* This is the term which I have used to describe the attempt at *manipulation of all communication in the environment.* Everything said or done can be observed and reported back to a cadre or faculty member, and the information used to specify further manipulations within the group. This type of closed communication system is very close to Orwell's vision of *Nineteen Eighty-Four*; but Orwell,[5] with the mind of a Westerner, saw milieu control accomplished through mechanical means, the two-way telescreen. The Chinese have here done it through a *human recording and transmitting apparatus*, extending their influence more deeply into the inner life of the individual person. There is a blending of external and internal milieux, as the student internalizes the attitudes, values, and beliefs of his environment.

What is the significance of this for psychiatry? In some of our own approaches we attempt to create what we consider to be a therapeutic milieu: in the past we emphasized the "total push" within the mental hospital and more recently we have begun to study not only the complicated relationships within the hospital structure, but also the wider milieux with which we must deal in preventive and public health psychiatry. My work with "thought reform" convinces me that we would do well to retain a certain degree of humility in our own milieu manipulations, and to keep in mind the dangers of imposing too forcefully our own values and prejudices. I believe that psychiatrists are beginning to deal with this question in the more creative type of milieux which their studious efforts have helped to develop in various treatment centers.

2. *Guilt, Shame, and Confession.* Thought reform pressures strongly stimulate both guilt anxiety and shame anxiety. I am here using the concepts developed in recent studies of guilt and shame:[6] guilt anxiety, consisting of feelings of evil and sinfulness with expectation of punishment, shame anxiety of feelings of humiliation and failure to live up to the standards of one's peers or of one's own internalized ego-ideal, with the expectation of abandonment. The

5. ORWELL, GEORGE. *Nineteen Eighty-Four.* Harcourt, Brace and Co., New York, N. Y. 1949.
6. PIERS, G. and SINGER, M. B. *Shame and Guilt.* C. C. Thomas, Springfield, Ill. 1953.
BASKOWITZ, H., PERSKY, H., KORCHIN, S. J. and GRINKER, R. R. *Anxiety and Stress.* McGraw Hill, New York, N. Y. 1955.

student develops a sense of guilt relating to the evils of his past life and further stimulated through his denunciation of his father; he develops a sense of shame through the manifold group pressures, particularly those related to ostracism and public humiliation. The experience here seems to confirm the view that both the sense of guilt and the sense of shame are likely to play important roles in any culture, and that we must reexamine some of our concepts of guilt and shame cultures. It may be, however, that the shame pressures which function so prominently in the operation of the process are drawn largely from Chinese culture, and that many of the guilt pressures stem from the Communist ideology and frame of reference which has its origins in the West.

In theorizing concerning the individual sources of this guilt, one thinks first of the traditional view, its restimulation from the store of guilt originating in real or alleged transgressions of parental authority during early life. But there is in addition the creation of what may be termed a *guilty environment.* In this atmosphere of accusation, self-accusation, and confession, *one is expected to feel guilty, and one must learn to feel guilty.* A sense of guilt becomes a form of adaptation as well as a means of communication in this milieu. The same is true of a sense of shame, and we may speak of a *shaming environment.* Similarly, confession becomes not only a means of atoning for guilt and shame, but also a vehicle for making "progress" and bettering one's standing. In the *purging environment*, self-debasement leads to increased prestige.

I believe that many questions concerning the nature of guilt, shame, and confession can be further explored through intensive studies of their occurrence in people of other cultures.

3. *Language, Theory, and Behavior.* In thought reform there is a loading of the language to an extreme degree. Such terms as "liberation", "help", "progress", "the people", "proletarian standpoint", "bourgeois", and "capitalistic" become morally charged — either very good or very bad — and they take on a mystical quality. Catch-phrases and semantic manipulations are so prominently developed that the student must find himself thinking and conceptualizing within their sphere. One of them described this to me as follows:

> *"Using the same pattern of words for so long, you are so accustomed to them that you feel chained. If you make a mistake, you make a mistake within the pattern. Although you don't*

> *admit that you have adopted this kind of ideology, you are actually using it subconsciously, almost automatically. . . . At that time I believed in certain aspects of their principles and theories. But such was the state of confusion in my own mind that I couldn't tell or make out what were the things I did believe in."*

Thought reform is based upon an implied psychological theory — not completely spelled out but very much present: that adult behavior, attitudes, values, and psychological reactions are determined by one's class origin. Negative qualities such as greed, lack of consideration for others, and the inability to adequately achieve the proletarian standpoint, are attributed to exploiting class origins. More positive qualities of cooperativeness, consideration, and "progressive thought" are ostensibly derived from working class origins. Most of us in Western psychiatry would feel that this theory has severe limitations in explaining human behavior, but in the thought reform milieu it can be made to "work". It is rendered effective by the total support of the milieu and by the discomfort experienced by those who would, through action or statement, bring it into question. In this way, a limited, or even a poorly conceived, theory can become not only an explanation of behavior but also a fulcrum for action.

In our psychiatric work, we are faced with somewhat analogous problems of language and theory. We too must consider the danger of loading of the language with concepts which become morally charged, and in their routine and unquestioned usage lose their original vitality and narrow the scope of our thinking. In evaluating our theories, we are not free of emotional involvements which influence our beliefs: where we disagree with prevailing points of view, we too may encounter pressures in the direction of guilt and shame anxiety, contrasting with the relief of conflict and reinforcement of a positive identity when we accept opinions held in our particular milieu. But equally irrational factors may also be related to the need to rebel against a particular point of view.

4. *Changes in Identity and Belief*. I feel that the thought reform pressures are primarily aimed at bringing about a shift in identity (applying the concept as developed by Erik H. Erikson[7]) in the

7. ERIKSON, ERIK H. The Problem of Ego Identity. *Journal of the American Psychoanalytic Association*, 4:56, 1956.
ERIKSON, ERIK H. On the Sense of Inner Identity. *Health and Human Relations*, New York, 1953.

participating students, both collectively and individually. Traditionally, in Chinese culture, one has well-delineated social roles which are usually defined within the family constellation: the stress was on duty and reciprocal help, but especially upon filial piety. But under the impact of the industrial age, and of strong Western influence, this structure has been under attack by vanguard intellectual groups for at least fifty years, and in the ferment which developed, the young intellectual found himself torn between such identities as that of the rebellious reformer, the uninvolved cynic, and the more traditional filial son. The Communists seek to resolve all existing confusion through supplying a common identity – that of the zealous participant in the new regime[8]. They can readily make use of that of the rebellious reformer, and without too much difficulty undermine that of the uninvolved cynic; but the identity of the filial son has the deepest emotional roots and is the most difficult to change. Thus, the denunciation of the father becomes the central symbolic act of the reform process. The student casts off the old symbol of family and institutional authority, to become an equally filial and loyal "son" in a greater family, that of the Communist regime. The shifts in identity and belief follow those which occur in any ideological or religious conversion: old identities first must become associated with guilt and shame, they are cast out by means of the confession or "emptying" process, and the "convert" emerges with a new or modified identity whose basic alterations have been supplied by the prevailing milieu. I would also emphasize that, in addition to coercive pressures, the process is furthered by powerful psychological appeals: the "great togetherness" already described, the rewards of catharsis and self-surrender in sharing the strength of a greater power, the bond of participation in a vast "moral crusade", and the overwhelmingly powerful psychological appeal of nationalism, which embodies all these other elements.

It is quite clear then that thought reform resembles, in many features, an *induced religious conversion*, as well as a *coercive form of psychotherapy*. These comparisons can be made profitably, but

8. BUNZEL, R. and WEAKLAND, J. H. An Anthropological Approach to Chinese Communism, *Columbia University Research in Contemporary Cultures.*

LA BARRE, W. Some Observations on Character Structure of the Orient: II. The Chinese. *Psychiat.*, *9*:215-237, 1946.

should not be put forth loosely. There remain important differences among these various approaches to "changing" the individual person. Psychiatry remains quite distinct from religious and ideological "conversion" experiences through a constant reexamination of its goals and its premises, the continuous and critical evaluation of its methods and of the personal involvements of its practitioners. I believe that these are principles to which this particular organization has been very actively devoted.

I would like to close with an emphasis which is perhaps already clear. The psychological forces we encounter in thought reform are not unique to the process; they represent an exaggerated expression of elements present in varying degrees in all social orders. The extreme character of thought reform offers a unique opportunity to recognize and study them. Every culture makes use of somewhat analogous pressures of milieu control, guilt, shame and confession, group sanctions, and loading of the language, in order to mold common identities and beliefs. The problem of any democratic society, including our own, is that of limiting these pressures and achieving a balance in a manner which permits its people to retain feelings of individual freedom, of dignity, and of creativity.

Moderator Lilly: Thank you, Dr. Lifton. This interesting paper is now open for discussion by the membership.

Dr. Osborn: Could I ask Dr. Lifton one thing? What tradition was there in the background of Chinese culture for an experience of this sort? I have recently been reading some of the literature and it appears in the relationship between the master and pupil, which sometimes to our way of looking is a rather vigorous sort, that this would not be entirely foreign to the Chinese background. There are many, many accounts of extraordinary amounts of intensity in this relationship. One of the best accounts I have seen tells of a pupil who after having been with the master seven years and beaten vigorously with a large stick on every possible occasion had become rather adept at getting out of its way. One day when the master was eating, the pupil saw the cudgel lying by his side. He picked it up and dealt a tremendous blow to the worthy man's head. With tremendous dexterity the master caught it on the soup tureen. The pupil then understood the great mercy and kindness of the master. This conclusion I think is quite astonishing to the Western mind.

Dr. Lifton: To consider the tradition for this movement, I think it is necessary to examine its two most important elements: the Chinese and the Communist. The forms of the process — confession, criticism, self-criticism — have long been found in international Communist practice. But the nuances of group and individual psychological pressures have, I believe, been largely contributed by the Chinese. I also think that the emphasis upon "reeducation" and "reform" is also very "Chinese", contrasting with the Russian emphasis upon confession, followed by the "purge". I believe that it stems from earlier Chinese cultural influences, particularly Confucianism, in which there was always tremendous emphasis upon "self-cultivation" and reform. It is interesting that the Communist leaders, although they condemn Confucius and the older philosophers as "idealistic", often themselves quote Confucius and Mencius as examples in "self-cultivation" for good Communists to follow. There are also elements in the process that go against Chinese culture: particularly the denunciation of the father, and public acts of criticism and humiliation. But it is important to remember here that the Communists are riding on a wave of rebellious counter-trends — severe criticism of traditional values, and especially those of the family — which began more than fifty years ago, long before the Communist take-over.

To sum up (although not finally answer the question) there are so many elements in the process which apply to things in various cultures that it is terribly hard to label a particular thought reform practice as definitely "Buddhist" or "Christian", although both of these influences are also present. In presenting some of this material before very diverse groups of people, it has been very interesting to observe the particular elements in the process with which they identify their own experiences. In many ways it represents what is universal in attempts to persuade and "change" other human beings.

Dr. Henry Brosin: In the same vein, to what extent is the exploitation of the Pavlovian theory implicit?

Dr. Lifton: My feeling is that there has been a lot of misunderstanding about this question. I have never seen any evidence that there have been any deliberate, conscious application of Pavlovian theory. Whether there is an implicit or unconscious use of Pavlovian theory would be hard to say. Through what I could discover, I believe that the process has evolved mainly in a pragmatic, trial-

and-error fashion, with the Chinese making use of their own (and Communist) political and cultural forms. We can, of course, interpret the process in various ways, whether psychoanalytic or Pavlovian. But I think that the absolute assertion that this is an application of Pavlovian theory is a kind of myth which has evolved in journalistic and other professional circles.

Dr. James G. Miller: I am a little puzzled as to what position you are taking about the similarity between the brainwashing that you have described and the religious conversion of the typical Fundamentalist group of 25 years ago. You say that they have a good deal in common as far as the fundamental psychological processes behind are concerned, yet at another point you say they are quite different and it is important to distinguish them. In what way do you distinguish them and in what way are they the same?

Dr. Lifton: I am not terribly familiar with the fundamentalist type of religion. I did compare religious and ideological versions, but did not attempt to make a complete statement about their differences, although I think they do differ. They are quite the same in the accusation and guilt-stimulation processes. In the general "conversion" process—one seeks a new identity which rids one of guilt by means of the confession or "emptying" process. I believe that they differ in the specific nature of some of the group processes, and also in the elaborate ideology and intellectual structure which Communism supplies. The distinction I was emphasizing was that between organized psychiatric methods and those of ideological and religious conversion—a distinction I think that we should maintain.

Dr. Lief: I have been impressed with the Chinese language. It lends itself more to an analysis of feelings and motives than English, for example, and I was wondering whether you found this to be true, and if true, was this a help or hindrance in the process of thought reform?

Dr. Lifton: I cannot speak as an expert here but I would say this: the Chinese language tends to be more symbolic and suggestive, and in this sense is a help in achieving distortions and minor shifts in points of view which are useful to the thought reform process. Whether or not this is better geared for expression of emotions I really don't know. I would say that it is quite possible.

I have developed an additional impression which I think is important in seeking some understanding of the source of this psychological know-how. The Chinese Communists do not appear to use any organized psychology in a Western sense, but I am struck by their cultural heritage in this respect, one which has always emphasized human relationships. I believe that the Chinese have become especially skillful in learning how to meet the psychological needs of other people and to manipulate them. One finds much evidence of this if one works with Chinese people, and reports in the literature have indicated similar impressions. Although this may not sound like a very scientific theory, I think that we see in thought reform the perversion of a cultural genius. I believe that all of this must be related to the language, but I do not know enough about the language itself to say more.

Dr. Mendel: I am wondering whether they had evolved any fixed size of group; the small group and the larger group.

Dr. Lifton: From everything I have been able to learn, the groups always seem to be about the size I mentioned, anywhere from six to ten men. This was at least true for the small group which was the place where the real work of thought reform occurred. There are other types of gatherings—large groups or big public meetings as well as individual interviews or admonitions—but most of the thought reform processes take place in this small group.

Dr. Cohen: From what you said I think they are very effective. What I would like to know is why our methods don't work as well as theirs do.

Dr. Lifton: Methods such as these seem to be most effective when the entire culture is supporting their purposes and their results. I think that this is the reason why thought reform by and large seems to work much more with Chinese than with Westerners: the Chinese intellectual must remain within the Chinese Communist culture which constantly reinforces and furthers his thought reform experience. The Westerner goes back to a world which creates different demands upon him. And the Chinese of course understand their own people better and can more readily communicate with them. Whether our own culture does or does not support our goals in psychotherapy, I would leave for others to decide. I would add that it is at this point very difficult to make any definite statement about the degree of success of the thought reform process.

Moderator Lilly: The next speaker will be Dr. Edgar H. Schein, Assistant Professor in the School of Industrial Management at Massachusetts Institute of Technology. He will speak to us on "Patterns of Reactions to Severe Chronic Stress in American Army Prisoners of War of the Chinese".

Dr. Edgar H. Schein: In this paper I would like to outline some of the constellations of stresses which prisoners of war faced during the Korean conflict, and to describe some of the reaction patterns to these stresses. I cannot present a *complete* catalogue of the men's experiences in a limited time. Therefore, I have selected those aspects which seem to me to throw some light on the problem of collaboration with the enemy. I will give particular emphasis to the *social* psychological factors, because the Chinese methods seem to emphasize control over groups, rather than individuals.

My material is based on a variety of sources. I was in Korea during the repatriation, and had the opportunity to interview extensively 20 unselected repatriates. This basic material was supplemented by the information gathered by three psychiatrists, Drs. Harvey Strassman, Patrick Israel, and Clinton Tempereau, who together had seen some 300 men. On board ship coming home, I also had the opportunity to sit in on bull sessions among repatriates in which many of the prison experiences were recapitulated. Back in the states I obtained additional details from Army dossiers on the men.

This interview material is supplemented with projective test data on some 200 men and objective test data on 750, obtained within one to two weeks following repatriation. The testing program was set up with Capt. Harold Williams. I want to thank him, Dr. Margaret Singer, Dr. Winfred Hill, and Dr. Ardie Lubin who have all worked with me on this project and have contributed significantly to it. I would also like to acknowledge the help of Dr. David Rioch and the Walter Reed Army Institute of Research.

The typical experience of the prisoner of war must be divided into two broad phases. The *first* phase lasted anywhere from one to six months beginning with capture, followed by exhausting marches to the north of Korea and severe privation in inadequately equipped temporary camps, terminating finally in the assignment to a permanent prisoner of war camp.

The *second* phase, lasting two or more years, was marked by chronic pressures to collaborate and to give up existing group loyalties in favor of new ones. While physical stresses had been outstanding in the first six months, psychological stresses were outstanding in this second period.

The reactions of the men toward capture were influenced by their overall attitude toward the Korean situation. *First,* many of them felt inadequately prepared, either physically or psychologically. The physical training, equipment, rotation system, and leadership all came in for retrospective criticism, though this response might have been merely a rationalization for being captured. On the psychological side, the men were not clearly aware what they were fighting for or what kind of enemy they were up against.

Second, the reports of the atrocities committed by the North Koreans led most men to expect death, torture, or non-repatriation if captured.

Third, the Chinese entrance into the war was marked by their penetration into rear areas where they captured many men who were taken completely by surprise. The men felt that when positions were over-run, their leadership was often less than adequate. Thus, many men were predisposed to blame the UN command for the unfortunate event of being captured.

It was in such a context that the soldier found his Chinese captor extending his hand in a friendly gesture and saying "Welcome" or "Congratulations, you've been *liberated*". This Chinese tactic was part of their *'lenient policy'* which was explained to groups of prisoners shortly after capture in these terms: because the UN had entered the war illegally and was an aggressor, all UN military personnel were in fact criminals, and *could* be shot summarily. But the average soldier was, after all, only carrying out orders for his leaders who were the real criminals. Therefore, the Chinese soldier would consider the POW to be a 'student', and would teach him the 'truth' about the war. Anyone who did not cooperate by going to school and learning voluntarily, could always be reverted to his 'war criminal' status and shot, particularly if a confession of 'criminal' deeds could be obtained.

In the weeks following capture, the men were collected in large groups and marched north. From a physical point of view, the stresses during these marches were very severe: there was no medicine for the wounded, the food was unpalatable and insufficient, especially by our standards, clothing was scarce in the face of severe winter weather, and shelter was inadequate and overcrowded. The Chinese set a severe pace and showed little consideration for the weariness that was the product of wounds, diarrhea, and frostbite. Men who could not keep up were usually abandoned or had to be helped by their fellows. The men marched only at night, and were kept under cover during the day, ostensibly as protection against being strafed by our own planes.

From a psychological point of view this situation can best be described as a chronic cycle of fear, relief, and new fear. The men were afraid that they might die, that they might never be repatriated, that they might never again have a chance to communicate with the outside, and that no one even knew they were alive. The Chinese, on the other hand, were reassuring and promised that the men would be repatriated soon, that conditions would improve, and that they would soon be permitted to communicate with the outside.

What made matters worse was the disorganization within the prisoner group itself. It was difficult to maintain close group ties if one was competing with others for the essentials of life, and if one spent one's resting time in overcrowded huts among others who had severe diarrhea and were occasionally incontinent. Lines of authority often broke down, and with this, group cohesion and morale suffered. A few men attempted to escape, but they were usually recaptured in a short time and returned to the group. The Chinese also fostered low morale and the feeling of being abandoned, by systematically reporting false news about United Nation defeats and losses.

In this situation goals became increasingly short-run. As long as the men were marching, they had something to do and could look forward to relief from the harsh conditions of the march. However, arrival at a temporary camp was usually a severe disappointment. Not only were physical conditions as bad as ever, but the sedentary life in overcrowded quarters produced more disease and still lower morale.

What happened to the men under these conditions? During the one to two week marches they became increasingly apathetic. They developed a slow plodding gait, called by one man a 'prisoners' shuffle'. Uppermost in their minds were fantasies of food: men remembered all the good meals they had ever had or planned detailed menus for years into the future. To a lesser extent they thought of loved ones at home, and about cars which seemed to them to symbolize freedom and the return home.

In the temporary camps disease and exposure took a heavy toll in lives. But it was the feeling of many men, including some of the doctors who survived the experience, that some of these deaths were not warranted by a man's physical condition. Instead, what appeared to happen was that some men became so apathetic that they ceased to care about their bodily needs. They retreated further into themselves, refused to eat even what little food was available, refused to get any exercise, and eventually lay down and curled up, as if waiting to die. The reports were emphatic concerning the lucidity and sanity of these men. They seemed simply to give up and accept the prospect of death rather than to continue fighting a severely frustrating and depriving environment.

Two things seemed to save a man who was close to 'apathy' death: getting him on his feet and doing something, no matter how trivial, or getting him angry or concerned about some present or future problem. Usually it was the effort of a friend who maternally and insistently motivated the individual toward realistic goals which snapped him out of such a state of resignation. In one case such 'therapy' consisted of kicking the man until he was mad enough to get up and fight.

Throughout this time, the Chinese played the role of the benevolent but handicapped captor. Prisoners were always reminded that it was their *own* Air Force bombing which was responsible for the inadequate supplies. Furthermore, they were reminded that they were getting treatment which was just as good as that which the average Chinese was getting. One important effect of this was that a man could never give *full* vent to his hostility toward the Chinese, even in fantasy. In their *manner* and *words* they were usually solicitous and sympathetic. Also, in their manner, the Chinese implied that conditions could be better for a prisoner if he would take a more 'cooperative' attitude, if he would support their propaganda for peace. Thus a man was made to feel that he was himself responsible for his traumatic circumstances.

Arrival at a permanent camp usually brought some relief from many of the physical hardships which I have just described. Food, shelter, and medicine, while not plentiful, appeared to be sufficient for the maintenance of life and some degree of health. However, the Chinese now increased sharply their efforts to involve prisoners in their own propaganda machine, and to undermine loyalties to their country. This marks the beginning of the *second* phase of the imprisonment experience.

The Chinese program of subversion and indoctrination was thoroughly integrated into the entire camp routine and it is likely that its aims were broad and inclusive. Managing a large group of prisoners with a minimum staff of guards, indoctrinating them with the communist political ideology, interrogating them to obtain intelligence information and confessions for propaganda purposes, and developing a corps of collaborators within the prisoner group were all carried out within a single framework of techniques. These techniques involved the manipulation of the entire social milieu in which the prisoners existed. What success the Chinese had, stemmed from this *total* control of the environment, not from the application of any one technique.

The most significant feature of Chinese prisoner camp control was the systematic destruction of the prisoners' formal and informal group structure. Soon after arrival at a camp, the men were segregated by race, nationality, and rank. The Chinese put their own men in charge of the platoons and companies, and made their own selections of POW squad leaders, usually on some arbitrary basis, to remind the prisoners that their old rank system no longer had any validity. In addition, the Chinese attempted to undermine informal group structure by prohibiting any group meetings such as religious services, and by systematically fomenting mutual distrust by playing men off against one another. The most effective device to this end was the practice of obtaining from informers or Chinese spies detailed information about someone's activities, no matter how trivial, then calling him in and interrogating him about it. Such detailed surveillance of the men's activities led them to feel that their own ranks were so infiltrated by spies and informers that it was not safe to trust anyone.

A similar device was used in obtaining information during interrogation. After a man had resisted giving information for hours or days, he would be shown a signed statement by one of his fellow prisoners giving that same information. Still another device was to make prisoners who had not collaborated, look like collaborators by bestowing special favors upon them.

If the men, in spite of their state of social disorganization, did manage to organize any kind of group activity, the Chinese would quickly break up the group by removing its leaders or key members.

Loyalties to home and country were undermined by the systematic manipulation of mail. Usually only mail which carried bad news was delivered to a man. If he received no mail at all, it was pointed out to him that his loved ones must have abandoned him.

Feelings of social isolation were further heightened by the complete information control maintained in the camps. Only the communist press, radio, magazines, and movies were allowed.

The undermining of the prison social structure is particularly significant because we depend to such an extent on consensual validation for judging ourselves and others. The prisoners lost their most important source of information and support concerning standards of behavior and beliefs. Often men who attempted to resist the Chinese by means other than *outright* obstruction or aggression, failed to obtain the *active* support of others, often earning their suspicion instead. This kind of social isolation is different from the physical isolation that is often associated with Russian confession extraction.

At the same time the Chinese *did* create a situation in which meaningful social relationships could be obtained through common political activity, such as the 'peace' committees which served as propaganda organs. As an additional outlet, Chinese interrogators or instructors offered some men close personal relationships by living with them for long periods of time and establishing an air of familiarity with them.

The Communist point of view was presented through compulsory lectures followed by compulsory group discussions, the purpose of which was to justify the conclusions given at the end of the lectures. On the whole, this phase of indoctrination was ineffective because of the crudeness of the propaganda, though its constant repetition seemed eventually to influence those men who did not have well formed political opinions to start with, particularly because no counter-arguments could be heard.

More successful was the Chinese use of testimonials from other prisoners, such as the false germ-warfare confessions, and appeals based on familiar contexts, such as peace appeals. Confessions by prisoners or propaganda lectures given by collaborators had a particularly demoralizing and undermining effect, because only if resistance had been *unanimous* could a man solidly believe that his values were correct, even if he could not defend them logically.

Throughout, the Chinese created an environment in which rewards such as extra food, medicine, special privileges, and status in the prison camp hierarchy followed cooperation and collaboration; while threats of death, non-repatriation, reprisals against families, torture, decreases in food and medicine, and imprisonment served to keep men from offering much resistance. Only imprisonment was consistently used as an actual punishment. *Chronic* resistance was usually handled by transferring the prisoner to a so-called 'reactionary' camp.

Whatever behavior the Chinese attempted to elicit, they always *paced* their demands very carefully, they always required some level of *participation* from the prisoner, no matter how trivial, and they always *repeated* endlessly.

To what extent did these pressures produce *changes in beliefs and attitudes,* or *collaboration?* I don't think the Chinese had much success in changing beliefs and attitudes. Doubt and confusion was produced in many prisoners as a result of having to examine so closely, their own way of thinking, but very few changes, if any, occurred that resembled any degree of *conversion* to Communism. The type of prisoner who was most likely to become *sympathetic* toward Communism was the one who had chronically occupied a low status position in this society and for whom the democratic principles were not very salient or meaningful.

In producing *collaboration,* however, the Chinese were far more effective. By collaboration I mean such activities as giving lectures for the Communists, writing and broadcasting propaganda, giving false confessions, writing and signing petitions, informing on fellow POWs and so on; none of which required a personal change of belief. Some 10 to 15 per cent of the men chronically collaborated, but the dynamics of this response are very complex. By far the greatest determinant is the amount of pressure the Chinese put on a particular prisoner. Beyond this, the reports of the men permitted one to isolate several sets of motives that operated, though it is impossible to tell how many cases of each type there may have been.

1) Some men collaborated for outright opportunistic reasons; these men lacked any kind of stable group identification and exploited the situation for its material benefits without any regard for the consequences to themselves, their fellow prisoners, or their country.

2) Some men collaborated because their egos were too weak to withstand the physical and psychological rigors; these men were primarily motivated by fear, though they often rationalized their behavior; they were unable to resist any kind of authority figure,

and were highly susceptible to being blackmailed once they had begun to collaborate.

3) Some men collaborated with the firm conviction that they were infiltrating the Chinese ranks and obtaining intelligence information which would be useful to the Army. This was a convenient rationalization for anyone who could not withstand the pressures. Many of these men were initially tricked into collaboration or were motivated by a desire to communicate with the outside world. None of the types mentioned thus far became ideologically confused; what communist beliefs they might have professed were for the benefit of the Chinese only.

4) The prisoner, who was vulnerable to the *ideological* appeal because of his low status in this society, often collaborated with the conviction that he was doing the right thing in supporting the communist peace movement. This group included the younger and less intelligent men from backward or rural areas, the malcontents, and members of various minority groups. These men often viewed themselves as failures in our society and felt that society had never given them a chance. They were positively attracted by the immediate status and privileges which went with being a 'progressive', and by the promise of important roles which they could presumably play in the peace movement of the future.

Perhaps the most important thing to note about the production of collaboration is the manner in which the social disorganization contributed to it. A man might make a slanted radio broadcast in order to communicate with the outside, he might start reading communist literature out of sheer boredom, he might give information which he knew the Chinese already had, and so on. Once this happened, however, the Chinese rewarded him, increased pressure on him to collaborate, and blackmailed him by threatening exposure. At the same time his fellow prisoners, often unwittingly, forced him into further collaboration by mistrusting him or ostracising him. Thus a man had to stand entirely on his own judgment and strength, and both of these often failed. One of the commonest failures was a man's judgment concerning the effects of his own actions on the other prisoners, and the value of these actions for the Chinese propaganda effort. The man who confessed to germ warfare, thinking he could repudiate such a confession later, did not realize its propaganda value to the communists.

A certain percentage of men, though the exact number is difficult to estimate, exhibited chronic resistance and obstructionism toward Chinese indoctrination efforts. Many of these men were well integrated, had secure, stable group identifications, and could withstand the social isolation and still exercise good judgment. Others were chronic obstructionists whose histories showed recurring resistance to any form of authority. Still others were idealists or martyrs to religious and ethical principles, and still others were anxious, guilt-ridden individuals who could only cope with their own strong impulses to collaborate by denying them and over-reacting in the other direction.

By far the largest group of prisoners, however, established a complex compromise between the demands of the Chinese and their own value systems. This adjustment, called by the men 'playing it cool', consisted primarily of a physical and emotional withdrawal from the whole environment. These men learned to suspend their feelings and to adopt an attitude of watching and waiting, rather than hoping and planning. This reaction, though passive was not as severe as the apathy described earlier. It was a difficult adjustment to maintain because some concessions had to be made to the Chinese in the form of trivial or well timed collaborative acts, and in the form of a feigned interest in the indoctrination program. At the same time, each man had to be prepared to deal with the hostility of his buddies if he made an error in judgment.

The *test material* which we have on prisoners was gathered some 1 to 2 weeks following repatriation. At that time the passive response which I have just described was still very evident in the majority of the group. Men who fell into the passive neutral group in terms of camp adjustment showed highly constricted Rorschach records and told short, bland TAT stories. On the other hand, there was a marked tendency for men who had *collaborated* to show *less* of this constriction, as one would expect, if one considers that these men had felt no need to withdraw from the environment. Thus, it is possible to separate collaborators from neutrals at a level considerably better than chance, by using criteria such as total number of Rorschach responses, number of human movement and color responses, reaction time, and number of card rejections.

In our sample of 750 *objective* test protocols we have a sufficient number of resisters to enable us to compare all three groups on several other variables.

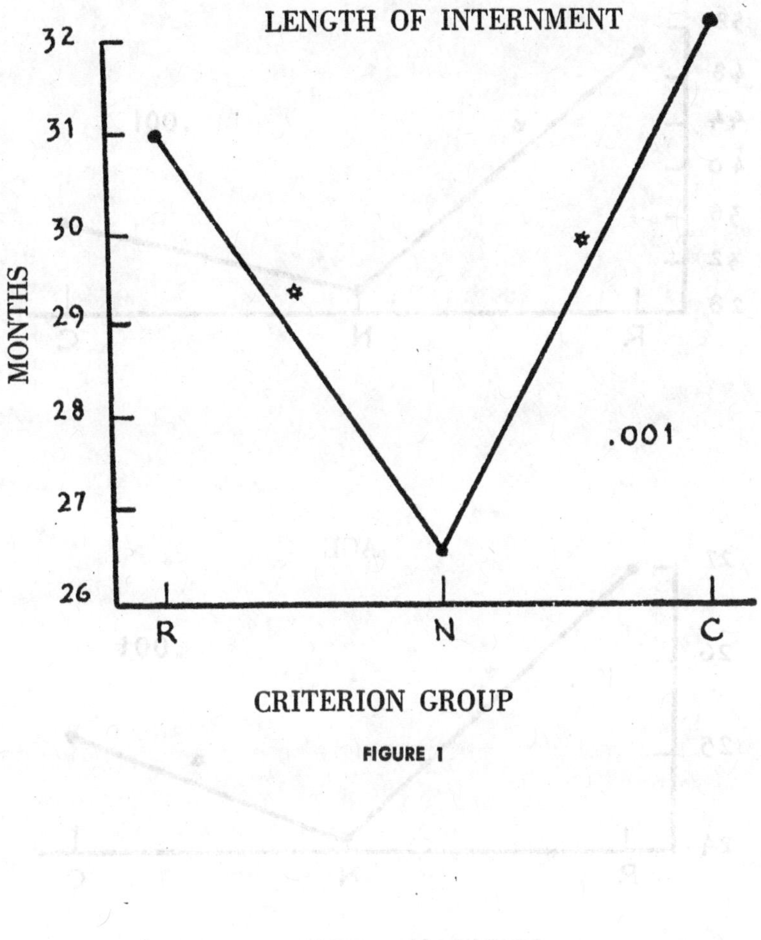

FIGURE 1

Figure 1 shows that both resisters and collaborators, the two extreme points on the graph, were interned for a longer period of time than neutrals.

*The difference between these two groups is significant at the .05 level.

**This indicates the overall significance level comparing all three groups by analysis of variance.

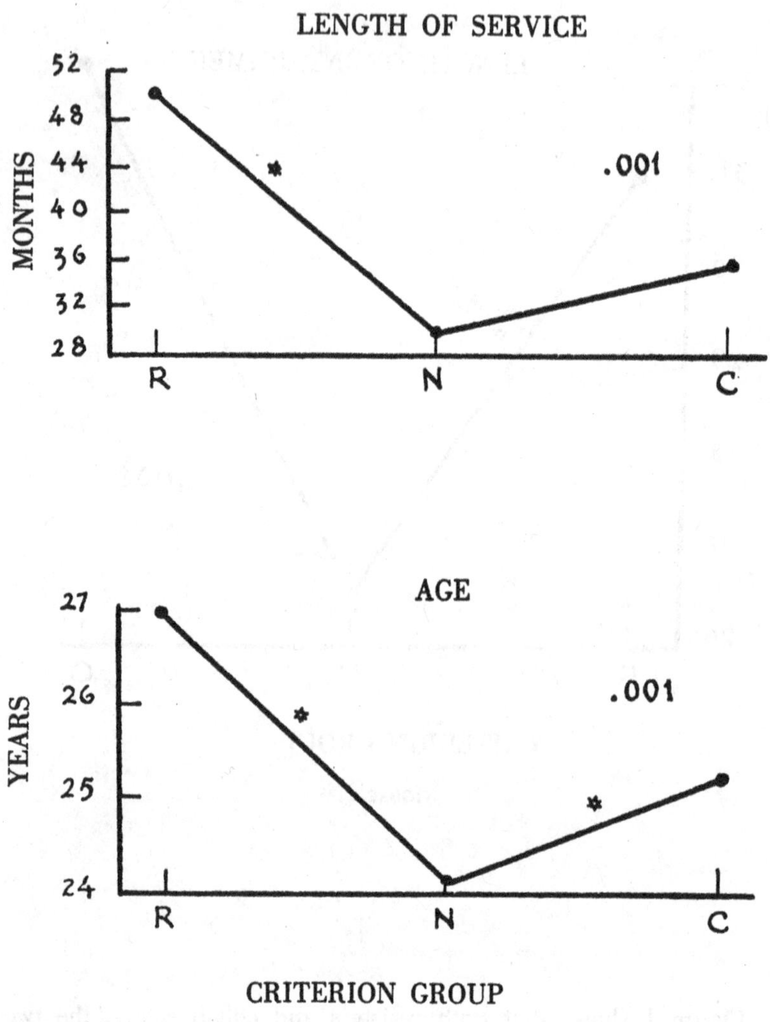

FIGURE 2

Figure 2 shows that the two extreme groups were in the service longer, and were older.

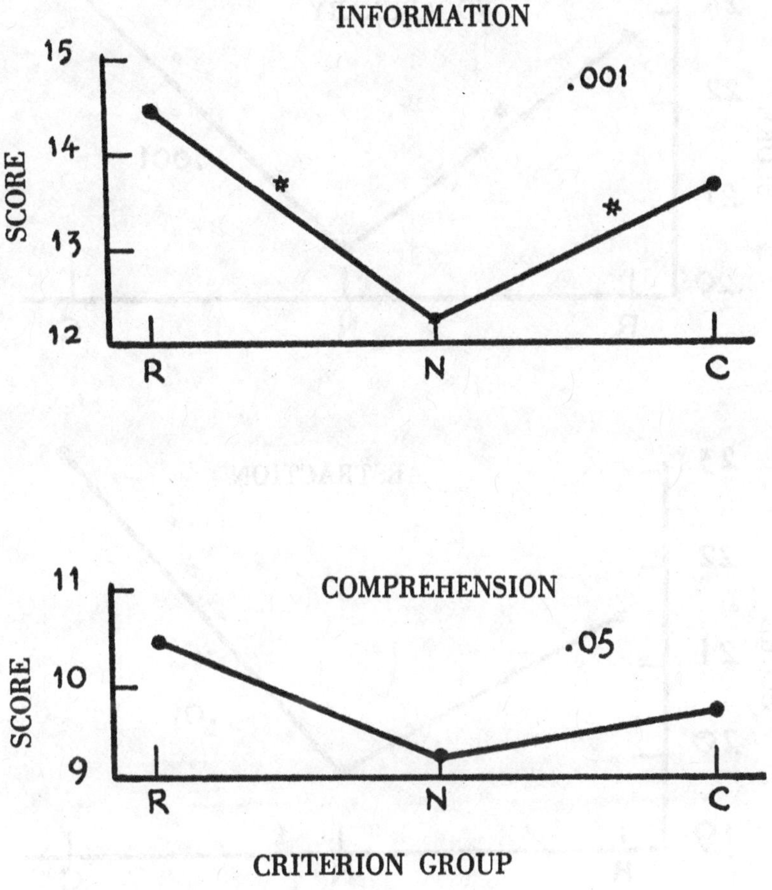

FIGURE 3

Figure 3 shows that the two extreme groups scored higher on the information and comprehension parts of the Wechsler-Bellevue intelligence test.

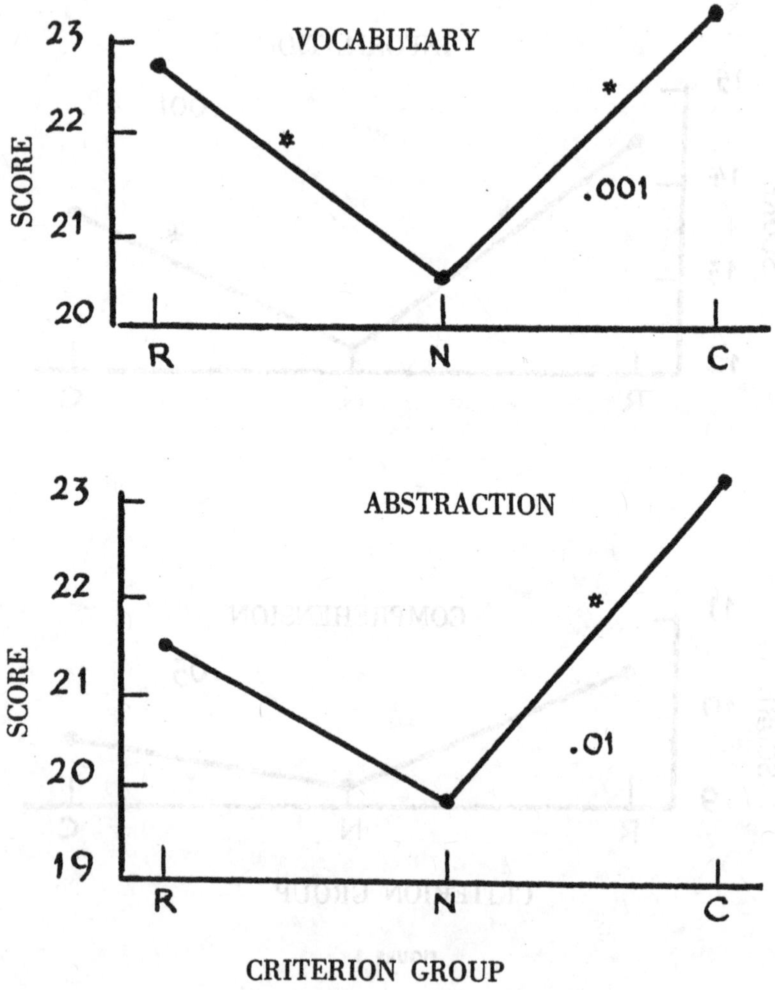

FIGURE 4

Figure 4 shows that the two extreme groups scored higher on the two parts of the Shipley-Hartford test of vocabulary and abstraction.

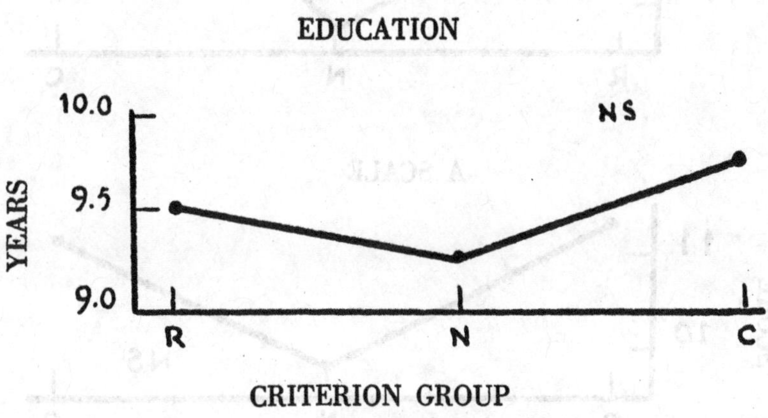

FIGURE 5

Figure 5 shows that the two extreme groups have a slightly higher level of education, as inferred from the number of school years completed.

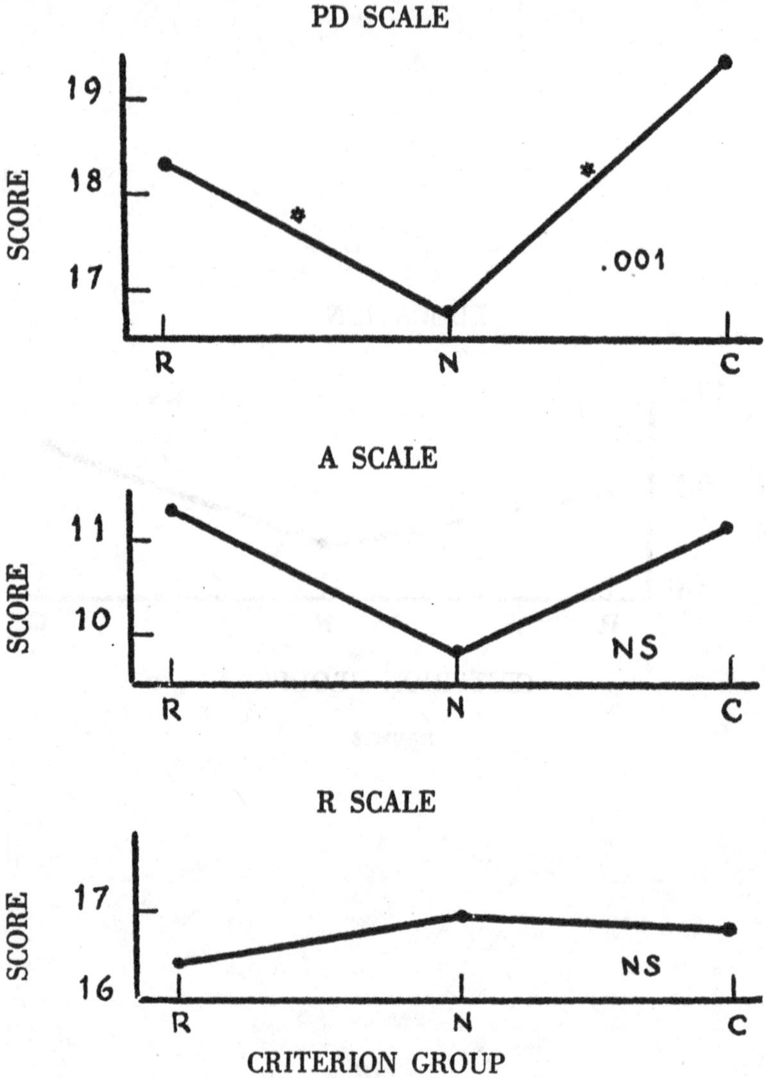

FIGURE 6

Figure 6 shows that the two extreme groups tend to have higher scores on the Psychopathic Deviate scale of the Minnesota Multiphasic Personality inventory. The scores on the anxiety and repression scales do not show a significant difference. Nor do the following variables discriminate any of the groups.

1) Occupation prior to army service.
2) Normal vs. broken home as defined in terms of the number of parents with whom a person grew up.
3) Rural vs. urban home background.
4) Location of home community geographically.
5) Religion.
6) Authoritarianism as measured by the California F Scale.
7) Rank, though the latter shows a definite trend for the extreme groups to have been higher than middle group.

None of these relationships are changed to any extent by controlling length of internment. However, it should be pointed out that the degree of relationship between our variables and the criterion of prison camp behavior is very small, even though statistically significant. The highest correlation ratio obtained was + .22 in the case of the Pd scale of the MMPI. Therefore, these results have no practical implications to speak of, though it is of interest to speculate what they might mean. You will have noted that in every case, the resisters and collaborators deviated from the neutral group *in the same direction.* This fact has led us to infer that the continuum which our tests seems to be discriminating is not *resistance-collaboration* but *action-inaction.* The chief contrast is between the neutrals, who defended themselves from stress with a wall of passivity, and the other two groups, both of which were characterized by some kind of positive action toward the Communists. The results just shown suggest that two complementary factors may have been operating to determine which men would respond actively and which ones passively to the stresses of prison-camp life.

One of these factors might be called *self-confidence.* Those men who were *older*, more *intelligent*, better *educated* and more *experienced* in the Army, may have felt more capable of taking some action. This action might have taken the form of 1) open resistance, of 2) pseudo-collaboration, which it was vainly hoped could be used as an undercover means of resistance, or of 3) genuine collaboration regarded as the best way of dealing with an otherwise hopeless situation. Those low on the variables in question might have been more hesitant to commit themselves either to open resistance or to collaboration, but rather, followed the passive middle road of the majority.

The other factor which we think may have been operating is *underinhibition of acting-out tendencies.* This explanation is based entirely on the Pd scale. This scale, as you know, was standardized on psychopathic deviates who are characterized by several adjustment tendencies such as difficulty with authority figures, delinquency, opportunism, and underinhibition of impulses. Since *both* resisters and collaborators were high on Pd, it seems reasonable to suppose that it is the underinhibition which is common to the two groups. I suggest, therefore, that both resisters and collaborators tended to be restless, under-inhibited individuals who would be more likely to do something active in a stressful situation, whether or not what they did was useful. Such men would be more willing to alienate either the Communists by active resistance or their fellow-prisoners by collaboration, while the more typical prisoners would try to avoid open breaks with either side.

Let me summarize. I have tried to outline the major stresses of imprisonment, and to show that a prevalent response to those stresses was passivity in various degrees. I have also tried to suggest that collaboration can best be understood in terms of the systematically created group disorganization in the prison camp. This disorganization prevented consensual validation, constructive group resistance, or sympathetic understanding and handling of the unfortunate prisoner whose initial collaborative acts were the product of having been duped or of showing poor judgment. Ideological involvement, I feel, was the result of a *predisposition* based on low status in this society.

From a personality point of view, the events in prison camp seem most intelligible if, instead of thinking about the personality dynamics underlying collaboration or resistance, we think of personalities who can handle stress by withdrawing from it versus personalities who must take some kind of action to remove it.

Moderator Lilly: Our third speaker is Dr. Louis J. West, Professor of Psychiatry, University of Oklahoma. He will speak to us on the "United States Air Force Prisoners of the Chinese Communists".

Dr. Louis J. West**:* A considerable amount of valuable material on so-called brainwashing has appeared in recent months[1,2,3,4,5]. I would like particularly to call your attention to the publications of Segal[6], Lifton[7,8], Schein[9,10,11,12], Hinkle and Wolff[13], and Biderman[14] which are now or soon will be available in print.

The recent symposium at the meeting of the American Psychological Association also contained much that was of value[15,16].

As a former Air Force medical officer and a current researcher on the topic of Prisoners of War, I shall attempt to present some material that may be of interest to GAP. Much of this material is derived directly from the work of Biderman[14] and Sander, to whom I wish to give full credit. I also wish to acknowledge the assistance of I. E. Farber, my collaborator in the POW studies now underway at the Oklahoma Medical Center concerning Prisoners of War and their reactions to various types of stress.

Of the Air Force personnel known to have fallen into the hands of the Communist Chinese and North Korean military forces, slightly more than half have returned. Two hundred and twenty were exchanged at Little Switch and Big Switch. Subsequently four fighter pilots and an eleven-man bomber crew have also been released. Of these 235 returnees, a number have been studied in considerable detail.

There are many good reasons for studying the Air Force prisoners as a separate group. Not only were they less prepared for the

*Professor and Head, Department of Psychiatry and Neurology, University of Oklahoma School of Medicine and University Hospitals, Oklahoma City, Oklahoma. Currently studying prisoners of war on a project supported by the Air Force Personnel and Training Research Center of the Air Research and Development Command. The views herein expressed are those of the author and do not necessarily represent official views of the United States Air Force.

1. FISCHER, CAPT. H. E., Jr. My Case As a Prisoner Was Different. *Life*, pp. 147-160. June 27, 1955.
2. HELLER, LT. COL. E. L. I Thought I'd Never Get Home. *Saturday Evening Post.* p. 17, August 20, 1955. P. 34, August 27, 1955.
3. SANTUCCI, P. S. and WINOKUR, G. Brainwashing As a Factor in Psychiatric Illness. *Arch. Neurol. and Psychiat.*, 74:11-16, July, 1955.
4. Communist Interrogation, Indoctrination, and Exploitation of American Military and Civilian Prisoners. *Hearings Before the Permanent Subcommittee on Investigations of the Committee on Government Operations, U. S. Senate, 84th Congress, Second Session.* June 19, 20, 26, and 27, 1956. U. S. Government Printing Office, Washington 25, D.C.
5. POW: The Fight Continues After the Battle. *The Report of the Secretary of Defense's Advisory Committee on Prisoners of War.* U. S. Government Printing Office, Washington 25, D.C.
6. SEGAL, H. A. Initial Psychiatric Findings of Recently Repatriated Prisoners of War. *Amer. J. of Psychiat.*, 3:358-363, 1954.

conditions of captivity in which they found themselves (being plunged literally from the heights to the depths very abruptly), but the enemy also considered them as a distinct population to be handled differently from ground force prisoners.

Flying over enemy territory in Korea with the constant hazard of forced landing or parachute escape from a damaged aircraft, the airman continually faced a unique survival situation. He had had no close contact with the enemy or his terrain. He was not physically toughened by the rigors of warfare on the ground. There was a violent contrast between his ordinary combat situation and the survival situation in which he suddenly found himself, far behind enemy lines and often suffering some injury received in the aircraft or in the process of getting down to the ground.

The enemy regarded the captured airman in a very special light. Our aircraft had flown far over enemy lines, often unopposed, and both military and civilian populations under Communist control were well aware of the highly effective destructive activities of U. S. Air Force operations. After February 21, 1952, when the Communists' world-wide germ warfare propaganda campaign went into high gear, the responsibility for this politically potent and highly propagandized "*germ warfare*" was placed by the enemy directly upon the flyers, who presumably were the instruments by which bacteriological weapons were delivered.

---

7. LIFTON, R. J. Home by Ship: Reaction Patterns of American Prisoners of War Repatriated from North Korea. *Amer. J. Psychiat.*, *110*:732-739, 1954.
8. LIFTON, R. J. 'Thought Reform' of Western Civilians in Chinese Communist Prisons. *Psychiat.*, *19*:173-196, 1956.
9. HILL, W. F., SCHEIN, E. H., WILLIAMS, H. L., and LUBIN, A. Distinguishing Characteristics of Collaborators and Resisters Among American Prisoners of War. *Presentation at the meeting of the American Psychological Association.* Chicago, September 3-5, 1956.
10. SCHEIN, E. H. The Chinese Indoctrination Program for Prisoners of War. *Psychiat.*, *19*:149-172, 1956.
11. SCHEIN, E. H. Some Observations on Chinese Methods of Handling Prisoners of War. *The Public Opinion Quarterly*, *20*:321-327, Spring, 1956.
12. STRASSMAN, H. D., THALER, M. B., and SCHEIN, E. H. A Prisoner of War Syndrome: Apathy as a Reaction to Severe Stress. *Amer. J. Psychiat.*, *112*:998-1003, June, 1956.
13. HINKLE, L. E., Jr. and WOLFF, H. G. Communist Interrogation and Indoctrination of "Enemies of the State." *Arch. Neurol. and Psychiat.*, *76*:115-174, August, 1956.
14. BIDERMAN, A. D. Communist Attempts to Elicit False Confessions from Air Force Prisoners of War. *Bulletin of the New York Academy of Medicine.* In press.
15. BAUER, R. A. Brainwashing—Psychology or Demonology. *Symposium address, American Psychological Association*, September 3, 1956.
16. MILLER, J. G. "Brainwashing"—Present and Future. *Symposium address, American Psychological Association*, Chicago, September 3, 1956.

There were other ways in which Air Force personnel differed from the ground force prisoners. The flyers were generally of higher rank; 70 per cent of the Air Force returnees were officers. The Air Force POW was more knowledgeable than his ground force counterpart; he had a higher degree of specialized training and technical skill; he had a better education. Fifty-three per cent of the Air Force returnees had received at least some college training, as compared with about 5 percent of the Army captives. Furthermore, air information always has a high priority, and data about aircraft equipment and training methods do not become obsolete as rapidly as do data concerning ground forces.

Thus, the Communists deemed Air Force prisoners particularly valuable for propaganda purposes and as intelligence information sources. For these and certain other reasons, the Communists chose to segregate most of their Air Force prisoners in special ways. Whereas officers and enlisted men were promptly separated among the Army captives, Air Force enlisted men were usually kept together with their officers. Many individuals were isolated for long periods of time. In addition to prolonged efforts to extract military information, extreme pressures were exerted in order to gain false propaganda confessions from the captive airman.

Sander, Biderman, and their associates[14] have studied the 235 Air Force returnees in considerable detail. Department of Defense teams debriefed all airmen at the time that they were returned. In addition, Air Force Intelligence (O.S.I.) conducted detailed interviews. At the Officer Education Research Laboratory, Maxwell Field, Alabama, personal interviews were conducted with a number of returnees. A follow-up attitude and opinion questionnaire was mailed to the first 200 returnees, with a 90 per cent response. It was possible for officers trained in clinical psychology and in psychiatry to participate in some of the interviewing, along with the responsible social scientists. Many interviews were tape-recorded and observed through one-way screens. A considerable amount of information has been derived from the detailed and continuing studies that were made of the repatriated airmen.

There were two aspects to the Communist exploitation of U. S. Air Force prisoners. First, they used them in ways that were quite independent of any acts of compliance on the prisoner's part. For example, they employed prisoners as hostages during peace negotiations; they used them to make the West lose face by marching defeated and bedraggled prisoners through the streets of Seoul; conversely they showed the world a picture of Communist leniency by exhibiting photographs of prisoners receiving good treatment.

It is with the second type of exploitation — Communist attempts to influence prisoners through systematic control and pressure — that we are particularly concerned. The Communists tried to get intelligence information through extensive written and oral interrogations. They tried to engage the prisoners in propaganda activities, including false confessions, peace petitions, special broadcasts and recordings, writing particular types of letters home, etc. And they tried to get the prisoners to participate in indoctrination sessions with a view toward influencing them to accept Communist ideas.

In the latter activity, the enemy met with little success. We know of no Air Force officer or enlisted man who was converted to Communism or who defected to the enemy cause. However, the enemy had a considerable degree of success in obtaining intelligence information and in forcing prisoners to engage in propaganda activities.

Of the various objectives that the Communists had in attempting to gain influence over prisoners, the most persistent and important objective appears to have been the attempt to make propaganda use of Air Force personnel primarily in connection with bacteriological warfare (BW) "confessions". Another important objective was to obtain military intelligence information. Other objectives were apparently held by the enemy to be of less importance.

From the prisoners' viewpoint, however, there was no regular or uniform sequence in which the Communists seemed to attack these objectives. There was no time when the prisoner could be sure that he was through with a particular ordeal. He could be hauled out at any time and be re-interrogated. Frequently interrogation for military information was a mere cover for getting the prisoner into the habit of compliance in talking. Interrogation toward the objective of propaganda use of prisoners might be carried on simultaneously or intermingled with interrogation for military information. Attempts at indoctrination of individuals in isolation or while undergoing interrogation could happen at any time.

Eighty-three Air Force prisoners of war who have returned (and at least one other who died as a result of efforts to coerce a confession from him) were involved in attempts to extort "germ warfare" confessions. Of these, 48 were subjected to a highly deliberate, systematic, centrally-directed campaign, carried out by the Chinese

Communists, to extort false germ warfare confessions. Eleven other Air Force prisoners of war were also put under intense pressure for confessions, although these cases are less definitely linked to the centrally-directed propaganda effort. Thirty-six of these men made some kind of confession. The Communists used 23 of these for propaganda purposes. The confessions of two Marine flyers were also widely broadcasted by the Chinese. As everyone knows, these confessions were publicized throughout the world. Films of the confessions of six of these men were shown as a part of this major propaganda effort. (See Table 1)

TABLE I

RESULTS OF COMMUNIST ATTEMPTS TO ELICIT "CONFESSIONS" OF BACTERIOLOGICAL WARFARE (BW) FROM USAF PRISONERS OF WAR

	Number	% of Total Interrogated on BW	% of Total USAF Returnees (235)
Interrogated on BW	83	100	35
Subjected to systematic "confession" extortion.	59	71	25
Clearly involved in centrally directed CHICOM propaganda effort.	48	58	20
Gave some "confession."	36	43	15
"Confessions" used for propaganda.	23	28	10

Some prisoners gave in rather quickly to the demands for a false confession. Fifteen per cent of all those pressured agreed to confess after one month of pressure or less. Others held out for long periods of time, two for almost a year. Nearly a quarter of those interrogated on BW still refused to confess after 24 weeks of intense pressure (compared with 35 days required for Cardinal Mindzenty's confession). It is difficult to determine in most cases how much of this variation was due to the differences between the strength and determination of the victims and how much was due to the skill and determination of the interrogators. The Communists clearly became more efficient as time went by.

The pattern of pressure by the Communists for getting false confessions, although varying in intensity, length, and sequence, was essentially as follows: Shortly after capture and initial interrogations, the prisoners were accused of having participated in germ warfare missions. For this reason, they were to be considered as war criminals, and were not entitled to be treated as prisoners of war unless they repented. They would be held in solitary confinement, and they would discuss their alleged crimes with the interrogators until they were ready to confess them. Then, as repentent criminals, there might be some hope for them. The total range of pressure is vividly described in the review of Hinkle and Wolff[13].

Of the 83 Air Force personnel subjected to coercion to confess to having engaged in BW, all were compelled to undergo a considerable degree of isolation. A number of other techniques were also employed in an effort to elicit compliance, but the use of isolation was one technique that appears to have been employed in virtually every case wherein a centrally-directed attempt was made to elicit a confession of germ warface. Clearly the Communists regarded isolation as a valuable means of increasing the influenceability of individuals in their control.

Another very common method was to attempt to get a great bulk of information about the prisoner and to prepare the usual extensive life history. A tremendous repetitive barrage of questions accompanied these maneuvers. There seemed to be a particular desire on the part of the captor to elicit a feeling or admission of guilt on the part of the prisoner for some act that he had committed at some time in his life; if not an act, then an attitude or compliance with some form of social injustice, etc. An effort was then made to generalize from the legitimate confession and the legitimate guilt in such a way as eventually to bring about a general feeling of guilt and a confession of some type that could be used for propaganda purposes.

The captors constantly attempted to focus the attention of the prisoner on what they defined as his predicament, his case, or his problem. He was constantly reminded of his complete dependence on his captors. In addition there was a clear-cut restriction of all types of sensory experience. There was also a systematic debility produced by a limited diet, prolonged interrogation under extreme tension, sleep deprivation, etc. There were constant attempts to induce anxiety and despair. The pattern of debility, dependency, and dread has been tagged "*DDD*" and analyzed elsewhere[17].

A particularly effective means of inducing pain and fatigue was to subject a prisoner to prolonged interrogation while forcing him to maintain a standing position. The prisoner nearly invariably tried to obey the strict command to remain standing. The chief coercion to make the prisoner maintain this position seems to have been in the form of contumely and minor physical abuse. It was very rare that a prisoner was able to perceive that the enemy was in effect making him torture himself. Thus a considerable conflict was aroused in terms of the prisoner's attempts to remain standing (hence continuing to suffer the severe pains that often accompanied this position after many hours) and his desire to obtain rest and relief. The interrogator seemingly remained aloof from this conflict, and merely continued the endless barrage of questions often so obscure as to make it difficult for the prisoner to understand even what was expected of him.

When, after weeks or months, a POW finally complied to the extent that he agreed to sign a confession of germ warfare, this was not sufficient. For a long time subsequently he was pressed to elaborate: "Who directed this activity? When did you engage in it? What kind of germ bomb did you use? What were the targets? How many missions did you fly that were bacteriological warfare missions?" and so forth, expanding the bulky documented confession and attempting to make it sound as plausible as possible or to link it to other confessions which had been obtained. Some of these confessions were used to lecture other POWs about BW. They were also used in the attempt to provide "*scientific*" documentation of the BW charges by bringing them before what the Communists called the International Scientific Investigatory Commission, (consisting of Communists and fellow-travelers from various countries) which was brought to Korea to conduct the so-called impartial investigation of these charges.

People who completed BW confessions were faced with continuing demands of various kinds by the Communists on the BW issue right up to the last day of their internment. Immediately before their release there was an attempt to make all of these confessions (which had many inconsistencies in them) jibe with each other. During the Big Switch repatriation each of the people who had completed one of these BW confessions was again interrogated and

17. FARBER, I. E., HARLOW, H. F., and WEST, L. J. Brainwashing, Conditioning, and DDD (Dependency, Debility, and Dread). *Sociometry*. In press.

forced to sign a new confession which had some inconsistent details of the old one taken out and new details put in. The POW was usually tried, found guilty, and sentenced to a prison term which was "leniently" changed to "deportation" at the time of repatriation.

Needless to say, many of these men attempted to include implausible material in their so-called confessions. They dreamed up weapons and munitions that were fantastic. They included information such as speeds and altitudes for various aircraft that were impossible. They tried to figure out the areas of technical ignorance of the interrogator and to incorporate details in their documents which he would not be able to detect, but which would be palpably false for any informed person.

Rewards for cooperation were symbolic rather than real and were unpredictably bestowed. For example, a man might be given a holiday meal to celebrate some Chinese or American holiday just before a new bout of interrogation. This was to symbolize the "good treatment" he might receive. The accomplishment of the "confession" frequently resulted in further symbols of good treatment being accorded to the POW who "confessed". However, his overall treatment was not markedly different from that of his fellows.

From the point of view of learning theory, the uncertain and frequently haphazard nature of the rewards could be expected to have two separable but related consequences. First, since rewards were not consistently associated with any particular mode of response in particular situations, any learning that occurred must have been of a very general sort, namely, understanding, anticipating, and complying with anything one's captors might require. Under these conditions, the significant cues reside in the attitude of the captor. What is learned is to satisfy the interrogator, regardless of the particular responses demanded. Second, once expectancy of reward and the skills necessary to the attainment of reward have been learned under these conditions, their very irregularity would tend to increase the persistence of both expectancy and skill. If one may generalize on the basis of many laboratory experiments with both animal and human subjects, partial and irregular reinforcement of the sort experienced by the POWs would make learning difficult, but once accomplished, both expectancies (classical conditioned responses) and skills (instrumental acts) would be extraordinarily resistant to extinction.

From the point of view of dynamic psychology, the factors involved in the compliance and resistance of any given individual can best be understood in terms of characterological personality features and the relative effectiveness of various ego defenses. It would be naive in the light of our present knowledge of individual cases to equate any ultimate adaptive modality under this type of extreme stress with any previously existing classification of personality. I shall postpone further comment on this until the discussion period.

It is difficult to determine which among various factors in each case of a false confession were the ones crucial to the individual's final compliance. The factors most frequently mentioned by "confessors" as crucial or final were: 1) fear of non-repatriation; 2) fear of death; 3) the feeling of not being able to hold out indefinitely under pressure; and 4) hope of being treated as "a regular prisoner of war". That there were other factors of an unconscious nature will be discussed subsequently.

It now appears that most of the threats of death and non-repatriation made by the Communists against those whom they had pressured for false BW confessions were bluffs. It seems likely that some of those who confessed would not have done so if they had realized what would actually have occurred had they continued to resist. The threat of interminable interrogation would have proved untrue in many cases. It appears that if some of those who confessed had held out for only a short while longer they would have been spared further pressure to confess. This is almost certainly true of the group of prisoners who agreed to confess shortly before the deadline for their repatriation. Some of the prisoners who were subjected to pressure for BW confessions thought of the cases of Mindzenty, Oatis, Voegler, and others. "If these people could eventually be forced to confess", they thought, "how can *I* hope to resist?" However, on the basis of Korean war experience alone, one might predict that attempts to elicit confessions would persist for 12 weeks or more in less than 50 per cent of the cases, and for 24 weeks or more in only about 15 per cent of the cases.

The experiences of Air Force prisoners of war in Korea who were pressured for false confessions enabled Biderman[14] to compile an outline of the methods that were used to elicit compliance from them.

TABLE II

EIGHT COMMUNIST COERCIVE METHODS FOR ELICITING INDIVIDUAL COMPLIANCE*

METHOD	VARIANTS	EFFECTS
1. ENFORCING TRIVIAL DEMANDS	Enforcement of minute rules and schedules. Forced writing.	Develops habit of compliance.
2. DEMONSTRATING "OMNIPOTENCE" & "OMNISCIENCE"	Confrontations. Pretending to take co-operation for granted. Demonstrating complete control over victim's fate. Tantalizing with possible favors.	Suggests futility of resistance.
3. OCCASIONAL INDULGENCES	Unpredictable favors. Rewards for partial compliance. Promises of better treatment. Fluctuation of captor's attitude. Unexpected kindness.	Provides positive motivation for compliance. Reinforces learning. Impairs adjustment to deprivation.
4. THREATS	Of death or torture. Of non-repatriation. Of endless isolation and interrogation. Against family or comrades. Mysterious changes of treatment. Vague but ominous threats.	Cultivates anxiety, dread, and despair.
5. DEGRADATION	Prevention of personal hygiene. Filthy, infested surroundings. Demeaning punishments. Various humiliations. Taunts and insults. Denial of privacy.	Makes continued resistance seem more threatening to self-esteem than compliance. Reduces prisoner to concern with "animal" values.
6. CONTROL OF PERCEPTIONS	Darkness or bright light. No books or recreations. Barren environment. Monotonous food. Restricted movement. Absence of normal stimuli.	Fixes attention on predicament. Fosters introspection. Frustrates all actions not consistent with compliance. Eliminates distractions.
7. ISOLATION	Complete physical isolation. Solitary confinement. Semi-isolation. Isolation of small groups.	Develops intense concern with self. Deprives victim of social support. Makes victim dependent on interrogator.

TABLE II (*Continued*)

8. INDUCED DEBILITATION AND EXHAUSTION	Semi-starvation. Exposure. Exploitation of wounds. Induced illness. Prolonged constraint. Prolonged standing. Sleep deprivation. Prolonged interrogation or forced writing. Overexertion. Sustained tension.	Weakens physical and mental ability to resist.

*Adapted from Biderman.

Table II shows a modified version of this outline. In studying this outline it should be kept in mind that it is still unclear whether these methods were undertaken knowingly to produce the precise effects described. The methods turned out to be not very different from those reported by persons held by Communists of other nations or in the management of ground forces personnel and civilian captives of the Communist Chinese. In this regard, the reports by Hinkle and Wolff[13], Lifton[7,8], and Schein[9,10,11,12] are particularly instructive.

In reviewing the individual accounts of the men who were subjected to systematic attempts by the Communists to extort false confessions, it becomes clear that there was no such thing as 100 per cent compliance or 100 per cent effective resistance. There are many examples of individual ingenuity, courage, and even heroism. In spite of debility, dependency, and dread; in spite of many threats against the prisoner's life; in spite of threats of reprisals against other prisoners and against the prisoner's own family through "Communist underground forces in the U. S."; in spite of dozens of tailor-made rationalizations; in spite of fears of deformity or chronic pain from untreated medical and surgical conditions; in spite of isolation and sleeplessness and deprivation and torture of many kinds; in spite of all the maneuvers of a wily and determined captor, every prisoner was able to draw upon sufficient inner resources to exercise a certain amount of resistance for a certain period of time.

Repatriates have often been called upon to explain why they *complied* with the enemy's demands to the degree that they did. Why did they *resist* the enemy's demands to the degree that they did? A list of reasons for resistance has been complied (in large part from spontaneous references in interviews). The list includes the following factors: 1) Moral and duty obligations; 2) Altruistic calculations in terms of national interest and the interest of fellow prisoners; 3) Self-interested calculations in terms of fear of "getting in deeper and deeper", and in terms of fear of official punishment sooner or later for collaborating; 4) Social pressures in terms of the relationships with other prisoners and fear of reprisals from them; 5) Emotional considerations, including feelings of pride, dignity, and self-respect; hatred of the enemy, of Communism, or of the specific individual making the demands; and a sense of outrage or righteous indignation that sometimes was the last remaining potent factor enabling a man to resist his tormentors.

There were additional important conscious and unconscious factors at work that can be understood only in terms of individual cases.

Some degree of cooperation was universal, since some degree of communication (and hence collaboration) was necessary to obtain any need or satisfaction. For example, prisoners felt that they would have to say something favorable in order to get a letter out. Everyone who did so in effect wrote and signed a propaganda statement available for use by the enemy. Furthermore, once a letter had been written there was apt to seem nothing wrong with making a recording saying the same thing. Then the Communists might suggest that it would be better to substitute for the term "Commies" the term "Chinese People's Volunteers", since that was their official name. Even if a man had put nothing at all into the body of his letter that might be useful as propaganda, his address itself was a propaganda slogan, i.e., "care of the Chinese People's Committee for World Peace". It was to that address that every parent and loved one of an American prisoner was required to send mail.

TABLE III
RESPONSES TO DEMANDS FOR FALSE CONFESSIONS: RESISTANCE AND COMPLIANCE*

COMPLETE RESISTANCE	Refuses to cooperate in interrogation.
	Refuses to engage in any discussion with interrogator.
	Refuses to affirm or deny accusations or respond to implicit accusations.
	Ridicules accusations; refuses to discuss them seriously.
	Responds with indignation to accusations.
DEFENSIVE RESISTANCE	Makes simple denial of accusation.
	Denies that captor has moral or factual basis for making accusation.

*After Biderman.

TABLE III (*Continued*)

	Makes statements and deposition to prove innocence.
	Makes statement that suspicion was reasonable, "investigation" fair and justified, but protests innocence.
DEFENSIVE COMPLIANCE	Makes statement of possibility that "crime" was unwittingly committed.
	Makes statement of "objective guilt"; i.e., that results were "criminal" irrespective of the motives.
	Makes ambiguous statements, containing no explicit admissions, but which constitutes a "confession" by implication.
	Agrees to comply, but fails to carry through; e.g., writes "confession," but refuses to sign it.
	Makes obviously unacceptable "sabotaged" confession; i.e., makes deposition with obvious inconsistencies, contradictions, or indications that it was obtained through coercion.
	Accuses associates, but maintains own innocence.
	Makes incomplete "confession," i.e., simple admission of acts without supporting details required to make "confession" convincing and without expressions of "repentence," makes statement rationalized as "harmless."
	Makes "compromise" deposition; bargains with interrogator for acceptance of "confession" of lesser crime, or for altering details of deposition to make it less offensive.
	Alternately "confesses" or retracts.
	Completes "acceptable confession," but refuses further cooperation; e.g. refuses to implicate others, to make recordings, films, or elaborations of "confession."
ACTIVE COMPLIANCE	"Confesses" to "criminal tendencies"; i.e. makes statement that his attitude was as criminal as if he had actually committed alleged crime.
	Makes "subtly sabotaged" "confession"; i.e., incorporates veiled communications to outsiders, but without making "confession" unacceptable to interrogator.
	Completely cooperates in all explicit demands associated with theme of "confession"; pretends to accept guilt.
	Strives to please captor; to anticipate demands; pretends repentence.
COMPLETE COMPLIANCE	Accepts "objective truth" of "guilt"; shows involuntary symptoms of remorse.
	Accepts "guilt" as literally true.
	Makes behavioral choices indicative of complete identification with and commitment to captor.

Table No. III indicates some varieties of behavior formulated to comprise a range of activity from complete resistance to complete compliance. Of the Air Force cases, behaviors at the extreme of *compliance* did not occur. At the other extreme, behaviors of complete *resistance* occurred only briefly and during the first stages of pressure or when the coercive attempts were unusually brief, unskilled, or prematurely terminated. In all cases where persistent and intensive efforts to extort "confessions" were made by the Communists, final outcomes were distributed through the range of intermediate possibilities. The breadth of this range is indicated by the variety of behaviors listed in Table III.

Among the Air Force prisoners pressured for false confessions in North Korea and in Communist China, there were cases of incredible fortitude and attachment to principle in the face of overwhelming pressure. There were also a few cases of surprising inability to withstand coercion. Depending upon how one chooses to draw the line, it is possible to say truthfully that *all* personnel resisted, or that *all* complied, for the behavior of every man involved at some point a mixture of compliance and resistance. We think it is fair to say that in most cases, including those who signed confessions, resistance was the dominant ingredient.

From the foregoing, it can be seen that the experiences of the Air Force prisoners were somewhat divergent from those of the Army prisoners. The Air Force captives were singled out for more intensive pressures and attempts at exploitation of individuals. They were much more frequently in solitary confinement and spent long periods under intensive interrogation. Air Force prisoners were generally in some form of isolation. This varied from complete solitary confinement, in which the prisoner saw nobody at all for long periods, to a less intensive extreme of isolation in which there was limited contact with other people. But most of the prisoners who were exploited in the centrally-directed bacteriological warfare propaganda campaign never saw an organized camp.

For these reasons, as well as others, it is not possible to conduct a meaningful statistical comparison of the behavior of 235 Air Force prisoners with the behavior of the much larger group of more than 4,000 Army prisoners. For example, there were some 13 "educational" courses that were taught to Americans in the large POW camps. Relatively few Air Force prisoners were subjected to these compulsory group indoctrination sessions. There were some voluntarily organized indoctrination groups among POWs subsequently classified as collaborators or "progressives". As far as we know, there were no Air Force personnel in such groups. The Air Force prisoners were almost automatically considered "reactionaries" and treated accordingly.

None of the airmen who eventually signed confessions, and who even thereafter gave lectures on BW, appeared sincerely to accept the status of a teacher of Communism or of a reformed criminal. The behavior of these airmen can best be understood as that of individuals who, having finally submitted to pressure to comply, attempted to maintain a status which appeared to be consistent with survival and for which it was possible to muster up rationalizations.

None of the 235 Air Force men who were returned by the Chinese Communists have been tried by courts-martial. A number met a board of inquiry; ten of these subsequently resigned or were separated under honorable conditions. This has been the subject of considerable discussion, inasmuch as the Army prepared at least 54 cases for courts-martial, more than 14 of which have already been presented, with 9 convictions to date. In this regard, I think it is fair to say that none of the captured airmen were "progressives" in the same sense that certain groups of other captives were. But these other captives were subjected to group pressures, which were in some ways different from the pressures exerted on the Air Force personnel. Thus some of the Army POWs appeared to give active cooperation to the enemy without being severely pressured to do so, a circumstance which is not too surprising in view of the size and unselected nature of the group as a whole. We know of no Air Force prisoners of war who engaged in voluntary pro-Communist oratorical contests, debating societies, dramatic productions etc. But there is much that remains to be understood about such behavior before a complete interpretation of it can be made, or final blame assigned.

Miller[16] pointed out some fallacies in the arguments of those who feel that blame is easily fixed in the cases of those who have undergone pressures, the effects of which are still not fully understood; I agree with Miller's conclusion that the relatively non-punitive approach by the Air Force toward those who signed false confessions is, at this stage of our knowledge, completely justified.

Moderator Lilly: Dr. Lawrence Hinkle has recently published a paper with Dr. Harold Wolff on indoctrination. Until quite recently their material has been classified by the Department of Defense. Dr. Hinkle has been invited to discuss the general problems.

Dr. Lawrence E. Hinkle, Jr.: I appreciate very much the opportunity to be here and to talk to the group at GAP about a subject of such great interest to all of us. Perhaps my excuse for being here is the fact that during the period from late 1953 until the early part of this year I was what you might call a "co-ordinator" of a group of some 20 investigators, both within and outside the government, who attempted to bring together the available information on the methods of interrogation and indoctrination that are used by Communist state police. This group was under the direction of Dr. Harold Wolff[1].

At the outset, I wish to pay tribute to the many selfless and able people who assisted in the gathering of the information upon which our report was based. For security reasons these people must remain anonymous. I cannot tell you too much about our sources, except to say that we did have access to information from sources available to the government; but I can give you some general outlines of these sources. The information about the details of the Communist arrest and interrogation systems and a great deal of the information about the purposes, the attitudes, and the training of those who administer these systems, were obtained from people whom I shall call experts in that area. The knowledge of the prisoner's reactions to his experiences was obtained by the direct observation of persons recently released from Communist prisons. Some of these observations continued for weeks, or even months, and were supplemented by follow-up observation periods months later. These included, in many cases, complete physical, neurological and psychiatric examinations, and psychological testing, as well as the testimony of friends, family, associates, and the like.

Among those who were studied intensively were military and civilian prisoners of diverse ranks and backgrounds, women as well as men, defectors, resisters, persons who were allegedly "brainwashed" and "not brainwashed", some people who admittedly co-operated with their captors and some who said they did not.

In supplementing this we made extensive use of the excellent information gathered by the United States Army and the United

1. HINKLE, L. E., Jr. and WOLFF, H. G. Communist Interrogation and Indoctrination of "Enemies of the State." *Arch. Neurol. and Psychiat.*, *76*: 115-174, August 1956.

States Air Force, some of which you have heard presented here today, as well as the material assembled for the Defense Advisory Committee on prisoners of war[2,3]. The very large and, I might say, very illuminating published literature was also drawn upon.

In general, it is our conclusion that the evidence from all of these sources is quite consistent, and that it provides a basis for confidence in the statements which we have made.

I want to give special credit to some of the men whose work you have heard presented here today. I think they have added significantly to our knowledge in an area where we constantly need more knowledge.

I cannot go into all of the things that we might say about our own work, but I do believe that the time has come when some conclusions can be generally accepted. The first of these is that the methods of the Russian and satellite state police are derived from age-old police methods, many of which were known to the Czarist Okhrana, and to its sister organizations in other countries.

DIAGRAM 1

BACKGROUND OF COMMUNIST METHODS

15th CENTURY BYZANTINE HERITAGE	1. Unrestricted Autocracy
	2. Internal intrigue and espionage
16th CENTURY	1. Permanent body of private retainers responsible only to Czar
	2. Central control of all aspects of the state
	3. Purges
17th-18th CENTURY	Central Directorate with mission to guard the internal security of the state
19th CENTURY	Most highly organized, effective and powerful secret police of any European state
	1. Sudden arrest
	2. Dossier
	3. Repetitive interrogation
	4. Isolation technique developed

2. Communist Interrogation, Indoctrination, and Exploitation of American Military and Civilian Prisoners, *Hearings before the Permanent Subcommittee on Investigations of the Committee on Government Operations, United States Senate, 84th Congress, Second Session, June 19, 20, 26, and 27, 1956.* U. S. Government Printing Office, Washington 25, D.C.
3. POW: The Fight Continues After the Battle, *The Report of the Secretary of Defense's Advisory Committee on Prisoners of War.* U. S. Government Printing Office, Washington 25, D.C.

DIAGRAM 2

BACKGROUND OF COMMUNIST METHODS

20th CENTURY CHEKA	1. Highly organized and refined methods 2. Communist ideology and logic 3. Abandonment of direct brutality 4. Development of persuasion techniques; exploitation of intimate interrogator-prisoner relationship
OGPU—NKVD—MVD (KGB)	1. Purges 2. Public trials 3. POW indoctrination (exposure to nothing but communist interpretation of history and current events)
CHINESE SYSTEM	1. Group pressures 2. Self and group criticism (Applied to non-party personnel and to prisoners) 3. Prisoner indoctrination Rote learning Autobiography and diary writing

During the 20th Century, first the Cheka, then the OGPU, NKVD, MVD, and now the KGB have systematized these methods. Nevertheless, they remain police methods. They are not dependent upon drugs, hypnotism or any other special procedure designed by scientists. No scientists took part in their design; nor do scientists take part in their operation. I confess to you that establishing a negative conclusion of this nature is difficult. I can only tell you that we have critically reviewed all of the information that we could get our hands on, and this is our conclusion.

DIAGRAM 3

A TYPICAL TIME TABLE
EASTERN EUROPEAN SECRET POLICE SYSTEMS (COMMUNIST)

Weeks			*Steps*			*Reaction of prisoner*
0	1.		Suspicion		P	Anxiety
1	2.		Accumulation of evidence		R	Suspense
2			Surveillance		O	Awareness of being avoided
3			Reports of informers		G	Feelings of unfocused guilt
4			Seizure of associates		R	Fear and uncertainty
5	3.		Seizure		E	Bewilderment
	4.		Detention		S	Hyperactivity
6					S	Diminishing activity
		I	Rigid regimen		I	Increasing depression
7	5.	S			V	Fatigue (pain)
		O	Increasing pressure		E	Humiliation, loss of self esteem
		L				Filth, mental dulling
		A		I		Despair
		T		N		Frustration tolerance
8		I		T		greatly reduced
		O		E	D	Great need to talk
		N		R	I	Utter dependence on anyone
				R	S	who "befriends"
9				O	O	Much more pliable
	6.			G	R	Great need for approval
				A	G	of interrogator
				T	A	Repeatedly frustrated
10				I	N	By interrogator's refusal to
				O	I	accept statements
				N	Z	By interrogator's alternating
					A	"help" and withdrawal of approval
					T	Increased suggestibility
					I	Confabulation
					O	Rationalization
	7.		Deposition		N	Profound relief
11						
	8.		Respite			
12	9.		Trial "confession"			
	10.		Punishment			

The essential feature of these methods is isolation and repetitive interrogation, the use of much personal history material; all of this carried out in an atmosphere productive of fatigue, sleep loss, and the various forms of physiological disturbance which can be produced by hunger, cold, unusual positions and the like. Prominent features of the reactions of the prisoner are anxiety, uncertainty, and intolerable discomfort. If this regimen is carried forward long enough it usually leads to mental dulling, confusion, loss of discrimination and despondency, associated with an intense desire to escape from the situation; and the ultimate result of this type of pressure is a state of delirium, associated with hallucinatory and delusional experiences. In this setting a "protocol" (or "confession" as our people customarily call it) is prepared. This is usually based upon what I call an "attractive rationalization", which is made possible by the relationship between the prisoner and the interrogator. It is obtained by a mixture of persuasion, pressures, and alternating rejection and reward on the part of the interrogator. The effects of this are made very much more potent by the state of demoralization and dependency in which the prisoner exists.

Prisoner of war interrogation has been described ably by Dr. West and Dr. Schein. We know that the attempts of armies to gain converts from their captives are nothing new in history. They have gone on for many, many years in the past, often with remarkable success. Such attempts were a feature of the Communist armies during the 1917 revolutions, and in the civil war of 1918-1920 in Russia. The modern methods utilized by the Russians were developed by the NKVD for the management of German prisoners of war in the latter part of the Second World War. These methods were later applied to Japanese captives. Information about them was transmitted from the Russians to the Chinese.

The Chinese, themselves, had already developed some of their own methods. As you will recall, following the break with the KMT, Mao Tse-tung's army retreated first to Southeast China, where it maintained itself in a hilly mountainous region for a period of some six or eight years before making the long march to the Northwest. Even at this time the Chinese were making active efforts to convert troops they captured and to indoctrinate the population which they controlled. Their methods, as Dr. Lifton has rightly pointed out, were based upon old Chinese methods of persuasion and pedagogy. Much of the rote learning and repetition which goes into them is taken directly from the Chinese traditional educational procedures.

In the period from 1936 onward, while the Chinese Communists were in Northwest China, they had the advantage of contact with the Russian Communists. It is quite evident that the information and experience of the Russians was transmitted to the Chinese Communists during this time.

In the development of their state police methods the Chinese Communists have also drawn upon the experience of the Russian state police, and indeed have been instructed by them. One finds occasional instances, especially in the dealing with prisoners of importance, in which the Russian methods and the Chinese methods are very much the same.

DIAGRAM 4

A TYPICAL TIME TABLE
CHINESE COMMUNIST SECRET POLICE SYSTEM

Weeks	*Steps*		*Reaction of prisoners*
0	1. Suspicion		Anxiety and suspense
1	2. Preparation for arrest:		
2 3 4	Denunciation by neighbors and associates covertly and at local group criticism sessions.		Awareness of being avoided Feelings of unfocused guilt
	Restrictions and annoyance by police.		
5	3. Seizure under dramatic circumstances Initial interrogation by 3 "judges".	VARIABLE	Fear, complete uncertainty as to fate
	4. House arrest		Reaction like that of KGB prisoner, leaving subject feeling defeated, humiliated, mentally dull, pliable and with great need for talk and approval.
±17 TO	5. Sudden transfer to detention prison Isolation resembling KGB procedure		
±20	6. Transfer to group cell Total absence of privacy		Emotional nakedness Unfocused feelings of guilt and unworthiness
	Rejected, Reviled, Humiliated, Brutalized — By fellow prisoners because of background and attitudes.		Helpless, degraded
	Public self- and group criticism Diary and autobiography writing		Increasing dejection, fatigue, sleep loss, pain, hunger, weight loss, mental dulling, confusion (occasional delirium)
	Constant reading, discussion and repetition of communist material, with total absence of other information		Increasing difficulty in discriminating between this material and that from earlier memory.
	Intermittent sessions with one or more interrogators		Attempts at self justification.

DIAGRAM 5

A TYPICAL TIME TABLE
CHINESE COMMUNIST SECRET POLICE SYSTEM

24	7. Preparation of "confession" (Some fellow prisoners sincerely helpful) Some respite from pressures	Hopeful, rationalizes, thankful for kindness and help and may acknowledge apparent dedication and idealism of his "teachers".
TO	8. Rejection of "confession" by interrogator	Hopes dashed.
	9. Resumption of pressures in group cell	Alternating hopefulness, frustration and degradation
	10. Preparation of new "confession"	
	11. Rejection of new "confession"	
100	(9, 10, and 11 may be repeated as many as 3 to 6 times over as many as 4+ years. Usual duration, 6 months to 2 years.)	
	12. Final achievement of "proper" attitude and acceptable "confession"	By rationalization, and tentative partial belief is able to conform and obtain group acceptance and approval
TO	Group acceptance and approval	Profound relief
	13. Continued study and discussion of Communist materials	
	14. "Trial" and "confession"	
250	15. Release, or punishment	Gradual readjustment of attitudes and behavior to the new reality situation.

However, in general it can be said that there are some significant differences between what the Chinese do and what the Russians do. The KGB, which is the present designation for the Russian state police, has as the goal of its procedure the production of a satisfactory protocol on which a so-called "trial" can be based. The Chinese have as an additional goal the production of long lasting changes in the basic attitudes and behavior of the prisoner. The Chinese use isolation, but it is not a necessary part of their handling of prisoners. More characteristically they make intensive use of group interaction; they put much greater dependence on the disorganization produced by the effects of doubt, rejection and hostility by a group, and by complete lack of privacy. They use public self-criticism and group criticism which, as Dr. Lifton has correctly pointed out, is derived from a Communist party practice that antedates the Bolshevik Revolution in Russia. The Chinese use self-criticism and group criticism as means of indoctrinating non-party persons, prisoners and the general population itself. The adaptation is Chinese, and a very effective one. The Chinese also use diary writing and rote learning, and they may greatly prolong the detention period.

There are some things that can be said to our comfort about all of these methods. First of all, none of them produce any detectable changes in brain function other than those secondary to organic brain damage. Secondly, they produce only variable changes in attitudes and behavior in those people who have been held in prison or other controlled environments and then released. These changes are not predictable in terms of the methods used; but, as Dr. West has accurately pointed out, and Dr. Schein also, the results are dependent upon many factors having to do with the personality, the character structure, and the immediate situation of the prisoner, as well as what was done to him. Change in attitudes and behavior produced by these methods are usually of much smaller degree than is generally supposed. In our experience they are relatively transient. After a period that can be measured in months the former prisoner tends to revert to attitudes roughly similar to those that he held prior to his imprisonment. Finally, these changes are, I think, entirely comprehensible as an aftermath of the experiences that the prisoner went through.

I believe it is safe to say that we know the methods that are used, and that neither we, nor those who use these methods, understand entirely why men behave as they do when exposed to them. This is the question before us at the present time.

Moderator Lilly: Thank you, Dr. Hinkle.

In the sense that George Orwell wrote a handbook for brainwashing I believe that the literature that is coming out at the present time, including that which we have heard here today, can be said to be a handbook on what brainwashing is rather than on what one fantasies it can be. I hope that this material does not help those who use the methods to sharpen up their technique to make them more effective. We hope instead it will bring worldwide discredit on any one who uses such methods.

Dr. Wedge would like to open the general discussion.

Dr. Bryant Wedge: I would like to congratulate the excellent panel for their sound discussion of this subject. One aspect of the subject which seems important in our planning but which was not discussed is the problem of means of defense against totalitarian indoctrination. I would like to summarize briefly some views about means of resistance derived from experience with repatriated POWs.

The experience is this: for ten days I spent the waking hours with the twenty-three repatriated POWs who had been exchanged in Operation Little Switch and who had been immediately transferred to Valley Forge Army Hospital as being the most thoroughly indoctrinated repatriates. At that time I was myself a patient which permitted a closeness of observation not otherwise possible. In subsequent months I was able to compare them with thirty other repatriates who had more or less successfully resisted indoctrination. While I certainly agree with much that has been said today about the nature of those individuals more subject to indoctrination than others (especially in regard to social isolation), I would particularly like to mention the issue of psychological means of defense against indoctrination of prisoners.

The process of indoctrination depends heavily upon the captors being able to convey an impression of omnipotent control. Hence the prisoner who is able to maintain a secret, internal, private *sense of psychological superiority* to his captors is immensely armored from indoctrination. Such a private sense of psychological superiority depends on the fact that every prisoner has unique knowledge and unique experience which is not shared by his captors. Particularly if the prisoner is in a group of other prisoners, he is able to develop methods of communication which exclude the captors and demonstrate their fallibility.

Some of the devices which were developed spontaneously in the Korean POW situation proved quite effective in maintaining the sense of personal identity which accompanies demonstrations of private secrets and undermines the myth of the captor's omnipotence. For example, many groups developed special code words which appeared complimentary to the guards, but meant to the prisoners that the captors were very nasty people. Often they misled their guards by teaching them American games with absurd twists of the rules and methods of play and would delight in the deception. At some points the prisoners took advantage of the rules under which they learned the captors operated to show some modest control of the situation. For example, when they discovered that the Chinese guards were forbidden direct physical punishment, some of the prisoners developed techniques of perpetrating petty annoyances which drove the guards to impatient fury from which the prisoners got tremendous teasing pleasure.

While the catalogue of devices for maintaining inner superiority could be greatly extended, I will mention only one other important means. This is the means of misleading by giving inexact information. So long as the POW feels relatively in charge of the kind of information which he reveals he is relatively protected from the serious effects of failure to maintain inner control. Unfortunately, the Military Service Code of Conduct for Prisoners of War instructs him to give only his name, rank and serial number so long as he is able to resist. This rule is almost impossible to maintain for any length of time under the conditions of captivity imposed in Korea. This rule deprives the prisoner of his ability to keep inner secrets or to mislead the enemy, no matter how slightly. While it is almost always possible to force a man to talk, it is much less easy to evaluate what he says, and knowledge of this fact may be greatly supportive to maintaining the private sense of superiority which enables a prisoner to resist indoctrination.

I feel, with Dr. James Miller, that this particular section of the Code of Conduct should be reviewed and altered in view of the kind of facts which have been brought out here today.

Dr. James G. Miller: I have found in talking to a number of my colleagues in the psychiatric profession that they have not been generally aware of the policy developments in our country relating to this problem of "brainwashing". Dr. Hinkle and Dr. Wolff and others whom you have seen, have testified before the Advisory Committee on Prisoners of War of the Department of Defense, attempting to aid that committee to resolve differences among the Armed Forces, differences with which our GAP Committee in co-operation with Government (Federal) Agencies or perhaps the Committee on Social Issues might well concern themselves.

The Air Force and Admiral Dan Gallery of the Navy took one position; the rest of the Navy and the Army took the other. The Army and Navy won out over the Air Force, and in August, 1955, President Eisenhower signed an executive order establishing the new code for prisoners of war which essentially forbids them from talking freely and directs them to use their moral stamina and patriotic force to withstand the various forms of brainwashing to which they may be submitted. We cannot discuss this at any length now. It is a complex and subtle issue but it is a matter with which GAP might be concerned. It has seemed to me—and I have had no direct association with it myself—that the representatives of our profession, including Dr. Hinkle and others, agreed more or less in testifying before the Advisory Committee that every man does have his breaking point. The report that was written to the Secretary of Defense was a highly literate and informed document which made obeisance to this viewpoint and then completely contradicted it in the final decision, accepting rather the traditional views held by Marine generals that moral strength can enable servicemen to resist any sort of brainwashing and similar views advocated by religious persons who testified before the Committee.

I think it is important to consider this as an issue in psychiatry, recognizing a potential future which may be decades off but which nevertheless is foreshadowed by developments like the work of Dr. Lilly[1] and Dr. Hebb[2] and others on sensory deprivation, work on psychopharmaceuticals which we now have and others which are undoubtedly to come, and work on electrical stimulation of the brain.

As Dr. Hinkle has said, these methods so far as we know have not yet been applied, at least extensively, in brainwashing. When

---

1. LILLY, J. C. Mental Effects of Reduction of Ordinary Levels of Physical Stimuli on Intact, Healthy Persons. *Psychiatric Research Reports 5*, American Psychiatric Assoc., 1-28, June, 1956.
2. BEXTON, W. H., HERON, W., and SCOTT, T. H. Effects of Decreased Variation in the Sensory Environment. *Canad. J. Psychol., 8*:70-76, 1954.

they will first begin to use them we do not know. It is quite possible, and frightening, that in some period not too far off some of these methods may be employed. (I am continuously using phrases to limit the potential meaning of this because it can be harmfully and unjustifiably magnified in the popular mind.) If so, the question of whether the military can order one of our prisoners of war to withstand these influences must be faced in the same way that we may ask whether it is legitimate for an officer to order a GI to stand at attention under the influence of ether.

There are complex moral issues which I think personally — and I suspect many of my psychiatric colleagues would agree — are best represented by the Air Force point of view, which at the moment is the minority viewpoint in the Department of Defense and does not represent the official policy of our country.

Moderator Lilly: Dr. West wishes to reply to Dr. Miller's question.

Dr. West: I would like to say one thing for the edification of this group in regard to the Code of Conduct. This is not intended in any way to support "Air Force arguments" against the views of any other group. In the military services the Code is now established — the decision about it has been made by the President — and unless the Code is modified all branches of the service will abide by it.

I am sure that most of you have seen the Code. It says: "1) I am an American fighting man. I serve in the forces which guard my country and our way of life. I am prepared to give my life in their defense. 2) I will never surrender of my own free will. If in command, I will never surrender my men while they still have the means to resist. 3) If I am captured I will continue to resist by all means available. I will make every effort to escape and aid others to escape. I will accept neither parole nor special favors from the enemy. 4) If I become a prisoner of war, I will keep faith with my fellow prisoners. I will give no information or (SIC) take part in any action which might be harmful to my comrades. If I am senior, I will take command. If not I will obey the lawful orders of those appointed over me and will back them up in every way. 5) When questioned, should I become a prisoner of war, I am bound to give only name, rank, service number, and date of birth. I will evade answering further questions to the utmost of my ability. I will make no oral or written statements disloyal to my country and its allies or harmful to their cause. 6) I will never forget that I am an American fighting man, responsible for my actions, and dedicated to the principles which made my country free. I will trust in my God and in the United States of America."[1]

You will note that the words "to the utmost of my ability" suggest that there are possible limits to the individual's capacity to resist indefinitely. Rather than to specify the total failure of resistance once the "name, rank and serial number" line has been breached, it seems to me that wise training procedures, (such as those used at the Air Force's Survival School) should emphasize the importance of continuing resistance – to the utmost of one's ability – no matter what concessions have been yielded as a result of force and coercion. This makes it possible for the prisoner to resist *in depth* rather than along a certain line rigidly prescribed. He should know many evasions and tricks, ways to outwit the enemy, techniques for maintaining his own integrity. The person who may become a prisoner should be prepared in such a way as to help him to sustain his ego in the face of the kind of assault to which we now realize a captive of the Communists may be subjected, particularly in the case of an Air Force prisoner. Our training procedures should be continually improved to teach every man how to survive with honor.

Moderator Lilly: Thank you Dr. West. Training for raising one's threshold against these procedures is extremely important; selection procedures may also be of great value in the light of finding the resisting groups.

Dr. Goldfarb: Because of the resemblance of some of these processes to what are generally regarded as psychotherapeutic processes, I wonder if the panel could tell us whether those who attempted to comply or resist, those who fell in one of the two extreme groups, had one or many interrogators successively and also whether there was any haphazard or planned attempt on the basis of the interrogation squads to establish relationships between the interrogated and the particular interrogators.

Moderator Lilly: Dr. Hinkle, would you like to comment?

1. U.S. Fighting Man's Code. *Office of Armed Forces Information and Education, Department of Defense,* Nov. 1955.

Dr. Hinkle: I find it very difficult to give any systematic statement about people who did or did not resist. If you study an individual case you can usually comprehend why he did what he did on the basis of the type of man he was, the situation he was in, and what was happening to him at the time; but you cannot divide men into "compliers" or "resisters" simply upon the basis of the methods used upon them. As a matter of fact, I doubt that you could really make too rigid a division on the basis of any one special personality characteristic either — this in spite of the fact, as Dr. Schein has shown us, there are certain discernible trends.

But you can say that among both those who resisted and those who cooperated have been people who have had one interrogator and those who have had several; and any one of a great number of things may have been done to them.

I would like to say a word about this business of a breaking point for every man. I think we all recognize the physiologic fact that by relatively simple means any man can be brought to a state of confusion, mental dulling, and lack of discrimination during which he can be made to comply with some demands of those who have him in their hands. In this sense, of course, every man has his breaking point. Yet even under these circumstances his compliance may be very limited, and not extend beyond the immediate situation. This is a far different matter from active collaboration in the absence of coercion, and is fairly readily distinguished from it. I would also say that most people — even the vast majority — can escape without active collaboration carried to a high degree.

I believe there is an awareness of the complexity of this among those who are concerned with the administration of the Code. I think that there will be a tendency to look upon the Code as an ideal to be attained. When persons are unable to live up to the Code, the circumstances will have to be considered.

PART FOUR

The Threat of Nuclear War

8
THE PSYCHOLOGICAL AND MEDICAL ASPECTS OF THE USE OF NUCLEAR ENERGY*

EDITOR'S NOTE

During 1957-58 several GAP members called attention to the psychological aspects of the nuclear arms race with particular reference to its destructive potential. This interest furnished the stimulus for planning an informal discussion on the subject by GAP on November 9, 1958. Unfortunately, the stenotype record of this discussion was too fragmentary to be published, even with liberal editing. However, Dr. Jerome Frank wrote an excellent article entitled "The Great Antagonism" which appeared in the November, 1958 issue of The Atlantic Monthly. In this presentation, he states some of the major issues, and investigates potential means by which the differences between the United States and Russia may be resolved. The interested reader may refer to this article for background information.

The symposium was presided over by Dr. Dana Farnsworth, and the moderator was Dr. George C. Ham. About twenty discussants participated.

Because very few GAP members had first-hand experience with the complex world of defense preparations as they applied to nuclear weapons and the allied fields of bacterial and chemical warfare, a friend of GAP with much experience, Dr. Franklin C. McLean of the University of Chicago was invited to give a brief historical introduction to the subject preliminary to the informal discussion by members from the floor.

Dr. McLean was well prepared for this large task because he had a long record as a distinguished investigator and scientist in the field of

*The papers that follow were presented at the meetings of GAP in November, 1958, and April, 1959, and were first published as Symposium #6 in July, 1960 .

physiology with many publications, particularly in this field of the skeletal tissues. Due to his eminence as a research scientist and administrator he was entrusted with many important projects and missions by the Atomic Energy Commission during and after the war. He has been the prinicipal investigator in classified projects relating to radiation effects upon biological organisms.

He was Director of the Toxicity Laboratories from 1941-43; Director of a Special A.E.C. Project 1948-51; Director of a special ASAF Project in 1951-54; Consultant to the Sante Fe Operations Office, A.E.C., 1947-49; Member Special Panel A.E.C., Washington, D.C., 1948-50; Deputy Chairman of the Joint Panel on Medical Aspects of Atomic Warfare 1949-53; and continues to serve in similar groups in the warfare office of the Assistant Secretary of Defense.

His most recent book (with M. R. Urist) is the outstanding text BONE: AN INTRODUCTION TO THE PHYSIOLOGY OF SKELETAL TISSUE, *University of Chicago Press, 1955. He has been honored by his government by the Legion of Merit (1954), Army Commendation Ribbon (1947), and War and Navy Departments Certification of Appreciation (1947).*

PSYCHOLOGICAL ASPECTS OF THE NUCLEAR ARMS RACE

Franklin C. McLean

On June 9, 1943, I was scheduled to speak on chemical warfare before a lay audience, as a part of a series entitled *Medicine and the War*. On the day before this, President Roosevelt devoted his press conference to a statement on chemical warfare, with the result that the subject headlined the newspaper and radio programs on the morning of the day I was to talk. One result was that I had to revise my manuscript from beginning to end between the early morning and midafternoon, when I was to speak. I mention this to emphasize how ephemeral everything I have to say today must necessarily be. The psychological aspects of the nuclear arms race may be subjected to complete revision overnight, by the actions or words of the representatives of at least two of the great powers on earth today. The best I can hope to do is to give some account of the current situation, and of the events and attitudes leading up to it.

President Roosevelt, in his press conference of June 8, 1943, used the concept of "massive retaliation", about which we have heard so much in recent years. He said, in part: "any use of gas by any Axis power . . . will immediately be followed by the fullest possible retaliation upon munitions centers, seaports, and other military objectives throughout the whole extent of the territory of such Axis country". He further stated that "the use of such (chemical) weapons has been outlawed by the general opinion of civilized mankind", and that "this country has not used them, and I hope that we never will be compelled to use them. I state categorically that we shall under no circumstances resort to the use of such weapons unless they are first used by our enemies".

Since chemical warfare was not used by either side in World War II, in spite of elaborate preparations for offensive and defensive chemical warfare by all the parties concerned, it would be easy to make a superficial case for the idea either that President Roosevelt's threat of retaliation acted as a deterrent to the use of chemical weapons by the Axis powers, or that the Allies withheld their fire for purely humanitarian reasons—President Roosevelt having referred to chemical warfare as "terrible and inhumane", and as "desperate and barbarous". The evidence, however, is to the effect that the United States did not use chemical warfare for two reasons: first, that it was not effective enough to be decisive, and that we had better weapons in the making; and second, that we did not want to assume the risk of involving England in the enemy's retaliatory raids should we begin it. From the other side, there is good reason to believe that Germany did not start chemical warfare, in spite of its state of preparedness and its discovery and production of more potent agents than were available to the Allies, because of an irrational fear of gas warfare on the part of Hitler, who is said to have been gassed in World War I. This is one instance, among others, in which Hitler's irrationality worked to our advantage, but it does not support the popular view for the failure of either side to initiate chemical warfare in World War II.

I have mentioned chemical warfare, at some length, and I shall have something to say about biological warfare, for the reason that both give us some opportunity to put the relevant psychological factors into proper perspective. While both chemical warfare and biological warfare are being kept alive by us and our allies, and presumably also by any potential enemies, they are not now the subject of constant attention in international affairs. This is not from any humanitarian reasons, but from the fact that atomic warfare offers a threat of such dimensions that the status of any possible competitors has assumed an insignificant place in our thinking.

My title, *Psychological Aspects of the Nuclear Arms Race*, seems simple enough at first sight. But I have read the comments of 67 members of GAP on the letter of Dr. Jerome Frank which initiated the interest of this organization in the subject, and I find that the title means 67 things to 67 different people. As Dr. Farnsworth stated in a circular letter dated July 17, 1958, "the opinions of GAP members cover a wide spectrum". It therefore becomes necessary to break the title down into its constituent parts. Many of those who have written on the subject tend to regard the nuclear arms race as a natural phenomenon, and to concentrate their attention on how to deal with it. Thus—and I am now speaking of members of GAP—we have proposals for the disposal of cities, for innumerable bomb shelters, and even for moving much of our industry to underground locations. Even while this is being written an official plan for the evacuation of large cities in the event of a warning of bombing raids is being made public. All of these proposals involve estimates of many billions of dollars in preparation for offensive and defensive nuclear warfare. Others are concerned with the psychological impact of nuclear arms testing, fallout, and the prospect of actual nuclear warfare on individuals. They think and talk in terms of apathy, denial, projection, and other uses by individuals of techniques of adaptation to the threats and perhaps to the reality of atomic warfare Their interpretation of my title would read *Psychological Reactions to the Nuclear Arms Race.*

I prefer, however, to regard the nuclear arms race—real as it is and real as its possible outcomes may be—as man-made, and to concentrate my attention on the build-up that has led us into the situation in which we find ourselves today. Perhaps I should suggest another title of my own, which might be *Psychological Factors in the Nuclear Arms Race.* I would prefer to examine the possibility of reversibility of some of the trends that have produced the threats with which we have to deal, rather than to regard the nuclear arms race as something that cannot be helped. I cannot pretend to have the answers, but perhaps I can ask some of the pertinent questions.

Atomic warfare was born of World War II. It was conceived in the minds of scientists, who proposed to President Roosevelt that a major effort be made to turn the energy of the atom into devastating weapons of warfare. Out of this came the first atom bombs, dependent upon atomic fission. They had great destructive capacity in comparison with other weapons known at the time, but they were relatively small in relation to what has since been accomplished by fusion. The realities of the situation today can hardly be exaggerated. The potentialities for destruction of human life and of the apparatus of civilization, both by almost incredible explosive properties and by the poisoning of the land and the air, to say nothing of water and food, are such that millions of lives may be wiped out in a matter of hours. The conditions of life on this planet, either short term, because of the immediate effects of the bombs and their radioactive products, or long term, because of the genetic effects to follow, will be radically altered, and perhaps, in large part, made impossible. The answer of the U. S. Atomic Energy Commission to concern over the effects of radioactive fallout (chiefly as strontium 90 resulting from the testing of weapons) is that while this is a real hazard to human life and welfare—and this in countries all over the globe, whether taking any part in the testing or not—the threat is infinitesimal in comparison with that of actual atomic warfare. All of this leads us back to the idea proposed a moment ago, which is that the only hope for mankind is to reverse the trends that appear to be leading us headlong into world-wide catastrophe.

Naturally, this point of view has not escaped attention, even from the first demonstration to the world of the destructive capacities of the atom bomb at Hiroshima and at Nagasaki, although the early efforts to keep atomic energy under control, for peaceful purposes, seem to have been forgotten by many of us. On August 6, 1945, President Truman announced that an American airplane had dropped on Hiroshima a bomb that "had more power than 20,000 tons of TNT", and went on to say that "it is not intended to divulge the technical process of production or all military applications" of this atomic bomb, "pending further examination of possible methods of protecting us and the rest of the world from the danger of sudden destruction". He went on to say that "I shall give further consideration and make further recommendations to the Congress as to how atomic power can become a powerful and forceful influence toward the maintenance of world peace".

Following some preliminary skirmishing, the United Nations Atomic Energy Commission was established by a resolution passed January 24, 1946, by the United Nations General Assembly without a dissenting vote. After two years of wrangling, the United Nations

Atomic Energy Commission was to all intents and purposes killed on May 17, 1948, by a vote of 9 to 2, with only Russia and its Ukranian state voting in the negative. The action taken was a confession of failure and a vote to suspend. On June 22, a month later, the Commission was buried in the Security Council, when Mr. Gromyko cast his 26th veto to kill the majority plan for international control. All that seems to remain of this is the United Nations Scientific Committee on the Effects of Atomic Radiation, which reported August 10, 1958, on the hazards from radioactive fall-out from bomb testing, without direct reference to the far greater peril from the possibility of atomic warfare itself.

While the United Nations Atomic Energy Commission was attempting to carry out its mission of prescribing for the international control of atomic energy, the United States carried out the Bikini tests known as Operation Crossroads, in the Marshall Islands in July, 1946. New atomic weapons were then developed, and in June 1947, President Truman approved a series of tests of these weapons—known as Operation Sandstone—carried out in great secrecy at Eniwetok, also in the Marshall Islands, during the months of April and May 1948. The announcement of these tests, made while the task force was on its way back to Pearl Harbor, and after the vote to suspend the deliberations of the United Nations Atomic Energy Commission, was regarded at the time as the official declaration of the nuclear arms race. The announcement included authorization for the U. S. Atomic Energy Commission for "steps it proposed to initiate at once for further nuclear development based on information gained from the tests". I had the now somewhat dubious privilege of observing some of these tests at first hand, and thus of participating in the official inauguration of the atomic arms race. What has happened since 1948, when efforts at international control were suspended, and the atomic arms race became official, is history familiar to all of you.

It seems hardly necessary to emphasize the fact that while we were negotiating for international control on the one hand, we were actively engaged on the other, in the development of new weapons. While I do not question the good faith of Mr. Baruch, our representative in the negotiations, I did not believe then, and I do not believe now, that our Congress would have approved the majority plan for international control as approved by the United Nations Security Council but vetoed by Mr. Gromyko. We felt much too secure at that time to give up our dominant position.

It now becomes desirable to look into some of the factors that transformed an effort to arrive at international control of atomic energy into an atomic arms race, all within the two short years after the agency to provide for international control was established.

First and foremost, there was the atmosphere of mistrust and suspicion in which the United Nations Atomic Energy Commission had to work. At the time the United States had a monopoly of atomic weapons and know-how, and there was never a serious proposal to relinquish our leadership. In fact Mr. Baruch, the United States representative on the Commission, stated that "before a country is ready to relinquish any winning weapons . . . it must have a guarantee of safety, not only against the offenders in the atomic area, but against the illegal users of other weapons—bacteriological, biological, gas—perhaps—why not?—against war itself. . . . If we succeed in finding a suitable way to control atomic weapons, it is reasonable to hope that we may also preclude the use of other weapons adaptable to mass destruction".

Mr. Baruch was in effect proposing that the Commission consider the limitation and control of all armaments, and in fact of war itself. We shall see later that the nuclear arms race to which our title refers is now indistinguishable from the broader armaments race, which includes every weapon of destruction that mankind can devise. The only reason we are ignoring chemical and biological warfare at the present time is that we are more concerned with guided missiles, jet bombers, and other means of delivering atomic warheads on targets, than we are in these relatively innocuous means of poisoning a potential enemy. In spite of Mr. Baruch's statement, the United Nations Commission never considered anything but atomic energy, although in Mr. Baruch's report entitled THE INTERNATIONAL CONTROL OF ATOMIC ENERGY there is a brief chapter on "Implications of Biological Warfare".

The desire of the United States to retain control of the situation at least until all possible safeguards were in effect, was made explicit in a passage in a report by the then Secretary of State, Dean

Acheson, and the Chairman of the U. S. Atomic Energy Commission, David Lilienthal, as follows: "The scheduling will determine the rapidity with which a condition of international balance will replace the present position. Once the plan is fully in operation it will afford a great measure of security against surprise attack; it will provide clear danger signals and give us time if we take over the available facilities, to prepare for atomic warfare. The significant fact is that at all times during the transition period at least, such facilities will continue to be located within the United States. Thus should there be a breakdown in the plan at any time during the transition, we shall be in a favorable position with regard to atomic weapons".

The Russian reactions to such proposals might have been anticipated. What was not anticipated was the Russian ability to implement its own points of view, by its success in the nuclear arms race, and consequently to be in a position to lead from strength. In the meantime, in October, 1946, Mr. Molotov said: "The American plan, the so-called 'Baruch plan' . . . is based on the desire to secure for the United States the monopolistic possession of the atomic bomb. At the same time it calls for the earliest possible establishment of control over the production of atomic energy in all countries, giving to this control an appearance of international character, but in fact, attempting to protect in a veiled form the monopolistic position of the United States in this field. It is obvious that projects of this kind are unacceptable . . ." He also said, in the same speech: ". . . it should not be forgotten that atomic bombs used by one side may be opposed by atomic bombs and something else from the other side. . ."

Many hundreds of thousands of words have been written about the failure of the United Nations Atomic Energy Commission, and about the efforts that still continue to bring nuclear energy under control—all of these going on simultaneously with all-out efforts to improve nuclear weapons and the means for delivering them on an enemy. For our purpose, that of defining the psychological factors that continue to dominate the nuclear arms race, these hundreds of thousands of words can be boiled down to two—*fear* and *aggression*. We were afraid, and still are, to stop making bombs and developing and testing new weapons, until a world-wide agreement has been reached and we are convinced that it can be enforced. We have convinced ourselves over and over—and as late as within the past few months—that international control is technically possible *provided* that the participating nations are willing to give up their sovereign rights to the necessary extent. There is as yet no evidence that any nation, including ourselves, intends to do just that.

In the meantime the alternative to international control—the nuclear arms race—continues to be inspired by the same fear and by aggressive impulses. We are back at the old concept of balance of power, a concept which has proved illusory more than once. We can feel secure only if we feel strong—and the same holds for any possible enemy.

The international control of atomic energy, even if it could be brought about and successfully implemented, is not synonymous with peace. Neither chemical nor biological warfare, nor any of the more conventional weapons, lends itself to international control, in spite of the pious hopes of Mr. Baruch. It may be assumed that if we could, by any miracle, get away from our preoccupation with atomic weapons, both we and our rivals, assuming that international tensions would still exist, would turn our energies into the most destructive channels that any of us could devise.

The very dimensions of the threat of atomic weapons seem at the moment to be the chief deterrent against their use. We have tactical atomic weapons, and presumably others have them too. These weapons could be useful in the Quemoy affair, but again fear dominates the picture—fear that if we use atomic weapons on a small scale, this will blow the lid off, and lead to all-out atomic warfare. It may be assumed that no one wants to deliberately engage in such a holocaust as is now possible, but the danger of drifting into this or of being drawn into it by accident or by actions of irresponsible persons is very real. Our Armed Forces are now geared to the use of atomic weapons, of all dimensions, and there have been suggestions that if we become actively embroiled in the Formosa-Quemoy area, the military may not be content to withhold the most effective weapons they possess.

This, then, is the present situation. Two potential antagonists, with their allies, are strong and are gaining in strength daily.

Each, in fear of what the other may do, and strongly motivated by aggressive impulses, is maintaining a threatening posture. The history of such situations is that they tend to lead, sooner or later, to open warfare, either by design or by inadvertence. Such open warfare, under present conditions, would quickly arrive at nothing less than a holocaust, out of which no one could emerge the victor.

Is this situation reversible? Can the world, in our time, be restored to a state of relative tranquility or peace, in which the armaments race, including the nuclear arms race, would recede, rather than grow more ominous each day? These are psychological problems. We have the technical capacity to monitor the development, testing and production of nuclear arms. Can the inhabitants of this planet put this to work, and would this be sufficient to ease the tensions with which we are compelled to live? And in this connection let us note that tensions other than the nuclear arms race are at large today. Africa, the Middle East, and all of Asia are embroiled in struggles that have little or no direct relationship to nuclear arms, but which contribute in large part to our state of unrest. We have noted that the nuclear arms race cannot be divorced from the armament race as a whole. And the armament race cannot be separated in our thinking from the rising tide of what, for want of a better term, is commonly called nationalism. The world is sick, and the nuclear arms race is only one symptom—a symptom, it is true, that may lead to the death of a patient.

Let us turn our attention to some attempts that have been made to answer these questions. One of the most serious and most recent attempts was made in a statement of the Third Pugwash Conference of Nuclear Scientists, meeting in Austria during the week of September 14—less than two months ago. The name of the conference is taken from that of a small village in Nova Scotia, where the first such conference was held. The statement was issued under the title "War Prevention and International Cooperation," and was published in the issue of *Science* dated 31 October 1958.

A section of this report carries the heading "Requirements for Ending the Arms Race". It starts with the statement: "The armaments race is the result of distrust between states; it also contributes to this distrust". It continues by noting with satisfaction that unanimous agreement was recently reached by scientists meeting in Geneva about the feasibility of detecting test explosions, and that the governments of the United States, the U.S.S.R., and the United Kingdom have approved the statements and the conclusion contained in the report of the technical experts. It expresses the "hope that this approval will soon be followed by an international agreement leading to the cessation of all nuclear weapon tests and an effective system of control". It sets this forth as "a first step toward the relaxation of international tension and the end of the arms race".

The section closes with the statement: "Recognizing the difficulties of the technological situation, scientists feel an obligation to impress on their peoples and on their governments the need for policies which will encourage international trust and reduce mutual apprehension. Mutual apprehensions cannot be reduced by assertions of good will; their reduction will require political adjustment and the establishment of active cooperation". It should be noted that the entire statement was unanimously adopted by scientists from 18 countries.

Another attempt to answer these questions has been published by your own Jerome D. Frank, in an article in the November 1958 issue of the *Atlantic Monthly*, under the title "The Great Antagonism". In this article Dr. Frank explores the possibility of applying psychotherapeutic principles to today's sick world. He begins by raising the obvious question: "Who is to be the psychotherapist?" and continues by asking: "Who has the confidence of both the United States and Russia, and is viewed by them as competent to resolve their differences"? He suggests that: "The industrially backward and relatively unarmed nations, small and large, who can only lose by a nuclear war may be able through the United Nations gradually to modify the behavior of the major powers". And of interest in connection with the statement from the Pugwash Conference, he states that: "Many nuclear physicists seem able to focus on the welfare of humanity regardless of the side of the Iron Curtain from which they come, and their prestige is great in all nations. That both Russia and the United States agreed to a conference to devise adequate measures of inspection of a test ban on nuclear weapons is a sign that both, at least provisionally, trust the other's scientists as well as their own".

After emphasizing the importance of keeping thinking straight in the present dilemma, and setting forth the relevance of the psychotherapeutic emphasis on improved communication, he calls attention to the need for a "change in our behavior toward Russia today, especially at the conference table," while noting that "beneficial effects of improved communication appear only slowly, (while) the danger increases rapidly". Finally he concludes with the following paragraph:

"If we and Russia can break away from the stereotype of each other as the enemy, we may be able to reach an agreement to stop testing nuclear weapons, with an arrangement for mutual inspection. Regardless of its effect on nuclear armaments, such an agreement, if it worked, would be of the utmost psychological importance. For it would be the first, and therefore the most crucial, step toward the establishment of mutual confidence. Then it would become possible to move further along the road to the ultimate goal: a general system for maintaining world peace and disarmament".

In this conclusion Dr. Frank is in agreement with the nuclear scientists. The conclusion, however, does include a big *IF*, and it is that *IF* that offers a challenge to your organization and to you as individual citizens and psychiatrists. It implies, if not a change in human nature, for which there certainly is no panacea, a change in human behavior which is perhaps more readily realizable. We are balanced between fear and our aggressive impulses. We can only make the most of such institutions as we can devise to maintain the balance, or better to reverse the current trend in international affairs. For this we need public opinion, as well as statesmen to man the institutions.

There are some encouraging signs, which means that the picture is not all black. The League of Nations failed to survive, and to prevent World War II, certainly in part because of our refusal to take part in its activities. The United Nations, in spite of one crisis after another, has so far managed to survive, and has certainly had a degree of success in preventing aggression. Whatever hope we may now have for a stable world rests in international statesmanship, of which the United Nations is the custodian. While the art of brinkmanship may have had some success, it is a dangerous practice—the line between safety and disaster is drawn too fine.

Working against success in arriving at workable international agreements is the isolationism that prevented our joining the League of Nations, and that still persists. This shows itself partly in insidious ways, such as in the pressures that recently led to the discontinuance by one of our major airlines in giving publicity to the United Nations. My impression is that isolationism is less powerful in the United States today than it was following World War I. If this is true, it is an indication that the climate of public opinion is changing for the better in international relations.

Whether we talk in terms of breaking the vicious circle, as Dr. Frank does, or of reversing the current trends, as I prefer to do, it is clear the world needs to take a long hard look at the possible, even probable, consequences of the armaments race, and to devise means to slow it down, or better to end it entirely. GAP has been eminently successful in helping to mold public opinion in other areas, and I see no reason why it should not do so in this situation. This is a problem in human behavior, with which psychiatrists are most familiar and best equipped to deal. Without suggesting how GAP may organize itself to exert its influence toward a better climate, I do want to end with a statement of my belief that this organization can find ways to advance the public interest in this respect.

EDITOR'S NOTE:

Due to the continued interest of GAP members in the problems associated with the use of nuclear energy, another symposium was arranged for the following meeting of GAP on April 5, 1959 on the **PSYCHOLOGICAL AND MEDICAL ASPECTS OF THE USE OF NUCLEAR ENERGY.** ***We were fortunate in being able to have with us three scientists notable in the area and a journalist who has done much work in alerting the public to the hazards involved. Dr. Marion E. Kenworthy presided and Dr. Henry W. Brosin was the Moderator.***

Dr. Brosin: **I shan't try to introduce this symposium in an extended way, because it is actually a continuation of our last one.**

All of us are certainly aware, at least vaguely, of the problems involved with regard to radiation and the psychological and medical aspects of the use of nuclear energy. Our group, and many others like it, is in serious need of information on this vital topic. As nearly as I have been able to gather from the various men who work in this field in its various aspects, we do not have available proper information through the normal media of communication. In short, we are pitifully ignorant, and it was with this thought in mind that the membership felt that another symposium on this topic was in order.

We have had the extraordinary good fortune to have men like Drs. Visscher, Livingston, Appleyard, and Mr. Lorentz give us

their views. They have spent many years, indeed if not their lives, in this area and can give us firsthand information.

Before our speakers begin, I would like to, if I may, give the "commercial". Many of you may not know that the World Health Organization TECHNICAL REPORT SERIES NO. 151 ON NUCLEAR ENERGY is available from Geneva. The psychiatrist in the group, which also had biologists (which as you know is a weak area in many of these study groups) was Dr. Alexander Leighton.

I am also happy to announce that Dr. Maurice Visscher, working under Minnesota Governor Freeman's Atomic Development Problems Committee, has published a very handsome and readable brochure entitled *Basic Data Regarding the Atomic Development Problems in Minnesota.** I am certain that all of you who have a more serious interest in the topic at hand, and want to spread the word and clear the air of the usual myths concerning radiation effects, will be happy that Dr. Visscher and his colleagues have published this report for public use.

Our first speaker is a distinguished man in the field of physiology, a professional biologist, and Professor and Chairman of the Department of Physiology, University of Minnesota. His accomplishments are many, and he belongs to the usual societies. In addition, Dr. Visscher has been the recipient of many honors which I will not take the time here to name.

It is more important that we listen to his findings and hear a synopsis of the serious work he has done in the last three years at the request of Governor Freeman. He will tell us the story of Minnesota with regard to the biological aspects of the use of nuclear energy, and the implications.

---

* Information concerning availability of this report may be obtained by writing to Dr. Robert Barr, Minnesota State Board of Health, Minneapolis 14, Minnesota.

SOME IMPLICATIONS OF THE FALL-OUT PROBLEM

Maurice B. Visscher

I gather from the statements that Dr. Brosin made, in discussing the desirable aspects of what I might say this morning, that one of the things you would like to have discussed are some of the questions concerning the biological effects of radiation generally, as well as the presentation of some current information concerning the fall-out problem.

I am sure that I have been asked to come here because I had something to do with the work of the Governor's Committee in the State of Minnesota dealing generally with atomic energy development, and I think as a preliminary to this presentation of mine, I should tell you what the objectives of the Governor's Committee in Minnesota are.

The Committee was set up not specifically to deal with fall-out problems, but rather to deal in general with atomic energy problems as they might affect a state. You are aware of the fact that the Atomic Energy Act both as it was originally passed, and as amended in 1954, gives responsibility for control of atomic energy developments entirely in the first instance to a federal commission. Nevertheless there is a feeling that sooner or later much of the control must pass to state and local bodies. Furthermore, there was the feeling, particularly in the individualistic state of Minnesota, that it was desirable that some authority as well as responsibility be taken by agencies other than federal ones, particularly in connection with protection against health hazards, which, in the American system of Government, is traditionally a state responsibility.

It was felt that the states should begin to look into what their responsibilities in the future might be, and what they might do now to begin assuming some responsibility and authority.

Among the other things that the Minnesota Atomic Energy Development Board has done was to recommend to the State that a very definitive radiologic code be established within the state. This code would go farther than other codes have in the past in the direction of requiring that any sources of nuclear energy to be utilized within the state would need to have state licensing and authorization, in addition to whatever licensing the A.E.C. might require. At the present time one of the power sources built on an experimental basis is going up at Elk River, under the auspices of one of the rural electric cooperatives. The state is in the process of trying to see how its control over the design of the reactor, and the conditions under which it is to operate, can be established and maintained. This, as some of you (who know about the legal problems involved) realize, is a new departure and is something that we think is quite important, since we think it is essential that local and state bodies take the basic responsibility for the health of their communities in these regards.

What preceded is by way of background to assure you that the Minnesota State Atomic Energy Development Committee was not concerned simply about the fall-out problem when it began its work. However, when we began thinking about the problems of environmental contamination, it was obvious to us that we needed to know what the existing levels of environmental contaminations were.

In assembling the fragmentary information which we had a couple of years ago, we found that the water supplies, including the Mississippi River, (which is the source of water for the major cities in the Minnesota area and a great many cities on down the line—thus is being re-utilized so to speak may times before it gets to the ocean) had high levels of gross beta radioactivity.

It turned out that most of this radioactivity was due to relatively short-lived isotopes, but when we became interested in the radioactivity in plant food sources as well as animal food sources, we found to our surprise and disappointment that the radioactivity from strontium 90 was rather high.

The strontium 90 content of wheat from various sources within the State of Minnesota, (which happened to be stored in the Institute of Agriculture because these samples were being retained for other purposes by scientists on the Institute of Agriculture staff) showed values expressed in terms of micro-micro curies per gram of calcium, in 1956 ranging between 74 as a low, and 169 as a high. In 1957 the readings ranged from 105 as a low and to 606 as a high; and in 1958 they ranged from 111 as a low to 213 as a high; indicating to us that in the first place there was a rising level, and in the second place the values were considerably higher than we would like to see them as levels in important food sources.

The amount of strontium 90 in any particular foodstuff is not equally important for the different foodstuffs. The important factor is how much of thc given food element is ingested relative to the amount of radio-isotope in it.

Actually, there is no entirely satisfactory way of expressing the relative acceptability of contamination in a particular foodstuff. The important problem from a physiological point of view is the total intake of the radioactive element.

Figures have been released by our State Department of Health for strontium 90 content of milk. Here the units are in micro-micro curies per liter of fluid milk, and the values in different cities in the state ranged from a low of 7 micro-micro curies per liter to a high of 24 in 1958.

The strontium in milk necessarily comes from the plant foods that cattle are eating, and one of the problems that comes up in connection with the study of the chain of events in the movement of these elements into the biosphere has to do with where the elements go in the plants that are carrying them. Milburn and Russell showed that when strontium is put on the soil as a spray more of it appears in the first cut of grass than in the second. Presumably most of the strontium applied to soil stays within the few upper inches, and a great deal of it is cropped off. This is an important point in connection with possible decontamination of soils where possibly plants can take the material out of the top soil and the first few crops can then be discarded. A larger share of the strontium in these experiments was found in the straw of barley than in the grain, and a larger share was found in the tops of sugar beets than in the roots. In Minnesota the highest levels of beta radiation in plant products were found in the leaves and stems of soy bean plants rather than in the beans or the berries of any of the grains or cereals that were observed.

When animals ingest food containing strontium 90, the ratio of strontium 90 to calcium in the bone that is laid down by these animals is not the same as the ratio in foodstuff. Comar and his associates have studied the ratio between the body and the diet for the strontium 90 calcium relationship. In man on a milk diet the observed ratio is .54, which means that in the human subjects studied, the amount of strontium retained relative to the amount of calcium retained, was about half. Only half as much strontium 90 would be stored in the bones of these subjects relative to the amount of calcium stored as there was in the dietary materials. It appears here that on different diets the "discrimination factor" is not constant and that it ranges between .1 and .7.

Unfortunately this discrimination factor is less favorable to those on milk diets. I say this is unfortunate because in growing children milk is a major source of all bone mineral, particularly calcium, and therefore most human beings are going to be confronted with the problems of the strontium content in their milk diets during growing years.

The situation with regard to the appearance of radio-active substances in the environment from fall-out in the United States is approximately this: We are approaching the stage in which the amounts of elements like strontium are at levels where they might be influencing some of the so-called threshold-effect diseases involving human beings.

I am sure most of you are aware of the fact that there are two types among the biological effects of low level radiation. These are the genetic effects and somatic effects.

So far as the genetic effects are concerned, there is no reason to believe that there is a threshold for action. There is, however, every reason to believe that the genetic effects are of significance with any and every increase in radiation intensity in the environment. It is not certain that there is a straight line relationship. This was thought to be true, but the recent work of the Russells has suggested very strongly that the rate of application of the dose of radiation is an important factor in the genetic response. In other words, a given dose applied over a short period of time will have more genetic effect than the same dose applied over a much longer period of time. The Russells' results, however, do not indicate that there is a threshold in any sense. They would only indicate that more rapid rates of application of a given dose have a greater genetic effect than do low rates of application.

On the contrary, with respect to the more typical somatic effects, some evidence has been given for a threshold. This seems to be true in the case of radium poisoning, in which bone cancer incidence has not been observed to increase with very low body burdens.

In dealing with non-threshold effects, it really makes no sense to talk about a maximum permissible dose, because what we are saying is simply how much of an effect we are willing to accept as worthwhile, in relation to other advantages that we may hope to gain or may actually gain from increasing our total load of environmental radiation.

This brings me to a main point in connection with the problem of maximum permissible doses and what may perhaps be a sensible attitude with regard to increases in environmental radiation.

It is of no particular importance to talk about the concentration of any particular radioactive substance in any particular foodstuff. What we are interested in is the total amount of such a substance that an individual is going to ingest over a certain period of time; and we are interested in knowing what percentage of what he or she ingests he or she is going to retain.

This brings up a number of physiological problems which are as yet unsolved. We do not know for a certainty how to control the discrimination between strontium and calcium in the body, nor do we know how to control the fraction of strontium that is ingested that will be excreted in the urine, for example. We do not know how to control how much will be secreted in the milk. There is work for investigators here. What we need to know from a practical viewpoint in considering the danger, or lack of it, in our fall-out problem is how much an individual is storing. Then we need to know today about the biological effects of particular radio nuclides, especially bone seeking nuclides, on processes like carcinogenesis; the amounts of bone seekers that are stored are not uniform throughout the entire bone structure. If, for example, one ingests a high level of radioactive nuclide over a short period, it will be stored in the bone at high concentration in the new bone formed during that time. There will be "hot spots" in the bone and as Angstrom has pointed out, these hot spots can determine whether or not the radioactive substance is going to have an effect in inducing bone cancer or leukemia. We are concerned with obtaining more information at the present time about the significance of local depositions of high intensity material, as well as information on overall composition.

What should our attitudes as scientists be toward the increase in radioactive material in our environment? Here are my feelings in the matter: First we should recognize that we are at the present time putting radioactive material into the environment at levels which will definitely have some effects of a genetic sort, and will, if the levels are raised greatly above present ones, have somatic effects.

Secondly, we should recognize that our problem is really one of deciding whether society can afford to continue to do this, in return for the other benefits that we may or may not be obtaining from this practice.

The scientists can undoubtedly do something to reduce the effects of fall-out. They can also see to it that the public is aware of the facts. They cannot prescribe the moral or political decisions.

Dr. Brosin: Our next speaker is Dr. M. Stanley Livingston, and he has a remarkable record; indeed a very distinguished career. I shall save myself and him the recital of his many honors, but to identify him for you somewhat, he is currently the Professor of Physics at M.I.T., and has been Director of the Cambridge Accelerator at Harvard University since 1956. He was the Chairman of the Accelerator Project at the Brookhaven National Laboratories from 1946 to 1948. Dr. Livingston was also associated with the distinguished E. O. Lawrence at the University of California in the original development of the cyclotron. As you can see he has kept very good company.

He is also the former Chairman of the powerful American Federation of Scientists and is now a member of their policymaking committee which is the Executive Committee.

He will discuss, among other things, how other scientists have reacted to the threat of damage from radio-active fall-out, other hazards of atomic and nuclear energy experiments, and the public reaction to them. Dr. Livingston will also discuss the growing responsibility of being a rebel against the *conventional wisdom* which has been so actively promoted in this field. With this background, I am very happy to introduce to you Dr. Livingston.

THE CONCERN OF SCIENCE WITH NUCLEAR DEVELOPMENTS

M. Stanley Livingston

I would like to speak today about my experiences as an atomic scientist, in which I have tried to take some responsibility in public affairs. I can give examples of the kind of activities going on within the professional and the non-professional fields of the physical sciences with regard to the problems induced by the cold war and the threat of nuclear weapons.

I am not an expert in politics, but only an amateur lobbyist. I am also very much of an amateur in psychiatry, although I do make some effort to understand some of the psychiatric implications. This is a report only of my own observations and I hope you will accept it as such.

Scientists have become involved in public affairs in at least four distinct ways. The first of these activities is that of the "rebel" scientists, an example being the Federation of American Scientists. This group was formed in 1946 by a few scientists from the Atomic Energy Laboratory at Los Alamos, Chicago and Oak Ridge, and soon others were rapidly drawn in. The motivation behind their activities has been to try to explain to the public and to government some of the implications of nuclear bombs and nuclear war. These scientists were a very concerned group of people. They had gone from their academic laboratories into government work during the war, as did many other patriotic citizens, and had done everything within their abilities to strengthen our country militarily. Some of them felt a moral repulsion to the use of science for war. Others did not like the decision to use the atomic bomb on Japan. Still others, however, accepted it as an unpleasant necessity, but wanted to minimize its future use in war.

I have talked with Dr. Arthur Compton and have read the story of his personal experiences in those days when the decision was made to use the bomb against Japan. It was not an easy decision to make. I respect those who had to make such difficult decisions, sometimes against their own humanitarian or moral judgments.

The Federation of American Scientists picked up this unrest, this disturbance, this feeling of guilt which scientists felt because of their connection with military weapons, and tried to transform it into an effort to improve the public awareness of these problems which would reduce the chances of a war in which nuclear weapons would be used. They acted in many ways. They tried to inform the public on new technical developments through newspaper articles and other publications. In government they advised legislators. Many were invited to congressional hearings and gave their advice and the opinions of concerned scientists.

Congressmen, by the way, have been very receptive to such testimony. The F.A.S. has made a series of technical studies on classification procedures, security clearance problems, radiation fall-out hazards, etc., and has presented these technical studies to proper authorities. They have criticized government policies, and have prodded certain agencies in the government. The F.A.S. has been a gadfly so far as the Atomic Energy Commission is concerned, in trying to get them to release and publish information which scientists believed should not be retained as classified. The F.A.S. felt that this type of information should be made available to the public, by way of non-government scientists who could analyze it and present it to the public. Decisions should be based on knowledge rather than on the *papa-knows-best* attitude which has dominated the policies of the Atomic Energy Commission through most of its history.

I can summarize the results quickly. I believe we failed completely in trying to persuade people to act intelligently on the basis of fear of unpleasant consequences. We sensed a closing-off; a withdrawal from the facts. People did not want to hear them. We sensed an urge in many, including newsmen, to find other activities and interests that would somehow make them feel more comfortable. The scientists themselves are widely split on this issue. The number in the federation is very small, no more than 2,000 out of over 60,000 professional physicists. The number of individual scientists who have tried to do something in public affairs is an even smaller number. As for the rest of the group, they choose to stay in their ivory towers and to proceed with their professional jobs. Some are still in government laboratories producing better bombs or better medical and biological information; by such professional concentration they don't have to face the responsibilities of what science has done toward increasing human problems.

Another consequence has been total failure in our attempts to influence the Administration, i.e., the executive agencies and the Atomic Energy Commission. Once in a while we got under their skin and they were forced to reply and release some information, but we were generally unsuccessful. It took a longer and broader effort through persuasion of legislators in Congress before very much of this kind of information could be pried out of the A.E.C.

But there have been some successes. I think the F.A.S. has been quite successful in informing Congressmen. Some of our more capable legislators have sensed the need for new approaches through legislation and have used the advice and thinking of scientists

The F.A.S. has also had some success in the international field. I hope this is not giving too much credit to the Federation of American Scientists. In 1954 the F.A.S. first called attention through newspaper articles to the international implication of fall-out radiation. We said the hazards were widespread, were not restricted to single countries, and must be considered as an international problem. This was called to the attention of the United Nations, and in the following year the General Assembly established a Commission for the Study of Radioactive Hazards and gave credit to the Federation of American Scientists for first bringing this problem to their attention. One of the few unanimous votes in the General Assembly of the United Nations was for the establishment of this Commission for the Study of Radiation Hazards. This Commission has since made its report. It has been a very important one on the documentation of the significance of radiation hazards. So much for the "rebels".

Let me now talk about the relations between individual scientists and the public. Here also a few scientists have done what they could to try to spread information more widely. We work with lay groups and give them scientific facts about technical problems. I have given many lectures to students, study groups, church groups, conferences, and panel discussions. Only a few other scientists, not too many, have made a similar effort. Here the response has been a steady and continuous spread of knowledge and awareness. This type of activity has culminated in the formation, about a year and one-half ago, of the Committee for a Sane Nuclear Policy. Norman Cousins and Thomas Pickett were the two major planners for this group. They enlisted representatives of all disciplines, including several non-government scientists, and set up a committee whose purpose was to inform the public of the hazards of radioactive fall-out, and the necessity of stopping bomb tests.

Perhaps the major thing the scientists contributed to this activity was to keep the facts straight, so that the newspaper advertisements were factual and contained valid numbers and estimates of the hazards. The committe policy on radioactive fall-out is sound and reasonable. The magnitude of radioactivity from fall-out and the probable build-up of that radioactivity due to past tests are now well established and generally accepted. The health hazards are also reasonably understood. Dr. Visscher has said that biological hazard can be estimated now within a factor of about 10, which is close enough at least to establish the basic facts. But these numbers can be presented in two ways. They can be presented in terms of the extremely small percentage of the total population of the world which will be affected, and which is less than one hundredth of one per cent. This is the way the numbers are usually presented by spokesmen for the Atomic Energy Commission and by others who consider the continuation of bomb tests essential. Or they can be presented as the total number of people who would be harmed, which is tens of thousands or hundreds of thousands of individuals throughout the world per year. They are the same facts, but presented differently.

It is not generally known, but it is true, that there is no longer any significant disagreement on the numbers between government and non-government scientists. The only difference is in their way of presenting the data, in order to make their particular points. You must be aware that scientists have different political opinions, as do all other groups, and the holders of the different views will tend to use the available data in different ways in order to prove different things.

The Committee for a Sane Nuclear Policy has spread rapidly. There are about 175 local groups throughout the country today. Some of the members are amusingly special in their interests. I have had occasion to discuss these special interests many times in executive committee meetings. Representatives of the housewife group, the mothers, for example, are concerned primarily with the radioactive dangers to their children's health, and just don't think anything else is important.

Then there are the pacifists who don't believe war should be allowed. We find them in any lay organization. They want us to concentrate on disarmament, by demanding that our government stop all armaments and weapons programs. They are opposed to all military plans and frequently seem to be opposed to government itself. Their most outsoken representatives, whom I call the "angry young men", want to do things immediately, and in big steps. Others who have thought the problem through recognize that progress can be made only one step at a time. The "angry young men" class is a powerful and vocal group, and are frequently present at public meetings. The reason they are so powerful is that most of the people who hear them don't know enough about the facts to see the total picture.

Then of course there are the sober and cautious individuals who are searching for real and practical answers. Maybe I am one of them. What, for example, are the real reasons for stopping bomb tests, and for searching for an agreement with the Russians? In my opinion, which by the way is the same as the stated policy of the United States Government, they should be stopped. However, we must develop an inspection system which is adequate to prevent cheating, and in which the probability of detection is so great that no country would dare to make clandestine tests. If we can get such an agreement, it will be an important first step in improving international relations; indeed, it will become one of the codes of international law. We can hope that it would be an example from which further law could be developed, and that it would eventually be extended to limit the spread of nuclear technology to other nations.

Three countries are now producing nuclear weapons; two or three others are almost ready to start. When the less responsible governments acquire the ability to make nuclear weapons then it will be a great deal more difficult to control the use of such weapons, accidentally or intentionally.

I concur with those individuals who feel it is important to stop nuclear bomb tests in order to reduce fall-out radiation hazards, but I also feel that unless we can solve the larger and longer range problems of the tensions between nations, with the ultimate establishment of more significant international law, the effects of radiation fall-out from bomb tests will always be a less significant issue. In my opinion, the fall-out hazard is well down on the list of reasons for stopping tests.

This is a summary of what I have observed in my work with nonscientific people. I think that much good has been done and I have seen a large amount of interest developing among laymen. There are many local organizations developing with the purpose of discussing these problems. With all of their extreme attitudes, it leads to some wonderfully interesting discussions.

Now let me go on to the third category, that of international science. Scientists have a tradition of international understanding and cooperation. Before the war we had many friends and trusted colleagues in other countries, including Russia. There is a long tradition of scholarship in Russia, as you all know, but the war pitted us against each other in the sense that we supported the war effort for our separate countries. The tradition of cooperation has been difficult to revive. It is slowly improving, however, and in the professional field I think it is on the way back.

By professional, I mean in this sense, such scientific activities as international conferences, which are being steadily reactivated. Conferences are getting larger and we are also rebuilding the earlier private professional interchange with scientists of other countries, but the significant problem is due to nationalistic pressures on the scientists themselves. Here there has only been one development of significance, the so-called Pugwash Meetings of scientists from many countries. The first was late in 1957, at Pugwash, Nova Scotia, at the estate of Cyrus Eaton; the second was at Quebec at Lac Bouchette in early 1958, and the third was at Kitzbuhel, Austria in 1958. I understand that you are aware of these meetings and have been informed of their significance. I know many individuals who attended. I have heard them describe their reactions to the discussions of international problems with the delegates from Russia and other countries behind the Iron Curtain.

It was not easy for the few American scientists who went to that first meeting to attend. This was soon after the McCarthy era in our country. It was at a time when scientists had real reasons for concern when talking politics with representatives of foreign governments. It might mean that their security clearances would be rescinded, so they might lose their usefulness in their own professional field. Those who did attend are greatly to be commended for their courage.

It happens that they did not lose anything. They were, in fact, highly commended. The second conference, held at Lac Bouchette, included a few government representatives of science, and the third one at Kitzbuhel had quite a few government scientists and representatives of the Atomic Energy Commission and of the State Department from our country.

It was found that there was a surprising willingness on the part of the scientists from the Russian orbit to talk about the technical difficulties having to do with such international problems as bomb tests, disarmament and inspection systems. Much was accomplished, since they were all reasonable people and did not allow the conference to discuss the divisions of political opinion which existed between the groups. Discussions were kept at the level of the technical possibilities, in such areas as inspection systems for disarmament. They did find large areas of agreement, and the meetings were tremendously valuable to our government. This preparation made it possible for our government to later set up the Conference of Experts in Geneva to study the bomb-test inspection problems after the U.S. Government finally changed its policy in this field. Thus we have the significance of Kitzbuhel and the other meetings. The scientists learned that they could talk to each other and could work out technical answers of value to their governments on the possible types of inspection systems and similar problems.

Propaganda at the meetings was well controlled. The conferences were not used as sounding boards for nationalistic propaganda. They were serious discussions, and there were also many private discussions behind the scenes at luncheons, at dinners and evenings in which a great deal more understanding was achieved then ever came out in the official reports. These papers are being published and some of them are now available. They are not impressive as a blue print for total world peace, but they are at least a start toward learning how to get along with scientists from other countries.

My fourth category has to do with scientists in government, working through official channels, either employed by government, or as members of advisory committees or as appointees to special responsibilities. The practice by government of using scientific advisors is not new. It existed during the war, and developed to a high level in government offices and laboratories, particularly in defense agencies, and thus it became a powerful tool. This bringing-in of experts from outside the government to survey, to criticize, to evaluate and recommend to the people who are the permanent employees in government is so valuable now that every government agency has its stable of stars. A scientific advisory committee is now a practical necessity, and many scientists of national repute in the areas pertinent to our government's work are now on one or another of these government committees.

I am not entirely sure how good this is. This practice has drained the very best people out of the private, non-government scientist group, and has put them into official capacities in one or another way. This has tended to make them considerably less outspoken, and they reserve their opinions for official reports. The reason why this practice has suddenly become more important than in the past is that the Russians sent up a satellite. This event shocked our people and our government severely, and they became worried. This technique is the government administration's answer to the sputnik.

One good result was that it stimulated the re-establishment of the President's Scientific Advisory Committee. This Committee had existed previously, but had not been called to action for years. Dr. Killian from M.I.T. was asked to be the Chairman of the reactivated committee. He became the President's Special Advisor on Science and went to Washington to do the job. He increased the list of the President's advisory committee, including some tremendously impressive people who are very clear thinkers and the world's top experts. Some of them have told me personally they have never worked so hard in their lives; that Jim Killian is the hardest *slave driver* they have ever worked under. They have really studied technical subjects and others intensively. They have brought in other advisory members to fill out special study groups until the total number involved in one way or another in this Presidential committee is now about 75.

They are called upon to make special studies and to make reports which are then evaluated by the total committee and presented to the President. I have heard Dr. Killian speak of his relations with the President in these matters and he says that he has always found the door open. The Presidential appointment secretary always gives an appointment to Killian or to representatives from his group within a day's notice. They have poured into the President's ear some very important information, thoroughly analyzed, including some studies which had never before been made.

This is the specific reason why the United States Government has changed its policy on bomb tests. Previously it had been receiving all of its scientific information through the Chairman of the Atomic Energy Commission and the President's Advisor on Atomic Energy Matters, who happened to be the same man, Admiral Strauss. Thus only one source of information for the President had previously existed.

Whether the President knew it or not, when he appointed the Killian Committee, he accepted into the government a broad ranging spectrum of advice which had never before been available to him. Much of this advice was diametrically opposite to that which he had been receiving earlier. I am tremendously impressed with the President's Advisory Committee and the work they have done. It is now government policy to search for an agreement with Russia to stop bomb tests, including an adequate inspection system. The bomb test ban negotiations in Geneva are now in recess.

The March, 1959 issue of *Fortune* included an attack against the scientists in government, and against the Geneva negotiations. Certain persons don't want the negotiations to succeed. This is still the policy of many people within the Atomic Energy Commission. They want the government to fail and want bomb tests to go on, but it is now the government's policy to work toward agreement.

I don't want to imply that the preceding is all that the President's Committee has done. It has studied many other problems, including the difficulty of how missile development is to be handled, and the inclusion of civilian interests. The Committee has also made studies of education for science, and has made recommendations. Changes are going on. The President's Advisory Committee is being called into the Pentagon, the State Department and into many other agencies, as well as the Administration Headquarters in the White House.

However, this is still an appointive system and the present high quality is due to the fact that the Russians scared us with a sputnik. The same system with the same authority acting previously led us into a bad mess. The basic question is: Is it safe? How long can we continue to have the best quality of scientific minds in government? When will it again be channeled by appointive manipulation to serve only the parochial purposes and policies of governmental agencies? I don't think I like this situation for the long pull. It is not at all obvious to me that this is the best way in which we should use scientists in government. The problem deserves a great deal of study.

I conclude that all of these approaches by which scientists have attempted to influence government are important in their different ways. They do different things. The most effective course is to influence the VIPS in government directly. It is always a temptation to operate through established authority. I have observed a general tendency that the more important the scientist, the more certain he is to try to work through the existing authorities in government. It is more effective for him to act through channels than to act through private or public groups. The smaller the scientist is in professional reputation, the more willing he is to talk to the public, and the less convinced he is that the *powers-that-be* are doing the right things. So scientists have a wide spectrum of opinion. I believe that all of these are necessary, and that they all have their place.

As a representative of a very small fraction of the scientific community, one who has engaged in such political activities over the past ten years, I certainly welcome what is going on now in the Group for the Advancement of Psychiatry. It sometimes seemed to us that we were getting nowhere in our efforts. What this meeting means to me today is that another professional group is reaching the stage where they are willing to accept some responsibility for studying this problem professionally and objectively, in order to do what they can to search for the alternate roads to peace, alternate to the use of force. I am very grateful for this. I am beginning to feel optimistic because I see much of this activity going on. I know of dozens and even hundreds of groups in the lay public who are starting to study these political problems and are getting profoundly interested. I have seen many student groups and have attended several student conferences. I find that students are intensely interested in the subject of international relations. They are beginning to recognize their responsibilities and to accept the challenge.

I also find a tremendous interest in other professional groups. The organized churches are searching for a way to be effective, although they have been almost completely ineffective in the past. The Friends' Service Committee of the Quaker group is one organization which has been really useful, but other groups are starting, too. The lawyers now want to start talking about international problems, and plan a symposium soon in which they will discuss the elements of international law and how they can help in their professional way. Newsmen are getting together. I attended a meeting last week of a group of science writers where Professor Jerome Wiesner of M.I.T. spoke. He is a member of the President's Scientific Advisory Committee, and was one of the members of an advisory group going to the Surprise Attack Conference at Geneva, which was another attempt at negotiations with the U.S.S.R. It failed completely and Wiesner told us the reasons why it failed. Professional scientists like Wiesner are now taking a real and direct interest in such international problems. They are realizing one by one that something other than military force must be found in trying to solve the problems between nations.

This is the reason I am optimistic. I sense a tremendous growth of this sort of awareness and responsibility throughout the country.

Dr. Brosin: Our next speaker is Dr. Raymond K. Appleyard, who did his basic training in the natural sciences at Cambridge University in England and then continued his work in physics and biophysics. We were fortunate that he was at the California Institute of Technology from 1951 to 1953 where he worked in genetics. He then joined Atomic Energy of Canada, Ltd. for three years as a research officer in biological research related to the fields of radiation and biology. In May 1956, he joined the United Nations staff as an Acting Secretary, and in 1957 became the Permanent Secretary of the Scientific Committee on the Effects of Atomic Radiation. He is an eminent scientist, well qualified to speak about the international implications of the radiation problem.

CONFUSIONS IN THE RADIATION FIELD

Raymond K. Appleyard

Like many who were trained as physicists but became interested in biology, I have been haunted by the radiation problem on and off for a good many years. The United Nations has been exposed to it for a rather shorter time, but the issue did arise there in a serious way, especially in the 1955 session of the General Assembly. At that time many governments were especially worried about the possible dangers of widespread radioactive contamination of the environment, and, moreover, the complexities of a very complicated technical issue had become mixed up with the very complicated complexities of a political dispute. The reaction of the General Assembly may perhaps be regarded in part as an attempt to re-separate the issues.

It set up in late 1955, a committee of 15 nations which was to examine solely the scientific aspects of the radiation problem and report on them. There was no question of recommending action or setting maximum permissible levels or anything of that nature. The report was to be factual, and considering the obvious problems of international coordination and relationships, it had to be prepared rather quickly.

What follows are mainly some personal impressions derived from participation in this work over a period of three years. But first, let me remind you from the start, that radioactive fall-out is only one facet of the problem. Certainly in the technologically advanced countries of the world there are many other man-made contributors to the radiation exposure of populations that greatly exceed the fall-out from weapons' tests. The problem is, of course, a very complicated one for scientists and for the public health authorities, for reasons of economics and of course, for reasons of politics. Perhaps politics especially because leaving on one side the exact magnitude of the effects, one can specify a moral or quasi-moral issue which is much bigger than the physical one. Of course it is not a new issue, but an old one which arises whenever one government or its agents causes the population under the care of another government to be exposed to a possibly dangerous agent, in this case radiation, without any possibility of the people irradiated influencing those who release the agent. Any Britisher who was brought up on the sad tale of *no taxation without representation* is aware of at least one closely related issue of its potential importance in the world. With the understanding that taxation, like radiation, is a potentially dangerous agent, most of us would agree.

I would like now to turn to direct consideration of the Committee set up by the General Assembly.

One interesting feature of this group, as compared to others who have studied the same field, is that the United Nations Committee consisted from the start of governments. Governments were the members. They had, of course, scientific representatives; and these men possessed a sort of dual capacity: one as the representative of the political organism, government; the other as an expert in some area or other of the radiation health field. Being a committee of governments, the United Nations group is a body easily able to deal with governments: indeed the material available to it has consisted of information supplied by governments and their agencies. Of course in order to evaluate this information, it has been necessary to view it against the background of general and current scientific literature.

With all its governmental complications, a feature of the United Nations work that has greatly impressed me has been the ease of obtaining voluntary assistance. It has been possible throughout to write to almost any competent or eminent scientist in this field and ask him to comment on a document, or to draft something to cover a knotty problem with which he was unusually familiar, and to get an immediate and wholehearted response, although he might know he would never receive any acknowledgement or any other form of attribution. Perhaps this is a tribute to the prestige of the United Nations, but I think it is mostly a tribute to the public spirit of the scientific community as a whole.

Now over the years there have been some public confusions about this field. One of them is a very simple verbal one. It was mostly public commentators who first started to talk about atomic energy when they meant nuclear energy, and they were certainly I think the first to talk about atomic radiation when they meant ionizing radiation. It is important to realize that this simple confusion of terminology can lead to confusion by generating a feeling that these are really one and the same problem, or that ionizing radiation problems are really just a part of the nuclear energy problem.

A second confusion which it is surprisingly hard for most people to understand, and which will have to be made comprehensible either by the people who work in the field or by closely related professional groups such as yours, is the whole issue of probability or statistics.

After all damage from radiation is quite often statistical damage. Radiation, as far as we know so far, can never fairly be said to cause an individual to get leukemia. It may increase the probability of a person getting leukemia. The same applies to mutations. It cannot fairly be said to cause one individual to transmit to one child one mutation, but only to increase the probability of that event. Therefore, if two identical individuals are exposed identically, even if one later gets leukemia and the other does not, I ask, would it in our present state of knowledge at least, be fair to compensate the one who got leukemia and not the other? After all, the radiation did the same thing to both individuals. As far as we know, it increased the probability of getting leukemia by the same amount. This kind of complicated issue is going to have to be faced in connection with public policy in the radiation field, such as the making of rules or the making of laws on the national and international scale.

Another confusion has been that rather old one in the public mind between the scientist, the technologist and the magician. This has perhaps contributed to the widespread feeling of the sinister nature of radiation, already over-accented by its invisible nature, undetectable except through complicated instruments, and by the accompaniment of possible delayed but perhaps inevitable late effects.

Among the scientific problems let us take first of all genetic effects, about which we know so little. We don't know whether there is a dose rate effect. We don't know what the relationship between dose and effect is at low doses for man. It is surprising, but radiation induced mutation in man has not been *observed;* it is only *inferred* because it happens in so many other species. It does not need much amplification of that statement to make clear that we have a long way to go before getting at a quantitative relationship between the dose and the effect which could be used as a good basis for controlling the hazard, or making policy decisions about it. The question has recently been much complicated by Dr. Russell's demonstration of a dose rate effect in gene-mutations of mice, which may turn out to be quite a general phenomenon.

Another side of the genetic problem is often overlooked, yet it may in the end prove a tough one to resolve. That is the question of what is the fate of mutations after they occur in a population? Really very little is known about this. Perhaps four per cent of human infants are born dead or alive, with defects of genetic origin. What keeps the corresponding genes in the population? Is it the recurrent supply of mutations? Or is it perhaps that although these defects are so serious when they occur, the genes which cause them have under other circumstances (perhaps much more common circumstances) some advantage in the population which keeps them there? If almost the whole of the current mutant gene load in the population were to be maintained by this curious mechanism of smaller advantages in some circumstances, the effect of, say a doubling of the mutation rate might be very small.

There is another facet of the radiation question which cannot be neglected. One may think of the possible effects of radiation as of two kinds. First there is the serious rare effect. If for example, the level of exposure is increased sufficiently, perhaps one irradiated individual in a hundred thousand will get leukemia and die. But there is also the possibility, which must be taken seriously and explored, of small common rather than serious rare effects. Perhaps that same increase in the general radiation level would cause almost everybody's life to be shortened very slightly or perhaps it would, over the generations, cause a very slight diminution in the average intelligence. These problems are going to be much harder to investigate. We are right at the beginning of them, yet potentially they could be just as serious as the others, and they must be explored before policy, where radiation is concerned, can be completely set on a solid scientific footing. Incidentally, many of these considerations lead us back to one particular field of work which may in the past have been a bit neglected and that is human biology. There are so many things of which we need measures that we don't possess. Perhaps, as it has in other fields, the study of radiation problems may here do some good. We don't, for example, have a good measure of the physiological age of a man. Lots of parameters have been suggested and tried, but we still don't have a good one. If we are going to tackle problems of radiation-induced ageing, we need one.

It is also my impression that we do not have any reasonable measure of what one might call constitutive, or innate intelligence. Yet there are radiation puzzles for which we need this too. The I.Q. is the nearest, yet perhaps the I.Q. only measures, if it measures anything, developed intelligence after a certain amount of education. What is needed for this radiation genetic problem is a good, reliable measure of constitutive or innate intelligence, and I believe we are very far from it. Perhaps the radiation studies will turn some useful attention in this direction.

There are many other such situations. A much more direct problem, on which I have yet to see any very constructive ideas, would be to find a measure of the total accumulated dose of an individual in middle life. One advantage of this would be a real easing of the problem of conducting needed human radiation surveys. Instead of thinking in terms of the average of a group living in a high background area, say 100,000 people, and comparing them with the average of another group living on a low background area, you could almost start to take people off the street, measure any property you like together with their accumulated radiation dose, and start to make useful correlations. We do not have such a parameter. As long as we don't, we have to go on with the rather discouraging search for areas of high natural background in which there live large enough populations who are well enough controlled demographically for us to try to examine what slightly increased radiation levels do to them.

The worst trouble is usually to find a similar control population. This difficulty for example, bedevils all of the proposals to use populations exposed to greatly increased cosmic rays because they live at high altitudes. In order to be sure not to be misled by any peculiar effects of living at somewhat lowered oxygen tension, you have to find a similar population with similar habits, etc., living at the same altitude but sufficiently different latitude to have a different cosmic ray exposure—a very difficult proposition.

The strongest candidate at the moment for a population to be examined because it lives in a high radiation background and is large, lies in Kerala in South India, where about 100,000 fisher-folk live on the monazite sands. Here there may be enough people to get some useful information, for the background is probably about six times the usual natural level of radiation exposure. It is a unique opportunity for such a survey, and, although no one can tell what may come out of the attempt, I believe all of us hope that the Indians can make a good job of it, and would like to help them where we can.

An area in which much is being done is that of prevention or cure of the results of exposure to radiation. Radiobiology in its widest sense has two tasks for the world at large. One is to estimate radiation effects, but the other is certainly to control them. That branch of the subject is moving so fast at the present time that one would hesitate to predict where we are going—not just in respect to mechanical aids such as possible chelating agents to remove radio-isotopes from the living organism, but of developments such as the recent demonstration for the first time of a dramatic change in survival of irradiated cells brought about by post-irradiation treatment. In this work, the experimenters reported that among cells they irradiated, only between 4 and 8 thousand survived, but by a particular post-irradiation treatment they were able to raise the survival to a value between 80 and 100 per cent. This is one among many new leads into a greatly widened field of work in understanding and perhaps ultimately controlling radiation effects.

The other recent development in the field of modifying radiation injury leads us back to the ground of international co-operation. It is, of course, the dramatic incident of last winter when six Yugoslavs suffered exposures in a serious accident, were flown to Paris and ultimately were treated by bone marrow injections from volunteer donors. On today's evidence it seems probable that this treatment, risky, experimental and in its pioneering infancy, may have helped five of the persons *over the hump* and saved their lives. If so, it may mark the beginning of another breakthrough in medicine and, of course, will feed back into biology as people search for ideas of improving it. If radiation and allied studies lead eventually to a major development in breaking down the immunological barriers to transplantation of tissues, the possibilities opened up are very obvious to the imagination. Indeed it can hardly be overemphasized that just as radiation research draws its nourishment from the broad roots of general biology in the very widest sense, so also it returns to the tree of knowledge worthwhile contributions extending far beyond its own narrow compass.

Dr. Brosin: Our next speaker is Mr. Pare Lorentz, who has an imposing list of memberships, decorations and awards, which need not be recited this morning. He is the author of three books which I will not sell for him this morning because they are not of immediate interest to the subject, but he has been working on a book on the radiation problem for the past ten years and we can all look forward to it.

I would like particularly to call attention to the fact that Mr. Lorentz has made some outstanding motion pictures, which were one phase of his activity during the war in the area of general motion picture work. He did *The Plow that Broke The Plains* in 1936, and *The River* in 1938, which was released by Paramount and received the World Prize in 1938 for the best documentary picture at the Venice Festival. These achievements are especially worthy of note, and I am sure many of you are familiar with these outstanding motion pictures.

He also did one film which is of very real importance to physicians, *The Fight for Life* in 1940, which received a number of awards and is included in the book, THE TWENTY BEST FILM PLAYS by Professor John Gasner and Dudley Nichols.

From 1938 to 1940 he was appointed Chief of the U.S. Film Service by President Roosevelt and was the National Defense Editor of *McCalls* from 1940-41. I won't try to recite here his distinguished war record and his postwar work.

Mr. Lorentz has been indefatigable and, as he says, enjoyed his trudging up and down the country becoming acquainted with many of our leading figures in this area in order to better understand the implications of atomic radiation from a civilian point of view.

THE COMING STRUGGLE FOR MORE RESPONSIBILITY

Pare Lorentz

Distinguished doctors, if all people with authority over atomic affairs had the distinction and the good will of the gentlemen who addressed you this morning, then most of our atomic problems would be solved.

I used to know a very salty, wonderful old Irishman named John Carmody, at one time head of the Federal Works Agency under President Roosevelt. In 1940 he was a chairing a private cabinet meeting on unemployment. We still had about 11 million out of jobs at that time. Suddenly the doors burst open and a very confused, seedy-looking gentleman wandered into the room. John brusquely said, "This is a private meeting. You must have the wrong place."

The bewildered citizen said, "This is the Department of Commerce Building, isn't it?"

John said, "Yes, but this is a private meeting, a cabinet meeting on the unemployed."

The little man brightened quickly, "I'm in the right place. You see, I'm unemployed."

It is my understanding you distinguished people, among other things, are dedicated to the attention of anxious people. I am in the right place, strange as it may seem to you. I am an anxious man. I will not take your time to discuss the anxieties I share with all of you, the concept of total war and total destruction. I see no way out any more than any other helpless citizen. I feel each time you have built an ultimate weapon, stored it or transferred it, you have increased by that percentage that much chance of total destruction taking place.

I would like to suggest, however, a problem to you that I believe does come under your competence. I would not wish to be rude to my friend, Dr. Appleyard, who is a sincere scientist. I wish, Dr. Visscher, we had more M.D.'s with your good will and concern. But I would like to suggest to you that we have been doing something in the world the last ten years of the highest immorality: that is, we have been poisoning our entire planet. I am not making it up. I am quoting from the National Academy of Sciences agricultural report of June, 1951.

The food supply of this world is not what it was ten years ago. I would like to suggest to you a problem that is becoming increasingly grave and one that certainly comes under your competence. If any of you in your community learned that a handful of men were introducing, systematically, typhoid into the water supply of your city, I am sure you would demand that this group be discovered, identified, arrested and committed to an institution of some kind. Yet, a handful of men in three countries of the world have for some years been polluting the entire planet. The word is poison. The only question is one of degree. Ten years ago this poison was not upon us. Now it is. These men will be long since dead before we know the extent of this poison, and, more important, its ultimate effect on all living things. More diabolical, even though medical statistics a half century from now may indicate a pattern of damage due to radioactive poisoning, that generation of medical scientists will not be able to prove definitely that disabilities, disease and deaths have been caused by the acts of this generation.

Dr. Crowe of Wisconsin wrote me a letter some time ago in answer to a scientific inquiry. The gist of his reply is: we really aren't going to know. This generation of scientists won't know, and even fifty years from now it is unlikely that a new generation of medical scientists will be able to specifically identify death and disease and disability as having been caused by this generation of men. This is the risk we take.

The atomic age was conceived in terror and born in secrecy, but three years ago at Geneva, Sir Christopher Hinton of the British Atomic Authority remarked that we have moved from a military to a time of commercial secrets. And in this country the period of transition has meant that a great deal of the control of the atom that was in the hands of a high-caliber group of scientists, engineers, and admirals, has passed into the hands of promoters and hucksters.

For the purpose of a book which I am writing, I have trudged about the country seeking information and I have interviewed most of the organized groups of our society. My intent has been to find out who really has ultimate responsibility and control of public health and safety in the atomic age. I have attended a great many management forums and heard these two phrases over and over, "We must learn to live with it. We cannot set the clock back". Perhaps so, but I do think it might be proper to inquire who is winding the clock.

The publicity campaign called *Atoms For Peace* for example, has resulted in one of the greatest American folk myths since the days of Lydia Pinkham's Compound.

The reason I say this is that the word "peace" means beneficent, kindly, harmless, helpful; yet there is no such thing as a peaceful use of the atom if you mean by that completely harmless, undamaging and benign. Hardly a day passes that you do not read about the wonders of the industrial atomic age.

Two weeks ago a Subcommittee of the Congress held hearings on the subject of Workmen's Compensation and Employee Radiation Hazards. To any who have any concern with this topic, I recommend this official government testimony. Among the witnesses was a Mr. George Foster, Vice President of the Industrial Nucleonics Corporation of Columbus, Ohio. He listed some of the miraculous uses of radioisotopes now being used in thousands of industrial processes to provide more automatic controls and accurate measurements. Among the users listed were the Federal Bureau of Engraving and Printing. They use the industrial atom for measuring the amount of glue applied to postage stamps. The industrial atom controls the amount of water in fruit juice concentrates and it controls the amount of dough in crackers on a straight line. Breweries are using radiation beams in inspection systems to see that beer cans are filled to just the right level.

The New York Central Railroad is employing cobalt 60 to measure the weight of freight cars. Of the 500 largest industrial corporations in the United States, over 250 are using radioisotopes for various purposes. All told, more than 1,200 industrial firms are now licensed to use radioisotopes. The total shipment by the AEC of these materials last year almost equalled the grand total shipped in the ten preceding years, and these users are not in one area but are all over the country and are licensed in every state.

During these same hearings, Dr. Lauriston S. Taylor, Chairman of the National Committee on Permissible Radiation, made a statement which I think will be of interest to you in the light of the foregoing facts. Dr. Taylor said, "Permissible levels of radiation exposure is not basically a scientific problem. It is more a matter of philosophy and morality and sheer wisdom. The problems center about a philosophy to which man might as well become accustomed; it may be called a philosophical risk. Some of the risks that are commonly accepted can be mentioned: virtually any mode of transportation from boat or bicycle to the airplane—but without these, life today would be very different indeed; smoking, a luxury that all could well do without—except that some other relaxing habit that would be just as dangerous would be found; many forms of medication to which there are dangerous individual idiosyncrasies or allergies".

Dr. Taylor concluded by saying that, as far as scientific data goes, the only answer to the question, "What amounts of radiation may man receive in either chronic or acute exposure without any harm to himself or his progeny? is *none*". But, he went on, "radiation and nuclear energy have become so important in a number of fields that it is obvious man does not plan to give up their benefits. The fields include medical treatment, industrial uses, research and production of electric power".

I submit to you that if any amount of radiation harms a man and his progeny, then in this day of extraordinary electronics I would assume that we could find a safer way to measure the amount of beer in a can than by using an atomic gadget. And, I would suggest it might be worthwhile for you to take a hard look at the great benefits we are presumably getting from the atom in medicine, industry and electric power. "We have," quoting Secretary of Defense McElroy, "weapons sufficient to kill half the people of the world many times over". The other side of the medallion is obfuscated.

No one is questioning research tools. Yet I argue that now we need research men much more than we need research tools. I fear we have had a spate of miracles. We have lost track of the main miracle, which is life itself.

I would also like you to think of a hospital where, except for x-rays, there are no radioactive materials on hand, except for purposes of research. From the maternity ward, to the distressing problems of the old, very few doctors would find themselves bereft of knowledge of medicine because of the lack of radioactive materials.

In industry I feel it is fair to say that we have more atomic gimmicks than we have legitimate energy. As far as electric power is concerned, in our country the atomic power plant is much more expensive than a conventional power plant and is indeed much more dangerous. The truth of the matter is we have invested 20 billion dollars in the atom and most of that money represents weapons of total destruction, and the peaceful benefits merely represent the crumbs brushed from the military table.

Yet, because of the daily publicity, you might rightfully suppose that the Atomic Energy Commission has complete authority over all atomic matters in our country. Yet start with ore and examine the radioactive technological industry until you get to waste. Any reputable brokerage firm can supply you with a list of names of companies engaged in the nucleonic industry. Examine the contracts for atomic power. When the AEC gave a license to the Consolidated Edison Company of New York City to construct a large scale atomic power plant, Chairman Strauss announced, "Consolidated Edison Company has given the AEC reasonable assurance of the safety of this plant". This may seem enough assurance to you but I think it might interest you that it isn't assurance enough to insurance companies because you cannot get insurance to indemnify yourself or your family against the possibility of radiation damage from a power plant accident.

The AEC as it is now is actually a promotional agency in charge of regulating and policing its own promotion, or, if you like to put it crudely, the AEC is in the embarrassing position of being a man who is both an arsonist and insurance adjustor.

The AEC really is in large part a giant holding company in charge of letting contracts. It has regulations regarding atomic materials and they are very strict, but when you seek out ultimate responsibility you find yourself in the middle of the game of "Button, button, who's got the button?"—the Government, the State, the City, the County, private industry—who?

I would like to have you think for a moment of waste disposal. Here again the laws are strict, but who actually dumps the stuff in the ocean finally? In our area the AEC has let contracts to five marine salvage companies. Almost three years ago we signed an agreement and said politically at the UN that we would subscribe to an international registry of waste disposal in international waters, and we would inform the UN of any disposal of any *significant* waste. So far we have sent no word to the UN. So we may assume we have disposed of no significant waste. When you get down to it, who is checking on waste as to whether it is significant or not: the weapons' manufacturer in Connecticut, or the tugboat captain from the marine salvage company?

The Congress has held very thorough meetings on this topic. If you are interested, I recommend the testimony of Dr. Abel Wolman of Johns Hopkins before the Joint Committee of Congress, who has for ten years been the leading man in the AEC employed to study our waste problems. According to Dr. Wolman, at the moment we have 60 million gallons of high-level liquid waste stored in tanks in the United States. By 1980, Wolman predicted that industry will have to find ways to store or deposit 100,000,000 gallons of highly radioactive waste materials. Dr. Wolman said the radioactivity in these gallons would be equal to 100,000,000,000 curies. He observed to the Congress that this is an awful lot of curies. Of course, they are all peaceful.

I think the most touching testimony I have heard before the Congress in years of listening to testimony about atomic energy was given last week by a fireman, and I think it might be of interest to you. His name is Leonard English, President of the Cleveland Fire Fighters Association. He represents the International Fireman's Union. He went down to Washington to get some information. He ended up on the witness stand. This is a part of his testimony:

"In the City of Cleveland, we have a large industrial community. About two years ago the Firefighters took upon ourselves to make a study of this particular hazard in the City of Cleveland. We were quite amazed to find out that the problem was as large and widespread as it is. We tried to educate ourselves and at the start we found there was a lot of resistance on the part of industry to give us information which we felt was necessary in order to do an intelligent job of community protection. A lot of people in the industry felt we were trying to stick our nose in their business and checking on something we had no business checking on. We found a lot of resentment. The resentment was due to the fact, originally, that some people were doing secretive work or research work that they did not want anybody to know about.

"We finally convinced them that was none of our business. We did not care what they were doing with the materials. We felt it was necessary to find out what the materials were, what we could do to try to protect the town. We then contacted the members of the AEC and they sent an inspector to talk to us and he sat down with our committee, and after we talked to the members of the AEC, a lot of doors were opened to us that were not opened originally.

"We have formed a committee in the City of Cleveland consisting probably of some of the top scientific minds in the town. Mr. Keith Glennan is a member of our committee. We have representatives from the Police Department, the Teachers Union, the scientists of our town, members of the City Council. We are sitting down to try to work out an intelligent method of protecting our town.

"We do not want to create community panic or concern on the problem until we are ready to move. The members of the Council are now going to have a meeting with the people in the trucking industry and the warehousing industry in possibly two weeks.

"We feel that in transient storage of material such as this, any number of trucking companies could leave material such as this in a warehouse in the middle of a large town. The packages are stored miscellaneously. There is no set place to put these materials. Invariably it happens that it is usually two or three o'clock in the morning when you have a warehouse fire. I don't know why, but that is the way it happens. In order to put out a fire, it is best to remove most of the materials that are burning so the fellows can put the fire out. In most cases the labels on these materials are cardboard or paint. In the case of a fire at two or three o'clock in the morning, the lights are gone, and you cannot see these things. The chances are good with the smoke and fire the markings would be burned off.

"We feel it is reasonable on our part to expect these people in the warehousing industry and trucking industry to put these materials in a certain place to allow our members of the fire department to know where this room would be and work out some sort of liaison program with the warehousing industry to do an intelligent job of community planning and protection.

"We also feel it would not be an imposition on the part of the users to register with the local fire department. I am sure the local health department would be concerned. We feel that local registration is possible. We also feel that local planning—and I suggested that to the gentlemen from the AEC this morning—on the part of the AEC would certainly help.

"I think it was the activity of the Cleveland Fire Department that got the State of Ohio going on this thing".

He goes on to speak about truck accidents with school children gathering, and he then states that he was given orders by the AEC to cordon off any wrecked airplane and not to make any attempt to put out the fire or rescue the people but to call the nearest AEC office. He pointed out that the nearest AEC office was in Chicago.

"On the local Cleveland level, we in Cleveland have had a propensity for such accidents, and fires. We had a fire in a school and as a result we lost 200 school children and now we open our school doors outward. We had a liquid gas fire, and changes in the liquid gas storage have been made. We do not want to see such a thing happen in the new field.

"There is a lot of good to come to mankind from the use of radiological materials. I am sure all of us will agree that there are thousands of people doing research work trying to find civilian application for this industry. But we do have industrial fires. In the first council meeting we had on this problem, there were two extreme reactions. One member said, 'Out with it, ban the use of these things in the City of Cleveland.' We had an extreme point of view from one industrial group which said 'This is no problem at all. Why worry? There are laws that cover these things.'

"The firefighters of our town are charged with public safety. We are going to do it until we find out what the answers are and do an intelligent job of protecting the people we are charged to protect."

This is a simple story of a simple man which resulted in the first community council now in the United States, where the scientists and the industrial group and all interested civil groups are sitting down to work out a plan for keeping a registry of atomic materials in the city.

Among the other organized groups from whom I have sought information has been the lawyers. As you might imagine they have had an interesting time listing all the splendid new legal activities that are going to arise out of the atomic age.

Some of these questions might personally interest you. What should be done for workers, particularly technicians and professionals who have had all the exposure they can stand for their lifetimes and therefore will be unable to make use of their special skills? Should rehabilitation be aimed at training these men in new skills, of comparable values? What are the benefits? What should be done about personnel, who, after they have received their lifetime allowance of radioactivity, can find equally well paid positions having no hazards but who then lose very important union seniority rights? Should routine examinations for possible evidence of radiation injury be required periodically, as well as when workers terminate their employment?

This is a report by Dean Stassen of the University of Michigan Law School, who is the Chairman of the American Bar Association Committee on Radiation Law. This report is two years old. So far no action has been taken on the state or federal level that I know of to either get a broader statute in the works or even have hearings in the Congress on any of the recommendations of the Bar Association.

Of all the groups in our society, organized medicine has seemed the least interested and least informed of some of the basic facts of the atomic age. The biologists and the chemists have spoken clearly and forthrightly for ten years, but then you don't see many biologists driving Cadillacs.

A couple of years ago the Surgeon General of the United States Public Health Service did establish a National Advisory Committee on Radiation. This committee now has become a permanent council. The chairman is Dr. Russell Morgan, Radiologist-in-Chief of Johns Hopkins, and last Thursday he and the Surgeon General, Dr. Burney, released their report. I would do a disfavor to Dr. Morgan if I tried to tell you about the long work that has gone into this recommendation. I do urge you to read it. It is the first recommendation transferring public responsibility for atomic health to the Public Health Agency.

The members of the council I will read quickly because some of you may wish to know them or wish to write to them:

Dr. Victor P. Bond, Brookhaven National Laboratory, Upton, Long Island

Dr. Richard H. Chamberlain, University of Pennsylvania Hospital, Philadelphia, Pennsylvania

Dr. James F. Crow, University of Wisconsin, Madison, Wisconsin

Dr. Herman Hilleboe, Commissioner of Health, New York State, Albany, New York

Dr. Hardin B. Jones, University of California, Berkeley, California

Dr. Edward B. Lewis, California Institute of Technology, Pasadena, California

Dr. Berwyn F. Mattison, American Public Health Association, New York, New York

Dr. Lauriston S. Taylor, Bureau of Standards, Washington, D.C.

Dr. George W. Thorn, Physician-in-Chief, Peter Bent Brigham Hospital, Boston, Massachusetts

Dr. Abel Wolman, Johns Hopkins Hospital, Baltimore, Maryland

Dr. Arthur H. Wuehrmann, University of Alabama, University, Alabama

The first sentence of the report is the key to what we will see in the coming weeks in Washington as the struggle to put total responsibility for atomic health totally in one place. The first sentence reads: "Primary responsibility for the nation's protection from radiation hazards should be established in a single agency of the Federal Government and this committee believes this agency should logically be the U.S. Public Health Service. It urges immediate legislation to achieve this objective".

Hearings have been called for May 4th. The Joint Committee on Atomic Energy seemingly is willing to work with Health, Education and Welfare. There seems to be very little prestige jealousy between the legislative committees and legislation will be introduced by powerful members of the House and the Senate. It is my hunch that not a great deal will happen. The President has appointed Arthur Flemming and Commissioner McCone and the head of the Bureau of Budget to issue a report to him.

I think that the new management of the AEC would like to get some of the radiation concern off its back. So I think we will see some sort of transfer of responsibility this year. But as this Council to the Surgeon General is a permanent body, and as after July 1 it will be widened to include all proper civilian groups, I think that we are on the way belatedly to put medical care where it belongs, that is in the hands of the people we have given this responsibility to since Mr. Washington's time.

As citizens and doctors, I have no recommendation to offer you. I would be impudent to give you one. I am, instead, inclined to tell you a little incident that happened two years ago during the so-called fallout hearings. Dr. Glass, Dr. Crow, Dr. Muller, Dr. Russell, Dr. Sturdevant, Dr. Jones—probably a pretty good representation of qualified biologists and geneticists—testified for two days. At the end of that time the Joint Committee had an informal session with the scientists and Dr. Sturdevant of California Technical was asked to give a summary. He turned to the Congressional Committee and said, "We as scientists cannot give you a scientific equation, X amount of exposure represents X damage, and we cannot tell you what you should do. But we can say this, if you don't do *anything*, then you have done *something*".

Dr. Brosin: We have heard four challenging and thought-provoking discussions about a new power in our society—nuclear energy. I might also add that we have been privileged to note conflicting opinions expressed by our speakers in some areas of thought.

There is one area, however, where I am sure all our speakers are in agreement: nuclear energy represents a great potential threat to mankind. The subject calls for the highest degree of understanding, knowledge, and common sense we can muster. Every member of the family of man—be he laborer, scientist, physician or Australian bushman—has everything to gain, and all, certainly, to lose.

9

PSYCHIATRIC ASPECTS OF THE PREVENTION OF NUCLEAR WAR*

"The unleashed power of the atom has changed everything except our ways of thinking. Thus we are drifting toward a catastrophe beyond comparison. We shall require a substantially new manner of thinking, if mankind is to survive." — ALBERT EINSTEIN.

I

INTRODUCTION

The emergence of weapons of unprecedented destructive capacity in our nuclear age has given a new urgency to mankind's ancient quest for a world without war. Peace, as an alternative to war, is not, however, a static or quiescent condition. It involves a continuing process of dealing with international conflict and tension by means other than war. The achievement of such a goal in our time embraces profound developments in many areas of diplomacy, politics, law, science, technology, and ideology. It also requires modification of many entrenched complexities of human nature and behavior at both individual and societal levels, a matter of special concern to psychiatrists both as clinicians and as behavioral scientists.

Central to the need for a "new manner of thinking," which Einstein foresaw, is the overriding new fact that existing nuclear arsenals are capable of devastating mankind and its civilization. This suddenly changes the meaning of many age-old "givens" in

*Formulated by the Committee on Social Issues, and first published as Report #57, in September, 1964. For publications in the general area of this report by its authors, please refer to Editor's Note on page 371.

The members of the Committee wish to express their great appreciation to Dr. Otto Klineberg, who gave invaluable assistance as a consultant during the early stages of this report, and to Dr. Fritz Redl, who was a consultant and full participant throughout its writing.

the conduct of human affairs. Recourse to war traditionally has been a way of protecting national security, interests, and ideals; now, however, nuclear war incurs the risk of national suicide. A nuclear war cannot be "won," in the conventional sense of the term. A psychiatric follow-up study by Lifton (1) of Hiroshima victims illustrates some of the new meanings that nuclear war involves. He reports that survivors of atomic bombing undergo a new kind of psychological and physical experience — one that transcends the "ordinary disaster" in several important ways. The universal psychological barriers to thought about death become much greater in relation to a nuclear disaster. The human imagination may be too limited to comprehend death on such an enormous scale, and may resist doing so; therefore it may be unable to "prepare" individuals for nuclear attack. Lifton concludes: "Since these consequences [of nuclear bombings] now inhabit our world, more effective approaches to the problem of human survival may well depend upon our ability to grasp the nature of fundamentally new relationships to existence which we all share."

Yet the pervasive backward pull of the familiar and habitual ways of thinking is strong, and widespread suppression and repression of the new implications of the destructive power at man's disposal is comforting, but perilous. The writers of this report, whatever their personal values, do not presume to be more qualified than other citizens to evaluate the intransigence or menace of an adversary nation. We cannot know with scientific certainty that "limited" wars are bound to escalate, or what proportion of a population might survive a nuclear attack, or in what condition. We *can* be certain, however, of the global enormity of the *risk* to life and health that nuclear war entails. This risk, with its immense psychological as well as physical ramifications, is a decisive reason for our feeling a professional obligation, as psychiatrists, to concern ourselves with the prevention of war. As other physicians have stated: "There are situations in which prevention is the only effective therapy. The physician charged with the responsibility for the lives of his patients and the health of his community must begin to explore a new area of preventive medicine, the prevention of thermonuclear war." (2)

Some psychiatrists, as well as other people, doubt the appropriateness of psychiatrists involving themselves in such a global issue as peace in their professional capacities rather than solely as citizens. One reason for such misgivings may be an adherence to a traditional conception of psychiatry that excludes its application to the large social arena. However, psychiatry has been greatly extending its scope through the major modern developments of Community Psychiatry, Preventive Psychiatry, and Social Psychiatry — areas in which clinical knowledge and insights are blended with content and methods selected from Public Health and Social Science.

But the participation of psychiatrists in areas of broad public policy has been opposed on other grounds also. Are psychiatrists qualified for such roles? Can *any* scientist exercise the necessary objectivity and detachment in politically controversial situations? Is not each discipline too biased in favor of its own approach to appreciate the complex totality on which conclusions must be based? Such questions are well taken. We believe, however, that the potential value of including psychiatric and behavioral science among the disciplines studying these multifaceted problems warrants the effort, with careful safeguarding against abuses.

As one form of safeguard in this report, we have not assumed that we could supply any definitive answers. Indeed, there can be none to problems of this magnitude. We can but make available whatever increments of understanding we achieve to those who bear the awesome responsibility of decision. Similarly, we recognize the need to stay within the limits of psychiatry when seeking to apply its insights and methodologies to broad problem areas. One of the most challenging technical problems that confronts psychiatrists who would extend their clinically derived understanding and approach to nonclinical situations is the management of their own subjectivity. This may be further complicated when the issues under study, like the war-peace dilemmas, have become interlaced with controversies that are emotionally charged.

Whatever the form of psychiatric approach to these widescale issues, e.g., research, consultation, and so forth, its aim is to deepen the understanding of the basis on which rest fateful policies in the conduct of conflict. The complex nature of these issues requires a pooling of knowledge, collaborative effort, and better communication at various levels, both national and international, between psychiatrists of different schools of thought and types of practice; between psychiatrists and other behavioral scientists; between behavioral and natural scientists; and between all of these and policy-makers, on the one hand, and the general public on the other.* One of the many advantages of such joint endeavors is that they tend to counteract one-sidedness, blind spots, and bias in any participating group or individual.

We realize that some thoughtful people may question some of the premises in this report in the light of international realities and conflicting ideologies. As psychiatrists, however, we are especially aware of the dangerous fallacies of thinking in absolute terms, such as the goal of absolute national security or a policy of absolute trust. In order to reach a position about complex matters of multiple causation it is necessary to strike a balance between many contradictory considerations. We hope to indicate, throughout this report, how various psychological problems interact significantly with social realities and how they mutually reinforce, alter, or lessen the influence of each other. As behavioral scientists we cannot but be mindful of how, throughout history, social realities have been based on a fusion of objective phenomena with aspects of human irrationality.

This report has been formulated by the psychiatrists of the Committee on Social Issues of the Group for the Advancement of Psychiatry, with the invaluable collaboration of its psychologist consultants. The writers involved all share a preference for the kinds of democratic institutions that stress open societies, human

* The 1963 meetings of the American Psychiatric Association and the American Orthopsychiatric Association devoted expanded program-time to issues of war and peace. Psychiatrists have been participating increasingly with other behavioral and natural scientists in national and international scientific meetings, such as those of the American Association for the Advancement of Science, Scientists on Survival, World Federation for Mental Health, and the International Pugwash Conferences on Science and World Affairs (Pugwash Coswa).

diversity, individual liberties, and civil rights. We also, however, share the conviction that the resort to war is no longer rational in an age of nuclear weapons. We do not assume unrealistically that the alternative is a world without conflict. On the contrary, we believe that conflict between groups as well as individuals is an inevitable aspect of human existence. Conflict, however, is not synonymous with war, or even with violence.

Among the 185 members of GAP a marked degree of heterogeneity characteristically prevails, both as to their political views as citizens and their professional competencies, areas of major interest, and theoretical frames of reference. Over and above such differences, however, is the whole Group's commitment to the psychiatric study of this topic as a relevant responsibility of our discipline.*

Our approach in this report has been mainly that of (1) marshalling data and findings from within our own and related behavioral science disciplines, and (2) ordering it interpretively in the light of our pooled scientific understanding and experience. We have not conducted research (other than bibliographical), for which this Committee's structure is unsuited, nor have we collected new data. One purpose of the report is to make available to colleagues in various disciplines the results we have obtained by subjecting a mass of material derived from diverse sources to the processes of psychiatric "filtration," assimilation, integration, and deliberation. We have sought to identify and examine some of the critical psychological questions of our topic, and to call the reader's attention to pertinent selections from the work of others. In certain sections of the report (as in Section IV) we have also offered some original conceptions of our own. A major hope and aim is that the report will help to stimulate a greater amount of research by psychiatrists. Many issues specific to peace-keeping need to be investigated, issues in which the emotional, irrational, and individual human factors are too apt to be either neglected or exaggerated.

---

* More than a decade ago, in THE SOCIAL RESPONSIBILITY OF PSYCHIATRY, A STATEMENT OF ORIENTATION *(GAP Report No. 13, 1950;* Chapter 1 in this volume), GAP first expressed views that are relevant to the present report also.

Editor's Note

Following is a list of publications in the general area of this report by its authors.

VIOLA W. BERNARD, with PERRY OTTENBERG and FRITZ REDL
"Dehumanization: A Barrier to Reducing International Tensions," in BEHAVIORAL SCIENCE AND HUMAN SURVIVAL (in press).

JEROME D. FRANK
"Breaking the Thought Barrier: Psychological Challenges of the Nuclear Age," *Psychiatry*, Vol. 23, 1960, pp. 245-266; also "Emotional and Motivational Aspects of the Disarmament Problem," *Journal of Social Issues*, Vol. 17, 1961, pp. 20-27; also "Human Nature and Non-violent Resistance," pp. 192-205, in PREVENTING WORLD WAR III: SOME PROPOSALS, ed. by Wright, Evan, and Deutsch, Simon and Schuster, New York, 1962; also "Group Psychology and the Elimination of War," *International Journal of Group Psychotherapy*, Vol. 14, 1964, pp. 41-48.

OTTO KLINEBERG
THE HUMAN DIMENSION IN INTERNATIONAL RELATIONS, Holt, Rinehart and Winston, New York, 1964; also "Tensions Affecting International Understanding," *Social Science Research Council*, New York, 1951.

HAROLD LIEF
"Contemporary Forms of Violence," in SCIENCE AND PSYCHOANALYSIS, ed. by Masserman, Grune & Stratton, New York, 1963.

ROBERT J. LIFTON
"Psychological Effects of the Atomic Bomb in Hiroshima: The Theme of Death," *Daedalus*, Summer, 1963, pp. 462-497.

JUDD MARMOR
"Psychological Obstacles to the Peaceful Resolution of the Cold War," in BEHAVORIAL SCIENCE AND HUMAN SURVIVAL (in press); also "A Psychoanalyst Looks at the Nuclear Arms Race," *Frontier Magazine*, June, 1963, pp. 14-18; also "War, Violence, and Human Nature," *Bulletin of the Atomic Scientists*, March, 1954, pp. 19-22; also "Psychological Problems of Warlessness," pp. 117-130, in A WARLESS WORLD, ed. by Larson, McGraw-Hill, New York, 1963.

ROY W. MENNINGER
"Attitudes Towards International Crisis in Relation to Personality Structure," in HUMAN REACTIONS TO THE THREAT OF IMPENDING DISASTER, ed. by Greenblatt, Grosser, and Wechsler (in press).

PERRY OTTENBERG, with VIOLA W. BERNARD and FRITZ REDL
"Dehumanization: A Barrier to Reducing International Tensions," in BEHAVORIAL SCIENCE AND HUMAN SURVIVAL (in press).

FRITZ REDL, with VIOLA W. BERNARD and PERRY OTTENBERG
"Dehumanization: A Barrier to Reducing International Tensions," in BEHAVORIAL SCIENCE AND HUMAN SURVIVAL (in press).

II

WAR AND THE NATURE OF MAN

One of the primary problems that confronts the behavioral scientists in considering the psychological issues involved in the nature of war is the widespread assumption that war is an inexorable consequence of the nature of man and that all efforts to eliminate it are therefore doomed to failure. The fact that wars have taken place from the beginning of recorded history, coupled with man's powerful tendencies toward violent, destructive behavior, has given persuasive support to the hypothesis that war must be indigenous to human nature. This presumption has gained further force from the conclusion that since war requires destructive acts from individual soldiers, it must be a collective expression of individual aggressiveness and hostility.

On closer inspection, however, the theory that wars, particularly contemporary wars, are the sum total of countless individual human aggressions is not a tenable one. Indeed, even if destructive aggression were indubitably an innate human instinct, it would not necessarily follow that war is inevitable. Modern warfare is a complicated institution, the result of the intermeshing of many factors—social, economic, political, and psychological. It requires a complex social organization, intricate planning and preparation, and great expenditures of resources. It demands a high level of scientific technology, highly organized armies, weapons and supply systems, recruitment and propaganda. It is not something one man can undertake by himself, no matter how hostile or aggressive he feels. Once such preparation has been accomplished, however, and once the wheels of the war machine are ready to turn, one man can indeed start it. But even at such a moment the complexity of the maneuvers involved and the precision needed for their execution require controlled, cool, scientific judgment and do not lend themselves to the direct expression of hate and anger. One of the paradoxes of modern war, in contrast to primitive battle techniques, is that, as its technology has advanced, aggressive feelings per se have become progressively less needed. The push-button weapons of the nuclear age require calm mathematical precision, not passion, for their discharge.

Since war is a social institution, it must be potentially capable of evolution, change, and eradication. In the course of history such other widespread social institutions as slavery, duelling, ritual human sacrifice, and cannibalism have been almost totally eliminated. Yet these institutions, in their time and milieu, also seemed deeply rooted in human nature and destiny. Moreover, we know from both history and comparative anthropology that societies have existed without recourse to war for many generations (3).

Nevertheless, the individual and group psychology of human beings, their hatreds, their fears, and their prejudices, do play a role in the complex network of circumstances that lead to wars between nations and therefore warrant further discussion.

War and Human Aggressiveness

The obvious existence within man of a *capacity* for violence has led to two major divergent views of human nature. One school views the tendency to such behavior as *instinctive;* the other interprets it as *reactive.*

Freud in his later instinct theory (4) advanced the thesis that man possesses a drive for destruction and hatred, derived from a "death instinct." He believed that the destructive expression of this instinct could be modified by fusion with the coexisting, antithetical "Eros" or life instinct. This amalgamation, he asserted, could express itself socially in two ways: in positive, meaningful relationships with others, and in mutual identifications that bring out significant resemblances between men. Freud was pessimistic, however, about the probability that mankind would ever fully achieve this amalgamation.

On the other hand, destructive behavior can be explained as a reaction to provocation or frustration without postulating any inborn autonomous propensity toward such behavior [5,6]. According to this alternative theory, destructive attitudes, actions, or impulses may be reactions to a threat to self-preservation or to a frustration of the creative drive, or by-products of the individual's attempts to achieve mastery of the outside world or control of his own body or mind. Both views assert, however, that whether and how man's capacity for violence is *expressed* usually depends upon environmental factors and is not simply an inborn phenomenon.

Actually, as von Bertalanffy has observed [7], although human aggressive and destructive tendencies based on biological processes may exist, the most pernicious manifestations of aggression, transcending self-preservation and self-defense, are often committed in the service of ideas and symbols. Moreover, as pointed out by Osborn [8], warfare as practiced by man has no parallel in nature; among the more highly developed animal populations of the earth, there has never been similar destruction within a species itself. One has to go to species as far removed from man as certain kinds of ants, Osborn indicates, to find anything comparable to human warfare. It may be pertinent to note, in this regard, that ants, like humans, have highly developed social organizations. The common element of complex social systems and warfare in two species that are biologically widely separated lends credence to the proposition that the phenomenon of war depends more on societal than on individual factors.*

One of the additional problems involved in many psychiatric discussions concerning aggression is that it is dealt with in such generic terms as to encompass a simple act of self-assertion and a violent act of homicide within the same broad category. It may

* Konrad Z. Lorenz, the naturalist, has suggested that intraspecies competition is the major factor that can lead to nonadaptive aberrations of aggression at the expense of its species-preserving functions. Unlike those beasts of prey which live in social groups, however, humans lack innate inhibitions against using their weapons of predatory aggression for intraspecies destruction. When two wolves fight, for example, according to Lorenz, the potential victor's fangs are powerfully inhibited, at what would be the moment of kill, in response to the other's ritualized signal of immobile exposure of his vulnerable jugular to the opponent. [9]

be useful to attempt to distinguish adaptive activity aimed at mastery from that which is primarily destructive in intent *(10, 11, 12)*. Efforts at coping with the environment in active, assertive, discovering, and creative ways, but without hostile or destructive intent, accordingly might be placed in the category of *mastery*. The term *aggression* might be more usefully restricted to activities that are motivated toward the removal or destruction of a perceived irritation or threat in the environment.

It would also be helpful, in this context, to make a distinction between the concepts of *force* and *violence*. Force is the more generic term, and implies the application of power to influence, restrain, or master an object; it may or may not be destructive. Violence is a specific physical form of force, the purpose of which is to injure or destroy the object. Under certain circumstances legitimatized agencies, such as the police and the United Nations, may threaten or resort to the use of violent force for purposes of social control.

War and Fear

Whatever validity there once may have been to the conception that wars were related to aggressive impulses in man, in today's world there is at least as great a danger from the effects of fear. Abundant clinical experience has shown that panic is a potent trigger for hostile behavior and that extreme fear of an adversary is as likely to provoke a violent act as is hatred of him (see Section III, "The Effects of Fear").

War and Other Aspects of Human Nature

Traditional wars have both served and stimulated many other human needs besides aggressive ones. Love and hate, courage and cowardice, self-seeking and self-sacrifice have all been entwined in the tangled and tragic pattern of war. As William James *(13)* has observed, the military spirit has stimulated human reactions such as altruism, courage, and devotion that have been valuable to society and that deserve to be nurtured, if only "moral equivalents" of war can be found that would afford expression for them without recourse to the "immoral" destructiveness of war.

Affiliative drives not only are capable of "fusing" with destructive drives to modify them, but may also contribute powerfully to an actual willingness to engage in destructive behavior. The increased effectiveness of a combat unit, when welded together by the affection of its members for each other and for their leader, often has been noted (14). The readiness to fight for the love of one's country or for the protection of one's family similarly reveals the role that love can play as an incentive to war. In general, man strives to conserve those things that are valuable to himself, whether by warding off direct physical attack upon his person, his family, or his home or by attempting to protect his values and his beliefs from corruption, disruption, or destruction.

War has served still another group of human needs: those involved with the pursuit of power and prestige. Its complex configuration has also included impulses toward self- or group-aggrandizement and the acquisition of material gain. There is also a "game" aspect to the conduct of wars, hot or cold, that carries a sense of excitement for many people. The maintenance of tension by courting danger may be a source of pleasure in itself.

Stereotypes Concerning War*

In the course of human history, deep-seated stereotypes have evolved around war that not only play a role in serving human needs, but also constitute an important psychological barrier to its elimination. The educational systems of all nations teach that war is right and proper under certain circumstances. War's destructiveness and violence are sanctioned in the name of a greater good for the group, and thus what the individual might view as wrong or immoral becomes, by group sanction, not only right but supremely right. "Manly" virtues such as heroism and courage are traditionally associated with being a warrior. Most of the great popular heroes of history have been soldiers. Monuments to war dead frequently quote Horace's classic phrase: *Dulce et decorum est pro patria mori* ("It is sweet and proper to die for the fatherland"). War is glorified as brave, just, righteous, and honorable.

* Some of the psychodynamic factors involved in the formation of these stereotypes are discussed in Sections III, IV, and V.

This glorification is usually so charged with overtones of patriotism that to look for alternatives to war may be regarded as unpatriotic. He who advocates the avoidance of war or the pursuit of peace risks being branded as effeminate, passive, cowardly, weak, dishonorable, and subversive. The enemy is described as vicious, despicable, inhuman, and threatening to all that one holds dear. Each side pictures God as favoring it, and His blessings and help in battle are invoked from the pulpit. The brutal realities of war often are glamorized and obscured in tales of heroism, glory, and victory. The warnings of an occasional General Sherman that "war is hell . . . its glory is all moonshine" go unheeded, and the excitement of martial music augments intrapsychic defenses of denial and repression.

However, such a conversion from the "peacetime ethic" of "love thy neighbor" to a "war ethic" that sanctions mass killing requires special training, indoctrination, and propaganda. The peacetime conscience of Western man, developed in a matrix of Judeo-Christian ethical values, rests on concepts of brotherhood and abhorrence of violence. Confronted with the military injunction to "kill or be killed," the soldier often experiences considerable inner conflict. In some battles during World War II and in Korea, a majority of combat soldiers did not fire their guns *(15)*. Also, in spite of the enormous social pressures and positive stereotypes about war, most societies have had to resort to conscription to raise large armies and to employ various mass propaganda techniques to "sell" war to their populations.

Some Differences Implicit in Nuclear War

But beyond all other considerations, there is serious reason to question whether any of the traditional stereotyped conceptions deriving from past wars are relevant to war in the nuclear age. Under the impetus of advances in military technology, the distance between the individual soldier and his "enemy" has progressively increased. As a result, warfare becomes a less and less satisfying outlet for the release of aggressive impulses or for combat heroism. In a push-button war involving nuclear missiles, there will be no direct contact between adversaries. The techniques of waging war are fast becoming as impersonal and mechanized as pulling a lever to start a production chainbelt. In such a setting, the best soldier is not the "hero" but the "automaton."

One sometimes hears the assertion that the threat inherent in modern nuclear weapons is grossly exaggerated and that throughout history the advent of every new weapon, from gunpowder to bomber planes, always has been accompanied by dire predictions about its ability to destroy mankind. Since these prophecies were always wrong, some argue that current predictions concerning the risk of global human extinction due to modern nuclear, bacterial, and chemical weapons are equally erroneous. The fallacy of this argument lies in a failure to appreciate the truly astronomical increase in destructive capacity that has been unleashed by the splitting of the atom. In 1944, the most deadly attacks in history up to that time—the fire-bomb raids on Japan—were able to kill an *average** of "only" 4,000 people at a time. Today, even a single *moderate* nuclear attack can kill 50,000,000 people. It is estimated *(16)* that current U.S.-Soviet nuclear stockpiles are equivalent to 55 billion tons of TNT. The American share, if converted to TNT, "would fill a string of freight cars stretching from the earth to the moon and back 15 times." In less than 20 years an increase of more than 12,500-fold has taken place in the destructive power of weapons, and with every passing year even this present fantastic annihilative capacity is multiplying. As President Kennedy said: "Russia and the United States each now have enough deliverable nuclear weapons to destroy the human race several times over" *(17)*. This is a genuinely qualitative change in weaponry that no longer permits even the possibility of victory to either side. A war that offers mutual annihilation as the only outcome can hardly be considered an adaptive solution to international conflict.

So great is this destructive capacity that virtually all national leaders, even when striving to heighten their people's will to fight,

* Reports differ. The number of persons killed in the various raids on Japan varied from practically none to more than 70,000 in the fire-bomb raid on Tokyo in 1945. Estimates of the number of people killed by the atomic blast in Hiroshima (20 kilotons, or 1/50 of *one* megaton) vary from 78,000 to 225,000.

feel constrained to stress their ultimate peaceful intentions. Indeed, the basic rationale of an arms race is that peace can be maintained only by continuously increasing and strengthening national armed might, in order to deter any adversary from resorting to war.

The authors of this report recognize that whether or not aggression and hatred are indigenous to human nature, conflict in one form or another will always be part of the human scene. The modes by which these feelings are expressed and the manner in which conflict is pursued, however, are highly variable, responsive to pressures for change, and amenable to controls that limit the degree of destructiveness.

In spite of man's proclivity for resorting to violence to solve problems or resolve conflicts, there is nothing in what we know about the nature of man that would prevent his learning to substitute nonviolent force for violent force in such matters. Indeed, the survival of humanity in the nuclear age may well depend on man's capacity to find and employ techniques less destructive than war in the conduct of international conflict.

III

SOME PSYCHOLOGICAL FACTORS CONTRIBUTING TO THE NUCLEAR ARMS RACE

In the next three sections we shall review some of the psychological responses of individuals and groups that may contribute to the continuance of the arms race and impede consideration of nonviolent approaches to conflicts between nations.*

The Effects of Fear

Within optimal limits, fear performs an adaptive function by motivating an individual to act to avoid impending danger. It may, in fact, be essential to survival. A relative absence of fear in a dangerous situation may lead to behavior that is maladaptive or even potentially destructive to oneself or others. Similarly, false reassurance and overemphasis on the constructive or hopeful aspect of a situation may produce an unrealistic sense of security and thus reduce the incentive for corrective action.

However, behavioral reactions in the face of external threat are not simply a function of the "quantity" of fear that a person experiences. The meaning of the confronting stimulus, the accuracy of one's perceptions about it, one's previous experience of pain or success in similar situations, and the degree to which adequate

---

* There is probably an intimate relationship between individual personality patterns and socio-political thinking, including reactions to a perceived enemy. THE AUTHORITARIAN PERSONALITY [18] and, more recently, THE OPEN AND CLOSED MIND[19], for example, contain suggestive material on this question. Various papers and monographs in recent years[20,21,22,23] have attempted to relate personality variables to attitudes about foreign affairs, but the great number of factors involved has made satisfactory generalizations difficult to establish. This report, therefore, concerns itself only with widespread patterns of psychological response, without attempting to delineate relationships of these responses to specific personality types.

assessment of the situation is distorted by fantasies about it, all have a crucial bearing on one's feelings, thoughts, and actions. The symbolic meaning of an event can be more threatening to an individual than the event itself. On the other hand, a sharper awareness of the reality of a threat *can* serve to mobilize more effective adaptive responses. Thus the scientists who worked with the first atomic bombs were moved to make vigorous efforts to alert the world to the enormity of the awesome danger that they perceived in the unprecedented destructiveness of these weapons.

Whatever its source, however, beyond a certain point an increasing intensity of fear may produce profoundly deteriorative effects on behavior, reasoning capacity, judgment, and other mental functions required for dealing with the perceived threat. Psychologists have long been aware of what has been called the *primitivizing effect of fear* (24). The reactions of human beings may become more archaic and less rational under conditions of extreme fear or panic. When fire breaks out in a theatre, for example, most people tend to rush for the main exits and to ignore more available but less customary exitways. This reaction is seen in exaggerated form in brain-damaged persons who, when faced with a problem they cannot master, undergo a "catastrophic reaction" with severe disintegration of behavior (25).

Excessive fear tends to destroy the *capacity for adaptive discrimination*. Under its effects people are more prone to fall back on conventional and habitual responses that are no longer appropriate. They are also less apt to search for new solutions to the threats confronting them. The impulse to resort to military violence in conflicts between nuclear powers constitutes such a customary reaction. Although it may have been appropriate to the conduct of international affairs in the past, it becomes maladaptive to the point of being suicidal in an era of intercontinental ballistic missiles and nuclear warheads of from 50 to 100 megatons.

When fears of the enemy are intensified by inflammatory propaganda or by political or economic reverses, tension in the populace as well as in government leaders may rise to unbearable heights. Under such stress, almost any course may seem better than none at all. Hence the cry so often heard for "action" and "getting it over with," even though such action might be self-defeating or self-destructive. This urge for "positive" action, for "doing something," carries with it the danger that it may pressure national leaders into making political or military moves that could precipitate a war.* Such impulses to act precipitously may be enhanced by the increased craving for certainty that is engendered by emotional tension (see p. 402). The immediate purposeful activities that war calls forth may appear more endurable than the uncertain risks of peace (27). It is worth noting, incidentally, that although such activity may not be motivated solely by hate, it can be fully as destructive as though it were.

Paradoxically, another common response to extreme fear is a type of *functional paralysis.* Normal, habitual motor activity may slow down or cease, rational thought may become less possible, and the organism may "freeze." This reaction of acute nonfunction in moments of crisis has its chronic counterpart. Continuing fear may lead to progressive restriction of activity, to hypercaution, and, eventually, to withdrawal and immobility. Several investigators of stress phenomena (28) have described the retreat into sleep of a threatened organism. One may speculate whether the chronic stress of cold war in a nuclear era may not stimulate in some people a similar kind of maladaptive withdrawal, inaction, and denial.

Fear also *shortens time perspective.* The fearful person may become so preoccupied with warding off an immediate threat that he may neglect to consider the long-term consequences of his behavior. National policies may also show this characteristic. Nations at times counter what they perceive as an immediate threat by an adversary with action that engenders long-term consequences that may be more serious than the initial threat. An

* During the Cuban crisis of October 1962, a psychiatric officer at an Air Force base observed among the personnel a great sense of exhilaration and desire to enter active combat in order to reduce the mounting tension. The constant simulated combat alert conditions were enhanced by the increased realistic danger, as was the psychological proneness to react under great tension even if such action were self-destructive. At the same base, minor and major suicidal gestures appeared to be a frequent symptom of personal distress even before the Cuban crisis (26).

example of this is the continuing and enormously expensive build-up of nuclear weaponry by the nuclear powers to the point of colossal "overkill" capacity.

Fear, however, does not operate only in the manifest ways thus far suggested. Anxieties of internal and irrational origin often are blended with fears of external dangers and may be concealed in well-rationalized statements whose plausibility seems above question. Statements ostensibly based on realistic assessments and offered as objective descriptions may, for example, emphasize the enormity of the evil, the severity of the threat, or the inevitability of catastrophe. The hidden motivation of fear may be evident only in the selectivity of the emphasis, the omission of contrary evidence, or the refusal to rationally examine the premises of the statements. One may infer a considerable degree of fear behind emotional prophecies of the imminent danger of nuclear war or the pressing perils of treason or subversion. From each extreme, the prophets of danger may eloquently and persuasively describe the reality they perceive. The statements of each include the distorting effects of fear as well as some aspects of reason. Because the sources of threat seem so far apart in content, however, the common element of fear contained in each view is seldom acknowledged by the proponents as a shared characteristic.

The extensive emphasis upon ever more powerful nuclear armaments in the effort to become more "strong and secure," despite the deadly risk that is involved, suggests that many people are motivated more by fears of weakness and helplessness than by fears of death. Universal experience with the helplessness of childhood appears to have engendered in most people a deep-seated dread of situations in later life that threaten to recreate it. On the other hand, the fact that people have not had the subjective experience of death, as well as the widespread unconscious illusion of one's own invulnerability (see p. 386), may contribute to the lesser psychological "reality" of annihilation, as compared to that of being defeated and forced to submit. Inveighing against the danger of nuclear annihilation, therefore, is apt to have relatively little effect upon people unless the fundamental problem of their fear of defeat or surrender has been faced and efforts to resolve it have been made.

Other Psychological Patterns of Response to Danger

One of the most basic of human psychological reactions to danger is the mechanism of *denial.* Denial is a term applied to various degrees of nonperception, nonrecognition, nonunderstanding, or nonacceptance of certain realities in order to cope with otherwise unacceptable intrapsychic conflicts, feelings, or memories. So it is that some individuals may simply be "unaware" of the destructive capacity of thermonuclear weapons, in spite of detailed descriptions of it in numerous news articles, books, and magazines. At a somewhat different level, people may recognize the existence of the weapons without acknowledging their enormous destructive capacity. ("One bomb is just like any other bomb.") At still a third level there may be an intellectual awareness of the destructive capacity of thermonuclear weapons, fall-out patterns, the radius of damage, and so forth and yet the feelings appropriate to this recognition may be absent. Here one may speak of the affect as being denied and, because of its separation from the associated thought content, consider it an example of the psychological mechanism of *isolation.*

One may also wonder, however, whether the word *denial* adequately describes the failure of emotional comprehension of an event that not only has never been experienced, but is unimaginable by virtue of its extraordinary magnitude. If an event is neither experienced nor imaginable, it is in effect without psychological meaning.*

Hiroshima and Nagasaki have been to date the only occasions

* Szent-Gyorgi(29) illustrates this point very cogently: "Here we stand in the middle of this new world with our primitive brain, attuned to the simple cave life, with terrific forces that are at our disposal, which we are clever enough to release, but whose consequences we cannot comprehend. Its dimensions are too far beyond our human dimensions. When my wife tells me, 'the water is hot,' I am careful; but if I hear that an atomic explosion has 15 million degrees of heat, it means nothing to me. I am deeply moved if I see a man suffering and would risk my life for him. Then, I talk impersonally about the possible pulverization of our big cities, with a hundred million dead. I am unable to multiply one man's suffering by a hundred million."

where the "baby bomb" with its capacity for overkill was used on civilian populations. Lifton *(1)* reported the effects on the A-bomb survivors and on himself: At first, the victim was utterly horrified by the strange scene of mass deaths, complete destruction, terrible burns, and skin stripped from bodies. Words and language were incapable of conveying the feeling fully. But then, each victim would describe how, before long, the horror of it all would almost disappear. One would see these terrible sights, human beings in the most extreme agony, and feel nothing. The feeling was just too much to respond to. Each person had all he could do to survive and possibly help his family to survive. The interviewer reported that, during the first few accounts, he was profoundly shocked, upset, and emotionally spent. But the effect gradually lessened and he could look at the interview situation "scientifically." For the survivors and the researcher the "task" gave a focus of concentration and a means of dampening disturbing emotions. Many people in Japan and elsewhere still cannot bear to see pictures of Hiroshima, and avoid the museums where they are displayed. In fact, their avoidance and denial of the situation sometimes even results in a kind of hostility to the bomb victims themselves or to anyone who expresses concern for these victims or for future ones.*

Relevant in this context is the *inadequacy of language in characterizing new phenomena* that are several orders of magnitudes larger than—and thereby different from—any previously experienced. One can either coin new words to describe them or continue to use old words with meanings that do not really apply *(30)*. The use of familiar terms to describe new phenomena not only characterizes them inaccurately but also may engender a false sense of security if the terms themselves are reassuring ones. For example, the words "defense" and "national security" arouse reassuring images despite the fact that the development of intercontinental ballistic missiles and hydrogen bombs has drastically

---

*** Closely related to these phenomena is another complex and composite defense mechanism that we propose to call "dehumanization." Because of what we believe to be its special significance in our modern technological era, however, we are dealing with it separately (see Section IV).**

modified their traditional meanings.* Experience often adds a crucial dimension of meaning to a word or a concept. The meaning of a word may differ profoundly for two individuals with different experiences with the phenomenon to which it refers. The word "war," for example, arouses quite different perceptions and reactions in a gold star mother, in the wife of a black market profiteer, in a front-line soldier, and in a rear-echelon staff soldier. Moreover, words that gain their meanings by reference to other words rather than by reference to direct experience are apt to lack emotional impact. Only the few persons who have witnessed thermonuclear devastation or who live on the slopes of volcanoes can fully appreciate the effects of an explosion of a million tons of TNT. Similarly, the words "nuclear radiation" generally arouse little emotional response because they refer to something that cannot be seen, felt, tasted, or smelled, in spite of its deadliness in large doses.**

An important element in the management of anxiety about death, already alluded to, is the myth of personal invulnerability: "It won't happen to me." In extension to the group this becomes "It won't happen to us." This illusion is strengthened by many subtle social factors, on the American social scene particularly; the advance of medical progress, economic prosperity, the improvement of general social welfare, and a sense of American historical tradition that suggests "we have always survived these crises—we'll get through this one too." In addition, most Americans have had considerably less experience with war itself than

* "Neither the United States nor the U.S.S.R. can prevent the other from wielding a society-destroying blow, regardless of who attacks first. Offensive military power has been made so varied and strong that all conceivable defensive systems can be overwhelmed or by-passed by the power of offensive nuclear weapons." (Senator George S. McGovern of South Dakota — Speech in the U. S. Senate on "New Perspectives on American Security" — August 2, 1963, *Congressional Record,* Vol. 109, No. 118).

**This intangibility can also play into a tendency toward magical thinking. Psychiatrists often see individuals who display a tremendous *overreaction* to the danger of radiation exposure, as in the fear of dental X-rays. This is generally a neurotic, phobic reaction in which the fear of radiation represents a displacement from a repressed, unconscious source of anxiety. Similar mechanisms may also be operative in some individuals who show an *obsessive* preoccupation with the danger of war.

the citizenry of many European and Asian countries. The cultural patterns of the glorification of war (as described in Section II) further contribute to the strength of the mechanisms of denial and isolation.

Adaptation and *habituation* are other reasons for inadequate response to a danger. Biological organisms cease to respond to stimuli, even harmful ones, if the stimuli remain constant long enough or increase only very slowly. By living daily with alarm in recent years many people have become so habituated and desensitized to the possibility of nuclear war that the prospect of from 50 to 100 million potential casualties has become stripped of feeling instead of stimulating horror.

IV

DEHUMANIZATION — ANOTHER PSYCHOLOGICAL FACTOR BEARING ON MODERN WAR

Much has been written in recent years about the social and psychological effects of industrialization, specialization, collectivization, urbanization, and automation. An effect that specifically concerns us here is one that we propose to call *dehumanization.* We believe it has a significant bearing on the psychological capacity of people to tolerate the implications of mass destruction in nuclear war.

The term dehumanization, as we are using it, encompasses two separate though related phenomena: (1) *object-directed dehumanization,* and (2) *self-directed dehumanization.**

(1) *Object-Directed Dehumanization.* By this we mean the tendency to view other individuals or groups as though they do not quite belong to the "human race" and to deny them some of the characteristics considered most "human." In its cruelest form, this type of dehumanization leads to the perception of those discriminated against as *sub-humans*—implying that they have not quite made the transition from animal to human being and that they therefore do not merit being treated as human. In another form, certain people or groups are perceived as members of the human race but as not deserving to be treated as such because they are *bad-humans.* Since such people are presumed vicious or bad, one is exempted from feelings of guilt or shame if he withholds from

* A more detailed discussion of some of the intricate intrapsychic elements that enter into the complex phenomenon of dehumanization was presented by three of our committee members, Viola W. Bernard, Perry Ottenberg, and Fritz Redl, in a paper entitled "Dehumanization: A Barrier to Reducing International Tensions" at the annual meeting of the American Orthopsychiatric Association, Washington, D.C., in March, 1963.

them the considerations or restraints that he would otherwise exercise toward human beings. Paradoxically, sometimes *super-human* properties are ascribed to some people or groups to justify discrimination or aggression against them. An example of this is the image of the "mad scientist" who is "all brain and no heart." The exaggeration of one set of human qualities at the expense of all others makes him different enough to be considered an ogre or a freak. Or—as studies of anti-Semitism have revealed with particular clarity—qualities of unusual smartness, shrewdness, and organizational skill may be attributed to a whole group of people in order to make them out to be public enemies whose very cleverness constitutes a menace to the rest of the populace. Indeed, sometimes contradictory qualities of subhumanness and superhumanness are attributed to the same group (Jews, Negroes, Orientals, and so forth). In all of these cases, the phenomenon of "dehumanization" protects a person from feelings of guilt about the way he feels about or acts toward other human beings. It also enables him to maintain attitudes and behavior that are more selfish, primitive, or even cruel than he would otherwise allow himself.

Somewhat more insidious and therefore less obvious, perhaps, is that form of object-dehumanization that leads to the perception of other people as *non-humans*, as mere items, statistics, or inanimate "consumable supplies." This carries with it a sense of *non-involvement* and *indifference* to the actual or potential problems of others. Thus, without any conscious malice or selfish motivation, one is enabled to write off the suffering, misery, sickness, or death of others as something that neither concerns nor moves him personally, and with which no identification takes place.

Object-related dehumanization, however, is by no means totally negative in its implications. Although we are primarily concerned with its *maladaptive* aspects in this report, there are certain conditions and life situations in which dehumanization, like most other psychological "mechanisms of defense," serves significant *adaptive* purposes. The effective mastery of many tasks in contemporary society, including war, requires some elements of object-dehumanization. Thus in epidemics, accidents, natural disasters, and other peacetime crises in which many people are sick, injured, or killed, psychic mechanisms against pity, terror, or disgust are called into play that divest the sick, the injured, and the dead of their human identities. Only then is it possible to perform efficiently the task at hand, whether it be first aid, surgery, rescue operation, or burial. In fact, certain occupations in present day society actually require "selectively dehumanized" behavior. Examples of these are law enforcement (police, judges, jail officials); medicine (physicians, nursing personnel); and, of course, national defense (military strategists, fighting personnel). Indeed, adaptive dehumanization seems to be a basic requirement of any institutionalized process. Almost every highly professionalized activity has some specific aspect that requires the elimination, at least temporarily, of those human affective exchanges that are not central to the task at hand. Although the official in the window who stamps the passport may be a warm and friendly individual personally, in the context of his job the passenger's happiness or anxiety lies outside his emotional vision.

(2) *Self-Directed Dehumanization.* While object-directed dehumanization makes "non-humans," "cases," or "figures in a numbers game" out of *other* people, self-directed dehumanization has a similar effect on the *self.* When an individual protects himself from a whole cluster of basically human affects and states of mind — fear, compassion, guilt, or shame — he also does something to his self-image. The defense of dehumanization leads him to compartmentalize his emotions and pauperizes his capacity to feel and act like a human being. While this mechanism may, in part, increase the efficiency of people in certain jobs, its effect on their total outlook on life and on their destiny can become as destructive as the effect on the victims of these dehumanized actions and thoughts. Becoming callous, disinterested in human suffering, and immune to almost all considerations except those of job efficiency can lead to the development of a self-image that is increasingly void of the very qualities that a person must have in order to remain "human" in the fuller meaning of the term. Thus the diminution of one's sense of personal responsibility for one's actions — (I am only following orders"; "I am only a cog in a larger machine";

"They (the government, my superiors) probably know what they are doing. Who am I to question it and if I did, what good would it do?")—tends to create a self-image devoid of the qualities of courage, autonomy, power, responsibility, and sacrifice that are usually considered part of a healthy self-image. It is not only an Eichmann who acquires such a distorted self-image. The complacency of the Northern white vis-a-vis lynchings in the South or, for that matter, vis-a-vis discrimination occurring right around his own corner; the placid acceptance of the deaths from starvation of thousands of men, women, and children in remote areas; the lethargy that prevents people from writing letters to their congressmen to protest blatant injustices, or that keeps them away from the voting booths even when vital issues are at stake—all these are reactions that empty a person's self-image of some of its most highly prized "human" properties in order to avoid conflict, anxiety, shame, guilt, or discomforting action. (We recognize, of course, that other psychological and reality factors also may account for such inaction.)

Yet we cannot deny that it would be impossible to be constantly and sensitively aware of all the misery and injustice in the world and still continue to function effectively. Nevertheless, when the mechanism of dehumanization prevents people from taking steps essential to the maintenance of the well-being of society, the preservation of human rights, and the prevention of mass-destruction, it must be considered maladaptive.

One of the greatest hazards in the process of dehumanization, as with all other psychological defenses, is that the more real the need or justification is for its adaptive use, the easier it becomes to miss the transition point at which what was intended as an ego-supportive device becomes destructive—to others as well as to the self. This can be demonstrated by an illustration somewhat less dramatic though no less unfortunate than the nuclear bomb issue. The same psychiatrist who will go to any length of effort, devotion, personal sacrifice, patience, and concession to human frailty when appraising the needs of a child he is treating individually may react with dehumanized indifference or unawareness to the inadequacies of a juvenile detention home or children's ward, or to the long waiting lists of those for whom the community cannot find funds or facilities. The defense of dehumanization protects him against the distress of horror he would otherwise feel: "These kids aren't treatable anyway"; "There is nothing I can do about it; the power to produce appreciable change is not mine." Up to a certain point, of course, this reaction is adaptive. *Where such a defense stops being professionally adaptive and becomes maladaptive is a fluid issue that needs to be defined specifically with full recognition of all details of the personality and community forces involved.*

It is clear that the "object-directed" and "self-directed" aspects of dehumanization are mutually reinforcing. The more people rescue themselves from fear, shame, guilt, and discomfort by making sub-humans, bad-humans, super-humans, or non-humans out of others, the more likely they are to lose some of their own inherent human qualities. The more a man acts on the basis of a self-image that assumes he is powerless, an impotent cog in a huge machine, the more likely he is to drift into a pattern of dehumanized thinking and action toward others.

Parenthetically, it is important to note that our use of the word "dehumanization" in the present concept is not derived from the traditional usage of the word "humane" and should not be confused with it. Adaptively dehumanized procedures are not necessarily "inhumane": the surgeon who protects himself from being swept away by sympathy with suffering in order to perform his operation efficiently need not at all become "inhumane" in the process. On the other hand, a well-intentioned but incompetent bystander may be deeply moved by sympathy with an accident victim or an animal in trouble, but his clumsy handling of the situation may turn out to be anything but "humane." Our term "dehumanization" is intended to describe a complex mechanism of defense. It is not to be confused with a sentimental appeal for compassion even where it might be indicated. Also, as with all psychological defense mechanisms, much of what we describe here under this term may occur entirely *out of the awareness* of the individuals within whom the process takes place. Whether dehumanization occurs consciously or unconsciously is an important problem in its own right, but that question does not bear on the meaning of the concept as we are trying to present it here.

One might wonder why the mechanism of dehumanization has not hitherto been given more study and emphasis in clinical psychiatry. The answer seems to be threefold:

First, dehumanization as a defense mechanism is not a self-contained unit. Rather it seems to be a composite of a number of the more familiar mechanisms of defense, such as denial and isolation, that are discussed in Section III. Therefore, when aspects of dehumanization turn up in therapy, they would usually be subsumed under one of the other mechanisms or special disturbances with which it happens to be associated. Thus, while the concept of dehumanization has not received the emphasis we think it deserves, the phenomenon as such, whenever it turns up in psychiatric treatment of sick people, would have been dealt with under a variety of different names.

Second, most defense mechanisms originally were not studied in relation to such issues as war and peace, national destiny, or group survival. Rather they have been viewed as part of the idiosyncratic pathology of individuals in therapy. In this respect the lot of "dehumanization" is not so different from that of all other mechanisms of defense. The mechanism of denial, for example, has been studied much more thoroughly with regard to its impingement on the adaptive functioning of individuals in treatment than with regard to its interference with realistic responses to political events (e. g., its role in the injudicious delay of emigration during the pre-Nazi invasion period in Austria).

Third, in those cases in which therapist and patient are involved in a productive therapeutic relationship, we can safely assume that neither would tend to any appreciable extent to express patterns of "dehumanization" directed at the sub-groups to which the other belongs. The patient, for instance, who would dehumanize the class, race, religion, or nationality of the therapist to any marked degree would hardly remain in therapy with him for long. Conversely, any therapist who would manifest attitudes of dehumanization toward minority groups, sub-groups, or out-groups to which the patient belonged, would hardly be likely to take or retain such a patient in treatment. Similarly, if patient and doctor belong to estranged or hostile nations, it is unlikely that they would join in a therapeutic relationship.

Thus, in cases of successful therapeutic work between therapist and patient, the following alternatives can safely be assumed: (a) Whatever use the therapist or patient may make of dehumanization in their personal reactions to political, national, or major social issues might tend to remain *unrecognized,* since both parties would be using the mechanism towards the same issues. (b) Whenever the therapist finds that the patient makes excessive or pathological use of dehumanization, this might become merged with the larger *issue of sickness and its treatment.* (c) In those cases where the patient uses dehumanization in a way that seems to be adaptive for him, the therapist, while not agreeing philosophically, might consider it to be *outside the range of clinical concern.* Most therapists consider it their responsibility to free the patient from pathological or pathogenic uses of defense mechanisms, but not to bring him around to their way of looking at the world at large. This factor of "clinical tact" indeed may be a major reason why the socio-political ramifications of a mechanism such as dehumanization have remained obscured for so long.

Maladaptive Aspects of Dehumanization

In the present context we are concerned with the process of dehumanization only insofar as it bears upon broad cultural, historical, and political issues. In relation to these problems, in our opinion, it assumes importance as a complex ego mechanism of defense against guilt, shame, fear, and external stress. Some of its maladaptive aspects can be outlined briefly as follows:

(1) *Increased emotional distance from other human beings:* Under the impact of this defense one stops identifying with others or seeing them as essentially similar in basic human qualities to one's self. Relationships to others are likely to become stereotyped, rigid, and unexpressive of mutual concern. People in out-groups are likely to be reacted to "en bloc," with feelings of concern for them being anaesthetized. In extreme situations one may fail to react to them as people at all.

(2) ***Diminished sense of personal responsibility for the consequences of one's actions:*** The "I am only following orders" theme makes it easier to treat others as sub-human, bad-human, super-human, or non-human without feeling guilty, ashamed, or afraid. Or one may focus only on one's own fragmented job and ignore all its ramifications.

(3) ***Increasing involvement with procedural problems to the detriment of human needs:*** There is an overconcern with details of procedure, with impersonal and de-individualized regulations, with the formal structure of a practice with a resultant decrease in the capacity or willingness to personalize actions in the interests of individual human needs and special differences. This, of course, is the particular danger inherent in the trend toward bureaucracy that accompanies organizational units when they grow larger and larger. The task at hand is apt to take precedence over the human cost; the individual is seen more as a means to an end than as an end in himself. Society, the Corporation, The Five Year Plan, become overriding goals in themselves, and the dehumanized man becomes a cost factor, a tool, an item, or an energy factor to serve the mass machine. Even "scientific" studies of human behavior and development tend sometimes to become dehumanized beyond the adaptive level.* Such words as "communicate," "adjust," "identify," "relate," "feel," and even "love" can lose their personal meaningfulness when they are used as technical contrivances rather than applied to individuals in specific life situations. In reaction to the new hugeness of global problems, patterns of speech have emerged that are additional reflections of dehumanized thinking. Segmented-fragmented concepts such as "fall-out problem,' '"shelter problem," "civil defense," "deterrence," "first-strike," "pre-emptive attack," "overkill" and some aspects of game theory represent a move-counter-move type of thinking that tends to treat the potential human victim as a statistic and to screen out the total catastrophic effect of the contemplated actions upon human lives. The *act* of strategy takes on an importance that is isolated from its inevitable

* Whorf[30] and other language experts point out that sign language (the language of science), as opposed to symbolic language, dulls perception and conventionalizes and stereotypes responses.

results, and the process of dehumanization operates to block out recognition of the awesome consequences that, if seen, would make the strategy unacceptable.

(4) *Inability to oppose dominant group attitudes and pressures:* As the individual feels more and more alienated in mass society, he finds it more and more difficult to place himself in opposition to the huge pressures of the Organization. Fear of losing occupational security or of attacks on one's integrity, loyalty, or family are more than most people can bear. As a defense against such fears and conflicts, one feels great relief in joining the party, the organization, or the club and in becoming only an inconspicuous particle in a larger scheme.

(5) *Feelings of personal helplessness:* The conflict between the acceptance of procedural red tape, performing one's own job, and trying to appreciate the total gestalt is an overpowering one, even for the most informed people. The mechanism of dehumanization serves to reduce the impact of this conflict. "The Government has secret information we don't have," "They know what's right; who am I to question what they're doing?",* "What's the use? No one will listen to me" are variations on this theme that one often encounters.

Increasing Importance of Dehumanization in Contemporary Society

The net long-term constructive or destructive implications of specialization, collectivization, bureaucratization, and automation lie outside the scope of this discussion. All this, however, has an immediate effect on people. The result, for a few, is a heightened awarenss of social impact; for many, it is a reduction in their sense of individual power. More than ever before, the world's fate rests on a few heads of state and their advisors who must make rapid and far-reaching decisions for which there are no precedents. The impact of this fact on the vast majority of people is to reinforce already existing feelings of anonymity, impersonalization, and de-

* In studying the differential public response to fallout shelters a 1963 survey[31] found a high correlation between such conforming attitudes toward "official" thinking and the favoring of a shelter program.

tachment from the decision-making process. At the same time the fragmented perception of his social role puts pressure on the individual to constrict his affective range to the mechanized task at hand.

Modern war, as a social institution, reflects these broad changes also. In addition to the factors of distance, time, and magnitude in modern technology, there are the push-button nature of weaponry and the indirectness of releasing rockets to sites halfway around the world with results outside our range of experience. When we look out of an airplane window the earth below looks like a toy, the hills and valleys like abstractions on a distant canvas. We do not picture ourselves, however, as we appear to people on the ground, as imperceptible objects within a moving speck in the sky. Yet, it is precisely this reciprocal awareness that is needed to keep in balance one's genuine size and vulnerability. This perceptual confusion introduces a machine-like, impersonal quality into our reactions. The thinking and feeling of most people has not yet come to grips with the sheer factor of numbers and with the frightening shrinkage of space that has resulted from our modern means of transportation and communication. The death of an animal run over by a car, a child stuck in a well, or any other preventable individual tragedy upsets our emotional equanimity. Yet the thought of six million Jews destroyed in Nazi death camps or of a hundred thousand Japanese killed in Hiroshima and Nagasaki may cause but moderate uneasiness and puzzlement. Arthur Koestler has put it poignantly: "Statistics don't bleed; it is the detail which counts. We are unable to embrace the total process with our awareness; we can only focus on little lumps of reality" *(32)*.

It is the combination of these unique social and situational factors that seems particularly to favor the use of this composite defense we have called "dehumanization," which in turn acts to produce more of the same. The new features of time, space, magnitude, speed, distance, irreversibility, and automation are somehow not yet "hooked up" in the psychology of human relationships. We are confronted with a *lag in our perceptual and intellectual development* so that the enormity of the new reality, with its potential for destructive and constructive human consequences, becomes blurred in our thinking and feeling. Particularly in relationship to the threat of nuclear war this defense acts maladaptively by neutralizing the customary psychological barriers that would otherwise be present to the destruction of millions of individual human beings. No other mechanism so fits the requirements of this unprecedented external and internal stress. Dehumanization, with its impairment of human involvement, allows us to play chess with the planets.

Results and Implications of the Increased Use of Dehumanization as a Defense

It is one thing to become aware of the reasons why people nowadays may have a special need to take refuge in dehumanization in ever greater degrees. It is another to assess correctly just what all this does, in the long run, to us and to our destiny. For like any other mechanism of defense, even its maladaptive use brings with it a momentary feeling of relief, an illusion of problems solved or at least postponed or evaded. Its full risks to our peace of mind, to our lives, and to the very survival of the human race need to be studied at a closer range and in greater detail.

Importance of "Re-humanization"

We recognize that intertwined with the dangerous trends to dehumanization we have described, there are also persistent, healthy impulses toward individuation in various sectors of our society — in art, in literature, and in the ceaseless strivings of men of good will everywhere toward goals of freedom, peace, and human dignity. The same technology that fosters conformity also enables an individual to make rapid and meaningful contact with an almost limitless audience. Ideas and events, for better or worse, can have immediate widespread impact.* The same budgets, organizations, and technology that can destroy mankind can also produce the most constructive achievements in world history. A push-button can set a holocaust in motion, and a transatlantic phone call can prevent one.

Nevertheless, we are placing special emphasis on the phenomenon

* Witness the world-wide emotional reaction to the assassination of President Kennedy.

of dehumanization in this report because we feel that the dangers inherent in this phenomenon are particularly pervasive, insidious, and relevant to the danger of nuclear war. To the extent that people continue to take refuge in patterns of dehumanized thinking they are protected not only from guilt and anxiety, but also from the need to take part in the kind of social action and/or administrative responsibility that could have a meaningful effect on their individual and social destinies.

There is urgent need that efforts be made to develop psychic antidotes of "re-humanization" against this phenomenon. Psychologists, psychiatrists, and educators must investigate what innovations in modes of thinking are needed, and how they may be brought about, to counteract the intensified callousness toward human worth and suffering resulting from the advances in modern technology and the push-button aspects of nuclear warfare.

V

SOME DISTORTIONS OF PERCEPTION AND THEIR CONSEQUENCES IN RELATION TO WAR

Real differences among people can provoke tensions that lead to open conflict. This may occur between individuals, between such groups as labor and management, and between nations. Objective differences are so much a part of normal human experience that they are too often mistaken for the sole factors in any given conflict.

Less apparent in such situations are the subtle operations of perceptual distortion that may potentially complicate any conflict situation involving human judgments. Conflicts that provoke strong feelings, such as fear, anger, and envy, are more likely to involve these distortions than relatively dispassionate conflicts. Conflicting parties who are deeply involved emotionally in the outcome are also more prone to perceptual distortions. Since issues of international politics, national sovereignty, and the threat of nuclear war provoke considerable feeling, it is to be expected that perception of these issues will be frequently distorted. The relationships that exist between affective states, perceptual distortions, and the actual "realistic" issues in conflict situations are often difficult to elucidate. Some of the more obvious distortions, however, are worth mentioning.

Ethnocentric Perception

A distortion deriving from the influence of the group to which a person belongs has been termed ethnocentric perception [33]. This refers to the tendency of members of a group to perceive and evaluate events from the standpoint of their own group's attitudes and interests. The virtues of one's own side are magnified and its faults are not seen, while the evils of the adversary are exaggerated and his virtues ignored. Thus, the identical behavior that is perceived as "standing firm" when exhibited by a member of one's own group is interpreted as "being pigheaded and obstinate" when manifested by a member of the opposing group.

The effect of mob hysteria on individual behavior is a well-known phenomenon, but the ways in which more subtle group pressures affect perception are often not so well recognized. This phenomenon was strikingly illustrated by an ingenious experiment performed by Asch (34). A subject was placed in a group of six to eight other persons, all of whom were asked to make certain perceptual or evaluative judgments. What the subject did not know was that the experiment was rigged, that all the others had been instructed to give *false* responses on a predetermined schedule. At first he found himself in agreement with them but then found his responses differing from *all* the others more and more often. Puzzled at first, he became more and more upset and began to doubt his own judgment. About one-third of the subjects tested in this way finally began to "see" things the way the others did. There is little doubt that this kind of unconsciously influenced perception occurs widely on both sides of the Iron Curtain, particularly as cold-war tensions increase the group pressures toward conformity. On the other hand, it is important to note that the effectiveness of such pressure depends on its relative unanimity. Thus in the Asch experiment, when even only one other person agreed with the (correct) response given by the subjects, only one-tenth yielded to the majority. This significantly confirms the paramount importance of preserving the right to express minority views as an antidote to group pressures toward conformity of thought and perception.

Group pressure to close ranks in the face of danger manifests itself in the view that all who are not "100 per cent with us" are "against us" and in a tendency to react to neutrality with suspicion and hostility. In extreme forms it results in the labelling of *any* criticism of one's side as "subversive" and "Communistic" or "revisionistic" and "Capitalistic," depending on the ideological position involved.

Stages of Social Perception

The development of social perception in human beings can be divided into three stages (24):

1. The most primitive and least mature is to project one's own frame of reference onto others and to judge their behavior on that basis. Thus it follows that "when Alter sees as 'straight' what to Ego is obviously 'crooked,' when he judges to be 'tasteless' what to Ego is obviously 'tasty,' and so on, he must be deliberately malingering, or evil."

2. In the second stage of development, one recognizes the "relativity" of the other person's frame of reference but not of one's own. "This is the level of understanding at which we account for disapproved behavior in others as being due to the conditions under which they happened to develop. Thus members of minority groups are 'pushy,' 'aggressive,' or 'immoral' because they grew up in an atmosphere of prejudice or without as much education as we've had." This approach enables one to be more tolerant and less punitive to differing points of view but leaves one still feeling smugly superior about the basic "truth" and "rightness" of his own.

3. The third and most objective stage—hardest to achieve and to maintain—is that in which one realizes the equally relativistic nature of his own frame of reference. In this stage he recognizes that his values, judgments, and policies are no more "natural" and no less relative to his cultural heritage and interests than those of another person are to *his* cultural heritage.

A major obstacle to achieving the third stage of social perception is the *homeostatic need* of all human beings to organize their perceptions to fit into pre-existent conscious and unconscious expectations, needs, and wishes, and to reject, minimize, or "fail to see" things that would upset their basic views about the nature of reality. This is an effort to keep the environment as constant and as meaningful as possible, and to avoid whatever might make it appear disturbing or unclear. This has been called the "intolerance of ambiguity" (35); others have referred to it as the "need for certainty." This phenomenon is likely to increase whenever individuals feel threatened and emotionally insecure. It tends to lessen to the degree that greater feelings of emotional security are present.

Problems of Communication

Information about an "enemy" may be systematically distorted by several additional factors (36). Not only is the perception of an event generally less detailed and less complex than the event itself, but it tends to be simplified still further in the process of being communicated to others. Perceptions of the external world often are determined mainly on the basis of information received from others rather than by direct experience. The more human links there are in the communication chain, the greater the simplification and distortion. This usually occurs in a characteristic way: aspects that are unusual, controversial, dramatic, and deviant tend to be accentuated at the expense of other less obvious but often mitigating details. In addition, communicators (such as foreign correspondents) tend to communicate selectively information that conforms to their own group-influenced preconceptions. This may be partly deliberate, insofar as they believe their jobs depend on giving their employers and their public what they want to hear. It may also, however, be a manifestation of the fact that memory of an event is influenced by the witness's anticipation of the audience to whom it is to be reported (37). On the other hand, not infrequently a reporter's account may suffer distortions through editorial deletions or suppression, for political and economic reasons, by those who control the news media.

Stereotyping

These and other influences tend to foster the formation of *stereotyped* conceptions, both of one's self and of the adversary. Values become *polarized.* Everything is regarded as black or white, never as any intervening shade of gray. All truth and morality is regarded as being on one side, all deceit and evil on the other. The motives of one's own group are assumed to be morally righteous, honorable, fair, and decent; those of the opposing group are always suspect. Thus Americans viewed the U-2 flights as justifiable defensive maneuvers; Russians considered them offensively provocative. Russians regarded their resumption of nuclear testing as a justifiable defensive step; to Americans it appeared as an aggressive threat to the existing stabilized deterrent system.

The same forces result in *exaggeration of differences and minimization of similarities* between two opposing groups. It has been suggested that "if a scholar from another century or another planet were to study the Soviet Union and the United States without the benefit of our existing statements of the difference between the two systems, he might be more struck by the similarities than by the differences. But ... the ideologies in both camps are so concerned with the differentiation of one system from the other that a discussion of points of similarity is resisted" *(38)*.

The tendency to see one's group as all good and the enemy as all bad is strengthened by the unconscious mechanism of *projection,* whereby a person disowns his own unacceptable impulses or attitudes by attributing them to others. At the group level, projection is manifested by selective inattention to certain questionable actions by one's own side and a focus, instead, upon similar questionable actions by the other—the "mote-beam phenomenon."

Stereotyping has still another aspect. The enemy is perceived not merely as evil, but also as operating in monolithic, consistent, rational, sinister, and purposeful ways. Each side minimizes or ignores the existence of conflicting parties and purposes within the opposing group. Also each party attributes to the other a sense of omniscience and rationality that he knows does not exist on his own side. "Thus some blundering bit of American policy is attributed to the subtle machinations of 'Wall Street.' Similarly, virtually every public action and utterance of a Soviet official is analyzed as a piece in a complex long-range strategy. Soviet leaders are also human beings subjected to pressure and fallibility and Soviet society is not the complete monolith that it is sometimes said to be" *(38)*. Indeed, intense factional disputes have been an almost constant feature of the international Communist movement.

Mutuality of Distortions

All of these distortions on both sides inevitably foster a *biased perception of what is fair and reasonable,* and thus render meaningful negotiations often difficult and sometimes impossible. Communication between the two sides even may increase misunderstanding as each fails to hear what the other is trying to say — a kind of *dialogue des sourds* ("dialogue of the deaf")—or else ethnocentrically distorts what is heard because of the differences in reality perception.

For example, a Stanford University geochemist (39) recently reported on the strikingly different connotation that the emotionally-laden word "freedom" can have for people in the Soviet world as compared to the West. The Russians "boasted of their freedom ... (and) seemed genuinely puzzled by the assurance of Westerners that true freedom exists only outside the Soviet world." The freedoms they considered important and felt they had were freedom of opportunity to get an education and to work at a job and freedom from economic insecurity.

The mutual distortions of groups perceiving each other as enemies may cause each to ascribe almost similar attributes to the other—a phenomenon termed the "mirror image" (40). A Russian-speaking social scientist on a recent visit to the Soviet Union was struck by the fact that the American and Soviet stereotyped perceptions of one another seemed to constitute mirror-images to an extraordinary degree (40). Following are two examples he encountered and described:

1. "*Their government exploits and deludes the people.*

   "*The American View:* Convinced Communists, who form but a small proportion of Russia's population, control the government and exploit the society and its resources in their own interest. To justify their power and expansionist policies they have to perpetuate a war atmosphere and a fear of Western aggression. Russian elections are a travesty since only one party appears on a ballot. The Russian people are kept from knowing the truth through a controlled radio and press, and conformity is insured through stringent economic and political sanctions against deviant individuals or groups.

   "*The Soviet View:* A capitalistic-militaristic clique controls the American government, the nation's economic resources and its media of communication. This group exploits the society and its resources. It is in their economic and political interest to maintain a war atmosphere and engage in militaristic expansion. Voting in America is a farce since candidates for both parties are selected by the same powerful interests, leaving nothing to choose between. The American people are kept from knowing the truth through a controlled radio and press and through economic and political sanctions against liberal elements.

2. "*Their policy verges on madness.*

"*The American View:* Soviet demands on such crucial problems as disarmament, Berlin, unification of Germany are completely unrealistic. Disarmament without adequate inspection is meaningless, a free Berlin would be equivalent to a Soviet Berlin, and a united Germany without free elections is an impossibility. In pursuit of their irresponsible polices, the Soviets do not hesitate to run the risk of war itself. Thus it is only due to the restraint and coordinated action of the Western alliance that Soviet provocations over Berlin did not precipitate World War III.

"*The Soviet View:* The American position on such crucial problems as disarmament, East Germany and China is completely unrealistic. They demand to know our secrets before they disarm; in Germany they insist on a policy which risks the resurgence of a fascist Reich; and as for China, they try to act as if it did not exist while at the same time supporting an aggressive puppet regime just off the Chinese mainland. And in pursuit of their irresponsible policies, the Americans do not hesitate to run the risk of war itself. Were it not for Soviet prudence and restraint, the sending of the U-2 deep into Russian territory could have easily precipitated World War III."

From these observations, one might conclude that it is easier for each side to recognize the stereotyped distortions of the other side than its own! It should be noted, however, that similar distortions of perception do not necessarily rest on identical bases of misunderstanding. Thus so-called mirror-images may really be asymmetrical because of differences in the social and political realities involved, and because of different meanings assigned to such words as freedom, justice, and so forth.

The Effects of Mutual Distrust

The mutual distrust that inevitably develops out of ethnocentric distortions of nations in conflict becomes itself one of the most serious of the obstacles to nonviolent conduct of the conflict. The behavior of individuals tends to "pull" reciprocal behavior from others, and behavior based on distortions may evoke behavior that makes the originally false perception come true. Thus a paranoid individual by his suspicious surliness may elicit hostility in persons who were originally neutral, thereby justifying his originally false perception of them. Similarly, the mutual perception by nations of each other as enemies encourages a process of mutual antagonism that increasingly validates the original perception. The expectation that no agreement can be reached because "the other side doesn't really want peace" and "can't be trusted" leads to behavior that brings about the anticipated failure. Thus it becomes a self-fulfilling prophecy. As long as neither side has any confidence in the other's keeping any agreement that is made, they cannot really negotiate in earnest. Since even an inspection system cannot be made 100 per cent foolproof, some degree of mutual trust or risk-taking will always be necessary.

Interrelationships Between Leaders and Their Followers

Discussion of the psychological obstacles to the achievement of nonviolent solutions to international conflict cannot ignore the significant interactions that exist between the political leaders of great nations and their peoples. Ideally, leaders and followers are in harmony and share the same objectives. The leader's freedom of action and clarity of judgment are enhanced by his knowing that he has popular support and that he can readily persuade his followers to endorse the course of action he recommends.

This state of affairs can be upset in various ways, however, especially when a group feels threatened. External pressures typically increase the cohesiveness of a group. On the other hand, if the group is large and complex, or its morale low, outside threats may cause it to fragment into subgroups with conflicting aims and mutual distrust. The interests of some of the subgroups may conflict with the welfare of the total group. The "military-industrial complex" about which President Eisenhower warned the country might be regarded as an example in point. The enormous commitment of personal status and material wealth to continuance of the cold war may impel members of such a group to oppose reduction of international tensions, despite the fact that it might be in the interest of the country as a whole. Also, conflicts between factions on a domestic issue may influence their voting behavior on foreign policy.

The emergence of conflicting subgroups inevitably raises doubts in the leader's mind concerning the cohesiveness or strength of purpose of his followers. To insure that their will to resist the adversary remains steadfast, or for such other reasons as the achievement of certain strategic objectives of foreign policy or the maintenance of his power at home, the leader may be tempted to use his control of communication channels to distort the adversary's actions. Such distortions are usually in the direction of exaggerating both the threat posed by an opponent and his weaknesses. Once such tensions, fears, and hostilities have been created in the minds of the population, however, they become forces that themselves limit the leader's subsequent freedom to act. Thus a constant dialectical interplay exists between national leaders and their followers that often makes both captives of a "vicious cycle" of increasing cold war tensions.

Other factors also may predispose groups under stress to take positions more rigid and extreme than those of their leaders. Group members, expecting to be outvoted, may advocate reckless actions for private ends only to find that, through the well-known phenomenon of contagion, the emotions they have whipped up have swung the majority to their views. This process is aided by the fear of each member of the group that he will appear cowardly or irresolute in the eyes of the others, leading to a competition of bravado that pushes the group to extremes.

The diffusion of responsibility also encourages more recklessness in the group than in the leader. No single member feels responsible for a majority decision to which he contributed only one vote. It is also easy for each member to believe that the potential evil consequences of the decision will fall on the others more than on himself. For example, in the event of nuclear war, as pointed out above (p. 386), most individuals tend to feel that though the missiles will destroy millions of others, *they* will survive.

Thus when national leaders negotiate in an atmosphere of fear and mistrust, they may be severely hampered by group forces that restrain them from going as far as they would wish or that impel them to take more extreme and intransigent positions than their better judgment dictates.

In this age of mass media, leader-group interactions are further complicated by the problem of multiple audiences. A leader's remarks intended only for domestic consumption are inevitably overheard by the adversary, who readily misinterprets them in the light of his own distorted perceptions. Conversely, "feelers" extended toward an opponent are also visible to home populations, especially when negotiations are conducted with full publicity. Efforts to bargain, compromise, or seek accommodation under such circumstances expose the negotiators to charges of disloyalty by their rivals at home—a predicament that has been aptly termed the "traitor trap" *(41)**.

---

* For a fuller discussion of the problems involved in negotiations between adversaries see Section VII.

VI

SOME PSYCHOLOGICAL CONSIDERATIONS CONCERNING DETERRENCE AND CIVIL DEFENSE

The operation of many of the principles discussed in the preceding chapters may be illustrated by examining the closely related policy constellations of deterrence and civil defènse and some of their implications. (In doing so we remain mindful of both the limitations and the assets of our psychiatrically grounded frame of reference.) As approaches to national security, these policies have been the subjects of heated controversy in this country, not only at governmental, military, economic, scientific, and political levels, but among the general public as well. Both pose dilemmas of far-reaching consequence.

Deterrence

Psychological factors are at the core of nuclear deterrence. Defined in broadest terms, it consists of a mixture of methods whereby one nation or group of nations seeks to control the actions of another by threat of nuclear reprisal. Several kinds of deterrence policies have been and continue to be developed and debated. These differ from each other in vital respects, including the optimal weapons and target areas chosen for retaliatory attack. Current deterrent policies comprise components from several types, including counterforce and controlled counterforce deterrence, stable deterrence, finite deterrence, and several others (42). Assumptions and predictions about behavior, however, are basic to all of these complicated and ever-changing strategies and therefore come within our focus. Such assumptions and predictions entail (a) convincing an opponent of the deterring nation's power and resolution to carry out its threats and (b) assessing the adversary's perceptions, strength, intentions, and reactions to a range of possible circumstances. Furthermore, when both possess nuclear arms, each "deterrer" is simultaneously the "deterree."

The two major nuclear rivals in the world today have pursued a course of mutual deterrence. How reliable, from the psychological standpoint, does this balance of power and terror seem to be for protecting humanity against nuclear catastrophe? In considering this question, a clear distinction must be made between deterrence as a short-term and as a long-range policy, between deterrence as a transitional expedient and as a permanent strategy. As a short-term transition toward better ways of curbing nuclear might, there seems little doubt that deterrence has been largely responsible for preventing the outbreak of nuclear war so far. This was demonstrated by the Cuban confrontation when, as Walter Lippmann points out[(43)], the neutralization of Soviet power by United States power succeeded in deterring Soviet use of nuclear weapons to enforce its purposes in Cuba. But the United States could not, without "incalculable risk . . . use or threaten to use nuclear weapons to enforce all of our own purposes in Cuba, . . . but only a limited objective." As Lippmann also indicates, however, the confrontation, which ended peaceably, might have gotten out of hand had the leadership on either side been more rash, with less "poignant personal realization of the meaning of nuclear war."

Throughout this report we have stressed some reasons why people generally do not more "poignantly" realize how the new magnitudes of weapons have qualitatively changed the meanings of war and violence. These reasons seem crucially pertinent to concepts and attitudes about deterrence. Deterrence as a long-range policy goal remains largely committed to the traditional belief that superior destructive power ultimately decides international disputes, although it is a step beyond the old-style policy of crude military preponderance in a shooting war. Nevertheless its long-range effectiveness seems questionable, since it rests on certain dubious psychological assumptions (as will be elaborated) and encompasses forces that tend to make the achievement of a stable peace increasingly difficult.

Between opponents capable of mutual destruction, each "deterrent" step that one side takes impels the other side to increase his deterrent capacity to the same level or beyond it. A spiraling arms race results, in which the contestants become involved in a vicious cycle of reciprocal tension-increasing behavior in their respective pursuit of security. This, in turn, combined with ever bigger and deadlier arsenals, heightens the risk of global disaster. In speaking before a Congressional Committee, Secretary of Defense McNamara* pointed out the growing improbability that either side could destroy enough of the other's strategic nuclear force without incurring devastating retaliation. In referring to mutual deterrence as a grim prospect, he stated: "It underscores the need for a renewed effort to find some way, if not to eliminate these deadly weapons completely, then at least to slow down or halt their further accumulation, and to create institutional arrangements which would reduce the need for either side to resort to their immediate use in moments of acute international tension. The United States and the Soviet Union ... have a great mutual interest in seeing to it that they are never used."

Perhaps the greatest gain to be derived from deterrence is the opportunity it provides of a warless interval during which man can employ his collective ingenuity to devise and institute steps toward more secure arrangements for dealing with conflicts. Deterrence then would have served as a transition in the process of world readjustment to the new level of destructive potential that has come into being. J. David Singer *(44)*, in an analysis of such a progression, has conceived of an over-all arms policy continuum in which deterrence precedes arms control and is followed by multilateral enforceable disarmament.

Because a stabilized deterrent system requires a two-adversary situation, the urgency of using the time that deterrence buys to establish safer forms of war prevention is heightened by the prospect that within the next decade a number of other countries are likely to obtain nuclear weapons. This may occur either as a result of a technological breakthrough on their part or by a "defensive" transfer from one of the great powers that now possess nuclear

* Statement on new military budget to the House Armed Services Committee, January 30, 1963.

weapons. If this should happen, some military strategists have expressed concern that there would be a possibility of a "catalytic war" in which, for example, a reckless leader of another power might set off a nuclear attack upon the United States or the Soviet Union in the hope that he might thereby precipitate a mutually destructive war of annihilation between them. In any case, with more fingers on the nuclear trigger the risks of war by accident, mistake, miscalculation, or unsuccessful brinkmanship are greatly multiplied, owing to human factors.

As behavioral scientists our main focus is upon the human factors in relation to deterrence; as psychiatrists it is upon their irrational and emotional aspects. A great deal of the theoretical and experimental work on predicting the psychological intricacies behind moves and counter-moves in deterrence seems to assume, unrealistically, that it proceeds between entirely logical opponents. As Michael has pointed out (45), there are fallacies in both extremes on a continuum: At one end, the significance of emotional, irrational, individual factors is ignored. At the other, the situation is perceived solely in terms of interpersonal dynamics, as if these were independent of their complicated social and political contexts.

For example, some careful psychological research (46) on the effect of threat upon interpersonal bargaining shows that threats are effective only if the opponent sees himself as weaker than the person making the threat. However, in considering the implications of this finding for the deterrence situation, we need to recognize the fallacy of assuming that one nuclear power with arms superiority can use deterrence to push another nuclear power to political extremes, all the while counting on the latter's "sanity" to withhold nuclear response. The danger is greater, according to this view, that he will choose the suicidal course of war. "Such actions may be madness," Michael states, "but if it is madness it is shared by those who are pushed and those who do the pushing" (45).

Grounds for misgivings about deterrence as a long-range way to prevent war include the fact that a stable deterrent system would exist only if the weapon systems on both sides could be held to relatively equal strength. In reality this is not likely to occur.

There is always the threat of a technological breakthrough on one side or the other that would upset the balance and increase the provocation for one or the other to attack pre-emptively, either out of increased confidence or increased fear. At the present rate of technological advance, it has been estimated, the power of the U.S. and the U.S.S.R. for mutual destruction will probably increase at least 100-fold during the next decade (44)! Inspection systems may not be capable of preventing this spiraling technological race, since the technology of inspection evasion can conceivably develop more rapidly than the technology of detection.

Another point to be considered is that a *stabilized deterrent system can work only if the populations of both sides are mutually vulnerable.* If one side or the other could develop an effective anti-missile system or undertake an effective program of civilian defense (see section on Civil Defense), thus in effect removing its population as hostages against the enemy's attack, this would have the effect of upsetting the balance between the two sides and might be regarded as a provocative step. J. David Singer (47), in an analysis of stabilized deterrence policy, refers to some of its dangers: "[A major] difficulty lies in the perceptual atmosphere which the traditional expectation of war and the new technology combine to create.... There is an infinite regression of expectations at work, so that each fears that the other might seek to exploit his vulnerability so as to prevent its own vulnerability from being exploited, etc. It is ... the reciprocal fear that the second will fear the first's attack, and hence decide to strike first, and so on."

In addition — and of major relevance to psychiatry — *the theory of stabilized deterrence presumes that there will be rational and responsible control on both sides of the decision to use the weapons.* This is a highly dubious assumption for many reasons, some of which we have already discussed. As we have indicated, the behavior of many human beings under stress of extreme fear or anger tends to become more impulsive and less rational. Since men differ greatly in their capacity to remain rational under stress, it is fortunate that the political processes through which political and military leaders of great nations are selected bring to the fore so many stable, well-integrated persons with high stress tolerance.

Unfortunately, however, history provides ample evidence that this is *not always* so. The spread of nuclear weapons fostered by policies of deterrence steadily increases the probability that crucial decision-making power will fall into the hands of those with limited tolerance for emotional strain *(48)*. As Charles Osgood has put it: "As the speed with which missiles can be delivered increases, the response-time for retaliation decreases; and as retaliation response-time decreases, so does the time available for rational thought and considered action . . . . This increases the chance that *someone* will be psychologically unstable . . . . Furthermore, we must accept the fact that there are people with suicidal tendencies who, in destroying themselves, have no compunction about destroying others. The stresses of prolonged mutual deterrence can be expected to increase the numbers of such people, in high places as well as low" *(24)*. Furthermore, irrationality may be expressed through a deceptive type of pseudo-rationality. Bland calculations in which millions of deaths are juggled may reflect disguised distortions of judgment due to unconscious defenses of dehumanization, as described in Section IV.

It is also worth recalling that the incidence of psychosis in the armed forces of all nations that have kept statistics is about 3 per 1,000 per year in peace and war. Tens of thousands of military personnel in the military forces of the United States, U.S.S.R., England, and France now have access to nuclear weapons. The number is increasing daily. It is true that strategic nuclear weapons can only be fired by the coordinated activity of several persons, but some tactical weapons can be fired by single individuals. One American bomber, the F-105D, flown by one man, can carry five nuclear bombs *(49)*. Furthermore, some nuclear weapons are in the hands of teams that exist in conditions of more or less prolonged isolation under stress, notably on the Polaris submarines. On the basis of research on the effects of such isolation situations, it has been suggested that these conditions may predispose to the emergence of group psychoses *(50)*. Liederman and Mendelson *(51)*, in reviewing some of the literature on the psychology of isolation, refer to a psychological study made on the response of a nuclear submarine crew.*

Recognizing many of these dangers, the American armed forces carefully screen personnel concerned with nuclear weapons and re-examine them at frequent intervals. The Air Force, for example, has announced that it re-examines its nuclear weapons personnel every six months *(52)*. These measures may reduce the danger but do not eliminate it. As psychiatrists, we know all too well how ingeniously the suicidal drive may circumvent safeguards. A skillful paranoid individual can conceal his delusions from the examiners, and a soldier may become psychotic between examinations.

The American armed forces are also devoting much energy and ingenuity to tightening command and control so as to reduce the risk of unauthorized firing of nuclear weapons. However, since there must be provision for the use of these weapons in combat conditions if communication with the central command post breaks down, the complete prevention of their being fired except on orders from the central command might render these weapons useless when most needed. Thus to the extent that there is room for local initiative, the danger of unauthorized use remains. That the irrational firing of nuclear weapons cannot be completely forestalled is tacitly recognized by this understatement of the Air Force: "Unauthorized destructive acts cannot be completely prevented" *(52)*.

Even if the danger of irrational reactions under conditions of heightened stress could be adequately guarded against, the probability that an accidental nuclear explosion may occur through either human or mechanical error grows ever greater the longer the arms-race tension continues. Our press has already reported a few such near-catastrophes, and it is more than likely that similar incidents have taken place on the Soviet side. Accidents themselves do not cause wars, but conditions of intense mutual distrust and limited decision time increase the likelihood that an accident may trigger a decision that will launch a holocaust. In the present situation of tension and conflict between the two great

* The contents of the report were still classified at the time this report was completed.

world adversaries, the ethnocentric misinterpretations, insecurity, suspiciousness, and dread on both sides would seem far less likely to lead to the stably poised, static "balance of terror" that many advocates of deterrence have envisioned than to a highly unstable, precarious, potentially explosive imbalance. In this state of imbalance, miscalculation, human error, or human breakdown under stress could accidentally trigger off the whole top-heavy dynamism, with incalculably tragic consequences for all mankind.

It should be added that a weapon discharged accidentally or by a psychotic could hit a target in the United States just as readily as one in the U.S.S.R. In an atmosphere of mutual suspicion and fear, this could spark a nuclear war just as easily as an attack on the adversary. As Herman Kahn has pointed out [(53)]: "For example, suppose one of our own Polaris submarines accidentally launched some missiles at our own country. Even if the submarine commander succeeded in informing us of what happened before the missiles landed, the accident could still cause a war. The Soviets might observe these missiles exploding, and if they did not know where the missiles came from, they might decide it would be too dangerous to wait. Even if the Soviets knew that the missiles had not accidentally come from a Soviet submarine, they might believe we would not wait to find out.

"We might ourselves be under pressure to attack even if we thought the Soviets knew nothing about the incident because we could not be sure they did not know. It might appear safer to pre-empt than to let precious minutes slip away while we tried to persuade the Soviets that we knew they were innocent . . ."

A final psychological difficulty with the philosophy of deterrence is that *it is based exclusively on punishment rather than on reward as well.* Punishment or the threat of it may inhibit an undesired form of behavior in individuals, but it tends to leave the underlying motivation unchanged and stimulates resentment toward the punitive agent. The result is that punished behavior reappears, perhaps even more strongly, after the threat of punishment is withdrawn. Reward reinforces the desired behavior and creates a favorable attitude towards the rewarding agent, thereby reducing the incentive toward the undesired behavior.

As applied to deterrence, this line of thought suggests that more emphasis should be placed on rewarding any behavioral steps of a potential aggressor that reduce the probability of war (54). In so doing, it is essential to take the antagonist's frame of reference into account and to recognize that what may seem to one side a trivial concession may be regarded by the other as much more substantial. The praise of American and Soviet astronauts by leaders of the Soviet Union and of the United States represents an example of "positive" deterrence. That is, it is in the direction of reinforcing efforts for the peaceful conquest of space and strengthening attitudes that favor cooperation in this task. This correspondingly tends to diminish hostile attitudes that are incompatible with cooperation.

Some steps were accomplished in 1963 toward de-accelerating the spiral of reciprocal tensions between the two nuclear powers. These included the limited test ban agreement and the installation of a direct telephone line between the two heads of State. Some lessening of tension at the international level in relation to these measures and to the weathering of the Cuban missile crisis seems to have been reflected in the general psychological climate in this country. It cannot be overlooked that these developments occurred within the continuing framework of deterrence. Although the evidence at our disposal leads us to stress its dangers as a future policy, we do not advocate thereby a disarmed world or foregoing the use of threat to prevent violence. Some form of centralized authority with coercive power is probably essential to most social systems. Armed power to deter aggression between nations would seem far safer, however, if it were exercised by an international governing body than by each nation or a coalition of nations.

Some Psychological Aspects of Civil Defense

Although all rational people hope that nuclear war can be averted, the risk of it remains great. Consequently, intensive thought and effort continue to be directed toward means of protecting the civilian population against such an eventuality. One "obvious" measure is to build shelters that offer some protection against fallout. A powerful psychological appeal of the argument for shelters is that they represent a form of insurance. Even in the case of a massive nuclear attack, any one person may well be in a part of the country where no atom bomb falls. In such areas the greatest peril would be from delayed radioactive fallout, against which a simple, inexpensive shelter would afford a high degree of protection. Moreover, since the fallout does not come down until several hours after the explosion, there would be time for almost everyone in the area to get under cover. Shelters would also offer protection from the delayed fallout of an accidental nuclear blast, if it were far enough away.

If it were possible to build shelters offering some protection against fire and blast — the greatest immediate hazards of a nuclear explosion — even more lives might be saved. The cost of such shelters, however, would be enormous. Thus, viewed solely as insurance, the civil defense program becomes involved in complex questions of how much protection for how many people at how much cost.

There is considerable disagreement in scientific circles as to whether any civil defense program can be effective against an all-out nuclear attack. The widely circulated government pamphlet* on fallout shelters was based on a postulated 5-megaton bomb attack — a postulate that is archaic in an era in which 20-megaton bombs are standard and 50-100-megaton bombs have been built. As Liederman and Mendelson point out (51), psychiatrists are especially aware how the communication of misinformation, or lack of information, frequently leads to impaired reality testing and consequent maladaptive responses. Public misinformation about the magnitude of nuclear danger confronting society, in relation to planning about shelters, prevents people from most effectively taking action that is beneficial to themselves, their families, and their communities.

Nor has there generally been adequate consideration of the prospects of survival upon emerging from shelters. According to certain estimates, a 10,000-megaton attack (which is well within the capabilities of the major nuclear powers) would destroy almost all livestock, forests, and crops. Survivors, weakened by hunger and radiation and without the protection of public health measures, would fall easy prey to disease (55, 56). A foretaste of

* FALLOUT PROTECTION — WHAT TO KNOW AND DO ABOUT NUCLEAR ATTACK, U. S. Department of Defense, Office of Civil Defense, December 1961.

what the short life of the survivors of such an attack could be like is suggested by Bettelheim's graphic description of what happened to the inmates of the Nazi concentration camps when they were reduced to desperation by conditions of extreme starvation and misery (57). Herman Kahn (58) has raised the question of whether the "living might not envy the dead." Furthermore, as pointed out by Grinspoon (59) among others, in most thinking about shelters the emphasis on physical safety has prevented a sufficient consideration of the kind and amount of psychic damage and symptomatology to be anticipated from the combined stresses of prolonged confinement, external peril, and post-shelter conditions.

The "insurance" aspects of a shelter program, therefore, cannot be considered independently of the "deterrence" aspects. That is, the degree to which shelters might increase the chances of survival must be measured against assessments of whether and to what extent they might increase the likelihood of nuclear war. For, although civil defense represents a response to the thought of nuclear war, it may be recognized with all its complexities as but one component of our total nuclear policy. Its primary significance therefore hinges on its bearing on the probability of war (60).

One school of thought holds that a shelter program contributes to the effectiveness of a policy of deterrence. According to this view, the effectiveness of a threat to retaliate depends upon its credibility as well as its magnitude. If the civilian population of a country is unprotected, it is less likely to launch a nuclear strike that would elicit a counter-blow. Hence, it is argued, the credibility of the deterrence is heightened by a shelter program, and nuclear war is thereby made less likely.

On the other hand, as we have already indicated, in an atmosphere of intense mutual fear and distrust, there is a great possibility that any steps that might effectively protect the bulk of the civilian population from a nuclear attack might be regarded as upsetting the balance of deterrent power between the two sides and might therefore *provoke* the very attack it is intended to prevent. Indeed, some have argued that—since the logistics of getting the bulk of our population into shelters is so complex that it might well be unworkable in the 20 minutes or so of warning that would be available against an enemy first-strike—the chief value of our civilian defense program would therefore rest with the circumstance in which *we* decided to strike first at a time of our own choosing. Under these conditions our population could have time to get into shelters and would be better able to sustain the enemy counterattack, which would have been at least partially crippled by our first-strike. In the ruthless logic of cold-war bargaining, a nuclear shelter program thus gives us what has been called "First-Strike Credibility" and presumably would strengthen our hand at the conference tables. But the dangerously provocative aspects of such reasoning are precisely what might provoke a fearful and distrustful opponent into a pre-emptive first-strike attack.

Thus evaluation of the deterrence and insurance aspects of various shelter programs reveals their enormous complexity.* At one extreme, a massive community shelter program against blast, fire, and fallout would increase the credibility of our deterrence and might offer significantly increased protection against a small nuclear attack. But it would tend to be viewed by other nations as preparation for a pre-emptive strike that would strongly tempt them to strike first. At the other extreme, a small-scale private fallout shelter program confined to areas remote from cities would not be likely to provoke such action, but by the same token would offer very little protection and so would not increase the credibility of our deterrent. The question would also arise as to whether such a program could be kept from inexorably developing into the first type, as city dwellers came to realize that it left them unprotected.

Psychological effects of shelter programs on the individual also present many facets. Some argue that building a shelter brings the consequences of nuclear war home, thereby increasing the sense of caution and so decreasing the likelihood of war. Others claim that a shelter program would increase the feeling that

* It is important, incidentally, to differentiate considerations relating directly to civil defense and its goals from those only indirectly relating to it. Thus the "ferment" surrounding civil defense activities such as the shelter program can activate into group formation and political discussion countless individuals who have previously shown no personal involvement. Such socio-psychological reactions, with both their positive and negative aspects, are nonspecific phenomena that tend to occur in relation to any program that personally affects large masses of people.

nuclear war is inevitable and might also give people a feeling of psychological security, justified or unjustified. The longing for reassurance as an antidote to the anxieties engendered by the risk of nuclear war is a powerful emotional inducement for distorting the facts* about shelters into illusory confidence in the safety they can provide. By contributing to wishful illusions about the ability to avoid the horrors of nuclear war and to convictions about the inevitability of its occurrence, shelters might increase a nation's willingness to take risks and so make war more likely.

Along the same lines, there is an aspect to the private fallout shelter program that is unlikely to be talked about but that may subtly enter into the underlying feelings of some of those who have built shelters. When an individual has built and stocked a shelter, he may tend to develop an emotional stake in there being a nuclear war — partly to justify his effort and his sense of superior foresightedness. Without being aware of it he might then feel, in effect, "Let there be a nuclear war. At least I'll survive; if others don't, it's their own fault." Thus such individuals, without recognizing some of their deeper motives, are apt to become members of the "get-tough-with-the-enemy-even-if-it-means-nuclear-war" group. The fact that a nuclear war would in all probability mean their own destruction too — with or without fallout shelters — does not affect this feeling because it stems not from rational considerations but from unconscious emotional ones.

The building and stocking of a family shelter *may* heighten a family's sense of solidarity and so contribute to its morale, but encouraging people to build private shelters has already proven to have unhappy social consequences. Since it is inherently an economically discriminatory program (really "adequate" fallout shelters are expensive to build), only the well-to-do can afford them. Thus there is danger of increasing tensions between the rich and the poor. But more than this, it has proven to be socially

* Even though the interpretation of factual information is susceptible to emotional distortion, such information is important to the shaping of opinions about the value of shelters. The public opinion survey cited earlier*(31)* found that the level of factual information about "nuclear age matters" was significantly lower among people who favored the shelter program. According to the survey, "the more people know about the cold war the less credible fallout shelters appear to be as a means of vitiating the effects of nuclear attack."

divisive in a much more pervasive sense. The very essence of such a program is "Each man for himself and devil take the hindmost." At the height of the private shelter program it was commonplace to talk of equipping each fallout shelter with a shotgun—to keep one's neighbors out. People who were building shelters often made great efforts to keep it a secret even from their closest friends. In 1961 newspapers reported that civil defense officials in Nevada and California advised their local citizenry to arm themselves with pistols to be prepared to fight off, not the enemy, but refugees from neighboring areas who might be seeking sanctuary in case of nuclear war. Although the authenticity of these reports was later questioned, the fact that they appeared to be widely believed or accepted as believable itself indicates the state of mind they portrayed.

Much of the earlier public clamor about the issue has subsided, however, since the community shelter program superseded the private shelter plan. The level of debate has become more sophisticated and informed, at least in many circles. Nevertheless, as was apparent from the testimony at hearings before the House Armed Services Subcommittee in the summer of 1963, widespread disagreement exists within all professions as to the basic feasibility and desirability of a large-scale shelter program.

On the face of it, a community-shelter program obviates many of the group-divisive dangers of the individual family-shelter program. The experience of Londoners during the blitz of World War II seems to demonstrate, in fact, that some aspects of such a program might even strengthen group cohesiveness. There are, however, certain important differences between what happened in London and what might happen in a nuclear war that should put us on guard against drawing analogies between the two. The bombing attacks during the London blitz went on from dusk to dawn, night after night, and often during the daytime as well. Between air raids, however, people could emerge to go to their homes or places of work. In a nuclear war, people will have to remain in shelters for a minimum of two weeks. This involves complicated problems of food and water storage, and of provisions for excretory function. With scores of people living together in very crowded quarters for a prolonged period under conditions of extreme anxiety and stress, there would be enormous psychological problems. Parents separated from their children or from one another, crying or bedwetting children, racial, ethnic, or interfamilial tensions, physical illness, deaths, panic reactions, and outbreaks of violence,—these are but a few of the problems that might occur under such conditions and that could be enormously disintegrative to group morale.

Thus, in their appraisal of some psychiatric considerations in the planning and utilization of defense shelters, Liederman and Mendelson [(46)] cite a study on adaptation to disaster. It found that "social disorganization is greater as the disastrous force is more rapid, the period of forewarning briefer, the disaster agent less well known, and less clearly perceived, the physical destructiveness greater, and the length of time in which the force acts is greater." As the authors point out, these are the probable conditions of nuclear attack.

The very process of building community shelters may raise problems that can be detrimental to group morale. For example, how will people be matched to available shelters? America is a nation on wheels. In case of nuclear attack will a stranger in an area be welcomed to a community shelter designed to hold a limited number of people? Will there be "separate but equal" facilities in nonintegrated communities? Once a community shelter program is undertaken in earnest, there is every reason to anticipate that questions and fantasies of this kind will increasingly occupy the attention of people, and that the consequence of this will be a steady increase in the kind of anxiety and group disintegrative reactions that we have already observed in response to the individual family shelter program.

A full-scale community shelter program will also require the predesignation of leaders empowered to determine which persons can enter the shelter and which cannot and to handle the problems of shelter living. It will also require pretraining the civilian population for such leadership and for shelter life. In short, to have any prospect of effectiveness at all, a community shelter program would have to be accompanied by radical changes in the American way of life, including, in all probability, the sacrifice of some of the liberties we would presumably be fighting to defend (61).

Thus it seems clear that the psychological and social implications of civil defense are considerably more complex than might appear at first glance. Various programs would differently affect the morale of individuals and groups and the probability of facilitating or inhibiting the outbreak of nuclear war. The strength of a nation depends not only on its armaments but on the group spirit of its citizenry. In view of their possible ultimate adverse effects on morale and their equivocal implications for military power, all civil defense programs would seem to warrant the most careful study before being put into action.

It is encouraging to note that behavioral science investigations of significance for civil defense are in progress and receiving attention in official quarters. One such example is the work of the National Academy of Science — National Research Council Disaster Study Group (62). However, a major obstacle to the researching of psychosocial issues related to shelters must be recognized. No past situations from which we can draw data or current experiments — such as simulated shelter living — are comparable in terms of all the crucial variables to the circumstances of shelter usage under nuclear attack.

The most basic reason for our position, as psychiatrists, that, on balance, current civil defense programs endanger more than they protect goes back to our central psychological theme: the fact of nuclear technology has transformed the meanings of war, but corresponding change in patterns of thought lags far behind, largely owing to psychological reactions of denial or inability to comprehend what has never been experienced. Unconscious denial operates not merely in an all-or-none way but with many subtle variations. It may be partial, limited to specific content, and may occur at different levels. Thus, one may face up to certain aspects of the nuclear situation, and indeed be preoccupied by them, while still denying, at a deeper level of emotional realization, the drastically changed actualities of modern war. The overcoming of such denial together with the actions and policies based on it is of vital importance to the issue of survival.

VII

SOME CONSIDERATIONS RELATED TO THE CONDUCT OF INTERNATIONAL CONFLICT WITHOUT VIOLENCE

In this section we shall attempt, within the confines of our competence and experience as psychiatrists, to examine some means by which conflict can be conducted and resolved without resort to violence. We recognize that these means, when they are applied to disputes between nations, acquire political ramifications that range beyond our sphere of proficiency. We hope, however, that some of the principles derived from our experience and the literature may be applicable to the broader arena of international discord.

Conflict as a Stimulus to Adaptation

As indicated previously (Section II), although warfare is not inevitable, human conflict in one form or another is. Moreover, the clinical experience of psychiatrists in dealing with intrapsychic as well as with interpersonal and intergroup conflict amply confirms that conflict has important adaptive aspects as well as destructive potentials, and that it is often the essential matrix out of which emerge constructive change and growth.

Periods of intense conflict are characteristically times of *crisis;* that is, situations in which the capacity of the organism to meet the challenge is in doubt. At such times of precarious equilibrium, new approaches, changes in the issues, development of new relationships, or shift of the conflict to another plane may be accomplished more easily than under less stressful circumstances. In the individual, such developmental crises as adolescence may be important in precipitating constructive or destructive developments (63). In group psychology crises may have an integrative effect in conflict situations by virtue of the fact that conflict keeps opponents in vigorous contact with each other (64) and mobilizes their energies in the direction of mastery of the presumptive danger. Groups characteristically manifest integrative tendencies under the threat of external attacks, and may, in fact, react with disintegrative trends when the external challenge is removed. Family crises have been identified as points at which interventions can produce favorable or unfavorable changes more easily than usual. In social and community psychiatry the same principle has been recognized in connection with the greater effectiveness of interventions at times of crisis such as epidemics, natural disasters, and economic depressions (65).

Undue focus upon rapid resolution of conflict may result in an unnecessary sense of failure when progress seems to be limited, thereby making further efforts even more difficult. Emphasis on conduct of the conflict as an ongoing process, and on *progress* rather than *resolution*, may be generally more realistic and constructive. Some conflicts can never be resolved with finality, since any solution demands excessive sacrifice from the antagonists. Pride and "face" often require extended conflict before there can be progress toward resolution. However, even when neither side is willing to capitulate, to make concessions, or to compromise, continued conduct of the conflicts may lead to greater clarification of the issues, to opportunities for each party to test the soundness and validity of different positions, and eventually to a better understanding of the factors responsible for the differences. Such relationships may require continuing conflict and striving toward solutions as toward an infinity that can be approached but never reached. One is reminded of durable marriages of incompatible persons in which the conflict itself is the method of communication that has become established between the marital partners (66, 67, 68).

The function of conflict and crisis as precipitants of change is illustrated by the international crisis over Soviet nuclear missiles installed in Cuba in 1962, which impelled American and Soviet diplomacy to achieve a significant step towards decreasing tension between the two nations. According to Krushchev,* the Soviet

* Press conference in Moscow, July 1963.

Union's confidence that the United States would stand by its word was increased by the fact that the United States had lived up to its agreement not to invade Cuba. Many commentators regarded this as an important factor in the limited test-ban agreement of July, 1963. Thus crisis situations, while potentially perilous, may alter the management of conflict in ways that are advantageous to all participating parties.

Conflict and Unconscious Motivation

Much individual behavior can be understood as an attempt to adapt to intrapsychic conflicts whose roots may be concealed from awareness. A conflicted individual's descriptions of his feelings often are characterized by rationalizations, displacements, distortions of various kinds, or even denial that the conflict exists.

Especially relevant to international conflict is the phenomenon — commonly observed by psychiatrists — of dealing with a conflictual dilemma by externalizing part of it. Although clearly evident in such pathological reactions as paranoid projections, this phenomenon is less commonly recognized in nonpathological life situations. For example, an individual faced with a difficult choice may, privately, see advantages as well as disadvantages to each alternative. In discussions, however, he may react to the other person's viewpoint with increasingly dogmatic opposition until he appears to be entirely convinced of the virtues of one way and the liabilities of the other. What has happened is that he has externalized one side of the problem in the other person, so that he can now take up the other side without further inner conflict.

This press toward polarities that is generally characteristic of arguments, disagreements, and conflict situations thus often conceals the fact that each party may recognize some validity to the other point of view but is driven to deny it by powerful inner needs to resolve ambiguity. Although externalization of the conflict may achieve some relief of inner uncertainty, it does so at the cost of persistent external stress.

Comparably, on the international scene, national leaders sometimes attribute domestic difficulties to external problems and pressures as a device for displacing blame and responsibility away from themselves onto an outside "scapegoat." Clinical experience suggests that many conflicts, however realistic they seem, have symbolic reference to issues arising from unresolved conflict situations encountered in the past that become "re-ignited" by parallel or similar situations in the present. Thus current attitudes of the Soviet Union and the United States toward each other are partly determined by the history of their interactions since 1917, although realistically this may be largely irrelevant to their present differences.

These illustrations of the operation of dynamic mechanisms that may be concealed or even unconscious and hence not readily available for analysis are reminders that virtually every conflict situation involves similar processes, no matter how "objective" the disagreement may seem to be.

Management of Conflict

We turn now to a consideration of various means for conducting, containing, and controlling conflict, as well as of more recent methods employed in group conflict situations. We will examine these methods *in relation to the threat of nuclear war,* without attempting a comprehensive discussion of the whole range of methods for resolving conflict. Furthermore, while we fully recognize the great importance of political, economic, and military aspects of conflict, we will focus on psychological aspects that are also important but often overlooked.

One of the basic dilemmas inherent in the current international struggle is that both adversaries have grown so powerful that the destruction of either side is no longer possible without the aggressor also being destroyed; nevertheless, the conflict between them continues to appear irreconcilable. It has been suggested *(69)* that historically the way out of such apparently insoluble dilemmas has been to critically re-examine the habitual modes of thought that led to the dilemma in the first place.

Thus some of the fundamental paradoxes in the field of natural science were resolved only when habitual "common sense" ways of thinking about space and time were transcended by new modes of thought in Einstein's theory of relativity. Similarly, many of the paradoxes of human behavior remained obscure until Freud's insight into the nature of the unconscious was able to clarify what habitual "common sense approaches" had been unable to. The dilemma in the current nuclear arms race is occasioned, partially at least, by the fact that both sides rely chiefly upon traditional strategies to conduct their conflict as they pursue divergent political ideologies. This traditional or "strategic" mode of thinking about international conflicts regards them as struggles in which the only possible outcome is total victory of one side over the other — a view that finds expression in the "Red or dead" formula that has such wide currency.

The leap in our thinking required to resolve this dilemma is to break away from the conception of all conflicts as "zero-sum games" in which one antagonist must lose what the other wins. We must recognize that some types of international conflict today can be resolved only by solutions in which neither side loses and in which sometimes both sides may win (70). The limited test ban treaty represents such a partial solution for the conflict represented by the nuclear arms race. As President Kennedy emphasized, in his judgment the U.S.S.R. was neither gaining nor giving anything away by signing the treaty. He added that it was the human race that was the gainer.

With this general point in mind, we shall now consider some aspects of the management of international conflict in today's world.

General Field Factors Common to Conflict Situations

Two significant sets of conditions between and within parties that influence their approaches to conflict situations are (1) the degree of trust or distrust and (2) the degree of communication or distance.

1. *Trust vs. Distrust.* Resolution of conflict or even its containment within nondestructive limits is generally dependent upon some element of trust. The concept of trust embodies the expectation that the behavior of another will stay within a spectrum of actions that will not be harmful. Mistrust, the expectation of dam-

aging results from an interaction, also covers a spectrum, ranging from an annihilative consequence to a neutral midpoint.

The degree of trust between opposing parties in conflict situations enormously influences their views of the conflict, their evaluation of the possible outcome, and the tactics they will use to defend their interests and pursue their ends. Complicating the trust-assessment process is the commonly held feeling that opponents are either trustworthy or not; that they must be either close friends or sworn enemies. Such a sharp dichotomy, based on feelings rather than judgment, ignores the broad gray zone between the extremes, in which opponents may be trustworthy in limited ways or in specific ways. The greater the mistrust, however, the more likely are the contenders to see the conflict in absolute terms and to react with intense emotionality. The issue becomes oversimplified ("death to the enemy!"), the opponent is viewed as satanic, and the risk of defeat is perceived as catastrophic, justifying the most extreme forms of self-defense, including pre-emptive attack.

A modicum of trust, even slight, enables the contenders to maintain more controlled views of the conflict. While they see the implications of loss as serious, the contenders no longer include the risk of annihilation as part of the outcome. The essential contribution of trust to a potentially deadly conflict situation is the mutual recognition that, however great their differences, the contenders nonetheless respect each other's right to exist. The consequent shift away from a "battle to the death" increases the likelihood that some of the points in conflict will be resolved. In this sense, trust may be understood as an ally of reason and an antidote to the irrational and the passionate.

With still greater mutual trust, the contenders are increasingly likely to see the issues with fewer distortions due to fear, and they are better able to understand the issue as the opponent views it, whether or not that view is acceptable.

Central to the maintenance of trust, and perhaps to its creation as well, is the development of a conviction that the adversary can be relied upon not to alter his actions in unexpectedly harmful ways. Such a conviction, however, can develop in the absence of any realistic basis for it. Contrariwise, even the most benign behavior may evoke suspicion in the presence of great distrust.

Among the factors that influence the development of unrealistic trust is an unconscious need to avoid conflict. This goal is achieved by identifying with the opponent so that he comes to be seen as having the same goals as oneself. On this often highly unrealistic basis, the overtones of conflict — or even the conflict itself — may not be perceived, and the opponent is evaluated as more trustworthy than he really is.

On the other hand, heightened suspiciousness, leading to a conviction that nothing about the adversary is reasonable, likeable, or reliable, may also have little or nothing to do with the reality of the conflict situation. This extreme position is exemplified by the paranoid person, though the evaluation of such a position is often complicated by the existence of a kernel of truth in even the most severely paranoid views.

Since the extreme positions of absolute trust and absolute mistrust seldom apply to real conflict situations, the problem remains to determine how much trust or mistrust a particular situation or adversary realistically warrants. One aspect of this involves making predictions about behavior and then testing them by challenges, concessions, offerings, and demands. The risk of this reality-testing process lies in a potential loss in position or face if the test fails. Such risks, if overvalued ("we can't risk a single concession . . .") may lead to progressively more intransigent positions until a deadlock is reached and resort to violence seems the only way to resolve the conflict. Not uncommonly, the unfavorable results from such testing operations are taken out of context (to the exclusion of successful tests forgotten or ignored) and held to show conclusively that the opponent is untrustworthy. In this selective fashion, evidence for self-confirming hypotheses is elaborated and fitted into the perceptual distortions and stereotypes discussed earlier, and trust-building efforts are rendered difficult or impossible. *Thus, although unrealistic trust usually is dissipated sooner or later by the behavior of the adversary, unrealistic mistrust tends to be self-validating.*

It is not necessary to depend blindly upon the benevolence of an adversary to achieve an agreement with him. One may even question his basic motivation or ultimate goals and still trust him to abide by a contract *when this is clearly in his own best interest.* In this way, the demonstration of a partial congruence of the self-interests of two contending parties may lead to at least limited agreement between them, even in the absence of mutual good will. Each bases his trust on the probability that the other will act in his own best self-interest. Though such agreements are sometimes precarious, since the definition of "self-interest" may shift, they may nonetheless provide testing opportunities that can subsequently lay a basis for more solid trust.

Some of these principles appear to apply also to international conflict situations. The limited test ban treaty of 1963, though long in coming, can be understood as the culmination of gradually increasing recognition by both the United States and the Soviet Union that continued testing, no matter by whom, was not in the best interest of either nation, because of the risks involved. In turn, it may provide a basis for further agreements by virtue of its trust-building effect.

However, resolution of conflict between adversaries need not depend upon mutual trust, or even upon the coincidence of self-interest, if each trusts the benevolent operations of a third party. Within a system of law, for example, the confidence of each party in the judiciary system promotes resolution of the conflict even though the adversaries may be ineradicably suspicious of one another. Comparably, opposing nations may find a path to conflict-resolution by trusting a mediating or arbitrating third party (see pp. 448-453).

2. *Communication vs. Distance.* The vastly increased volume of communication made possible by modern technology has not only changed the conditions of conflict but also created new opportunities for its resolution. Because hostility tends to disrupt communications (71), it can be assumed that conflicting groups are not communicating as adequately as they should and that improved communications may often help each group to correct its own distortions about the other. It must be borne in mind, however,

that increased communication between adversaries does not automatically reduce tension between them. Indeed, being forced to remain in contact may even heighten hostile feelings between them. "Understanding may not remove the issues at stake, nor does it affect the power relationships. In some cases fuller understanding of the opponent's ideology and intentions may even heighten the conflict"(72). Thus, as considered below (p. 436), in some conflicts temporary withdrawal may be advisable.

On the other hand, informational gaps about an adversary may become filled by tension-increasing false perceptions, stereotypes and phantasies that become indistinguishable from reality. To the extent that increased information replaces fantasy with fact and clarifies each side's perception of the other, the "enemy" becomes more differentiated and therefore more manipulatable. This may mutually relieve anxiety (73).

Communication becomes more effective when it is personally transmitted, but even in these circumstances distortions in reception may impede understanding. One observer, after assessing the experience of escort-interpreters of the Department of State with visiting foreign leaders, concluded that (a) visitors interpret their observations in terms of powerful preconceptions; (b) information is perceived in terms of one's own national communications system and experiences; and (c) more genuine understanding can be achieved by becoming familiar with the visitor's expectations and habits of communication and thereafter presenting information in a form that is familiar and meaningful to him (74). In some instances entire groups have developed characteristic traits in their communication patterns that are easily identifiable aspects of their culture. The Ute Indians, for example, typically say what they anticipate their listeners want to hear, instead of presenting their own ideas. Communications between members of the same societies take place in the matrix of shared customs of speech, forms of courtesy, and a common ideology. When this matrix is absent, frustrating misunderstandings may arise. If the communicators belong to societies that are not on a friendly footing with one another, these misunderstandings can lead to mutual accusations of obstinacy and bad faith, further impeding the communication process. It is very easy to violate canons of good manners in a strange country, thereby affronting its people (75).

The chief hoped-for gain from improved communications is the reduction of mutual fear and hostility. At the simplest level, progress toward this end involves refraining from emitting threatening communications that frighten the opponent, since this increases his hostility. On the positive side, communications should be fostered that reduce the likelihood that an act will be misinterpreted as hostile when it was not so intended. The development of the "hot line" between Washington and Moscow is an application of such an idea.* Similarly, public announcements of satellite launchings tend to prevent the danger of one being mistaken for a missile launching and of thereby precipitating retaliatory action against an attack that in fact had not occurred.

Communications that increase mutuality of group feelings or from which both sides benefit may serve to reduce intergroup hostility. Conversely, forced cultural isolation and lack of "people-to-people" contact increase the danger of mutual dehumanization and perceptual distortions. It has been demonstrated that cultural and technological interchanges, exchange scholarships, scientific conferences, and similar activities can help to "rehumanize" the potential enemy and to reduce the secondary tensions resulting from conflict that arise from other causes. The Peace Corps has been particularly successful in this respect (77). This is largely because of its policy of familiarizing its volunteers with the customs and language of the country in which they are to work, and because of its emphasis on "person-to-person" interactions with the local residents.

Some Alternatives in the Management of Conflict

To facilitate our inquiry we have chosen a model of conflict situations that examines the alternatives open to one, two, and three parties, where each party may be composed of one or more

* A subject for much-needed study is the question of the kind and speed of communication between heads of government that is most conducive to tension-reduction. While it is obvious that too little or too slow communication can be an obstacle to conflict-resolution, there is some evidence that too rapid or too frequent communication also incurs a risk of accident or misinterpretation (76).

units. While admittedly oversimplified, this model offers descriptive classification of conflict management that ranges from relatively uncomplicated actions to more complex ones.

Actions Taken by One Party in Conflict Management

1. *Avoidance and withdrawal.* Although maintenance of communication by contending parties is usually prerequisite to resolving their conflict, there may be times when the antagonists can advantageously reduce or break off contact with each other. Many situations in which nonviolent maneuvers have been successful have involved the possibility that one or both parties will withdraw. Indeed, in some instances it is the threat of withdrawal that acts as a major force toward obtaining conciliation. The steadily increasing density of population, however, makes avoidance less and less available as a means of managing interpersonal conflict.

Similarly, the progressive "shrinkage" of the world makes withdrawal less and less available as a technique of managing international conflict. As human societies are deprived of the tension-reduction values of certain forms of withdrawal, the needs for other methods of conflict management are enhanced.

2. *Assertive use of nonviolent behavior.* Under this heading we shall briefly consider psychological aspects of certain modern methods of conducting organized group conflict that are based on the renunciation of violence. Nonviolent methods of conducting conflict deserve serious study by behavioral scientists on at least two counts: (1) they have highlighted certain generally neglected psychological principles that may have wide implications for controlling violence in the conduct of all conflict; and (2) they are evolving to meet new conditions, so that some of their techniques may ultimately be found appropriate to international conflict [48].

We recognize that for many people the term "nonviolence" has emotionally charged connotations that may obscure communication. We are not referring, however, to any specific pacifistic slogan or formula, but are using the term here in a general sense, meaning simply "without resort to violence."

In considering nonviolent modes of conducting conflict, it is well to remind ourselves of the distinction between behavior and motivation. The terms "violence" and "nonviolence" as used here refer respectively to the presence or absence of destructive behavior as the means of conducting conflict. They should be distinguished from such a term as "aggression," which refers to the motives that give rise to behavior.

In conducting conflict there is a spectrum of nonviolent behavior with respect to its degree of overt activity or passivity. At one end of the spectrum there is a higher ratio of passivity to activity in certain forms of passive resistance; "sit-ins" or "lie-downs" are illustrations of this, although a considerable degree of activity is involved even in these, in the very act of going to the demonstration site, carrying signs, and expressing verbal protests. Toward the other end of the spectrum the activity-passivity ratio is reversed. This is instanced by the expert peace teams in India, who intervene actively and assertively where conflict threatens and who attempt, by Gandhian techniques, to divert the conflict into nonviolent channels (78).

The degree and nature of the forces that *motivate* the assertive use of passive behavior in conducting conflict also extend along a spectrum. Thus, at one extreme, nonviolent behavior may stem primarily from an individual's defensive struggle against the pressure of his own destructive impulses. For example, some participants in sit-ins seem to gain vicarious gratification by provoking their opponents to act out their own (i.e., the participants') suppressed impulses to violence (79). At the other end of the spectrum nonviolent behavior may be based on convictions, values, and intellectual appraisals expressive of ego strength and a high level of personality integration.

The relationships between the respective motivational and behavioral spectra are very complex and warrant much more investigation. There is ample evidence that no simple one-to-one correlation exists between them.

Sporadic examples of the assertive use of noncooperative, nonviolent behavior have occurred throughout history. In recent years, however, following the trail-blazing examples of Gandhi in India and South Africa, these methods have become widespread and have succeeded in apparently very unpromising circumstances. In the United States they have been used chiefly in campaigns for civil rights, starting with the bus boycott in Montgomery, Alabama.

On initial consideration these approaches do not seem to be immediately applicable to international conflict. They have been used only within societies by groups that could not hope to prevail by violence, and their effectiveness has depended on continuous personal contact between members of the opposing groups—conditions that are not met in conflicts between nations that are geographically separated and heavily armed.

It is questionable, moreover, whether a group that appears to have no compunction against killing others could be constrained by nonviolent methods. For example, it seems unlikely that the Jews could have successfully used nonviolent resistance techniques against the Nazis. It must be added, however, that in such situations violent methods would not hold much promise either. In some circumstances, a group cannot overcome its adversary by any means. However, in contrast to violent approaches that increase the cohesiveness of the opposing group, nonviolent methods under some conditions heighten the disruptive forces within the group. Thus if these methods can be appropriately modified in this type of predicament, they may hold out more hope for success in the long run.

A final major limitation to the general effectiveness of nonviolent approaches is that they have succeeded to date only in a context of some shared values between the adversaries. As described in Section IV, one method that people use to free themselves from the inhibition against slaughtering their own kind is to dehumanize their adversaries by viewing them as without morals or as supremely wicked. Those who employ nonviolent methods generally seek to restrain their opponents from violence by insisting on their common humanity. They try to exemplify the opponent's ideals and values as dramatically as possible and to evoke them in their own defense. In both India and the United States, for example, the ideology of the dominant groups rejects punishment without trial, condemns mass killings, and values dignified, controlled, self-respecting behavior. Nonviolent fighters exploit these values to the full and by their behavior make it very difficult for their opponents to dehumanize them. Many reporters have commented on the contrast between the dignity and restraint of the Negro students in sit-ins and the rabble-like behavior of the whites. The powerful impact of the mass march on Washington in the summer of 1963 was due in large part to its dramatic demonstration that Negroes were capable of the highest degree of self-control, thereby effectively combating one dehumanizing feature of the stereotype that they are at the mercy of their impulses.

Such behavior, in effect, makes an ally of the aggressor's conscience. If he resorts to violence, he violates his own moral standards and humiliates himself before both his own group and his adversaries. This aspect of nonviolent compaigns calls attention to the desirability in a conflict of determining what introjected values of the aggressor may thus be appealed to.

In addition to attempting actively to *inhibit* violent behavior in the adversary, nonviolent fighters *avoid stimulating* it by refraining from a display of fear or counterviolence, or from attempts to humiliate him.* Instead, they show respect for the adversary and attempt to direct their attack at his behavior rather than at his person or his motives. One fights the deed, not the doer; the antagonism, not the antagonist.

Techniques of nonviolent action try to restructure the field of conflict so that the contending positions become steps to a larger goal. To this end, they involve a continuous search, even in the midst of conflict, for interests shared with the opponents and efforts to make them visible; and an emphasis upon constructive moves rather than purely negative ones *(78)*. Gandhi did not just protest the salt tax, he marched to the sea and made salt *(80)*. King placed the Montgomery bus boycott in the context of an effort to benefit all the citizens of the city *(81)*.

* An exception to this, which also illustrates that nonviolent methods, like violent ones, cover a wide spectrum and can appeal to many different values, was the behavior toward the Nazis of the Danes and Norwegians. Apparently they powerfully unsettled the occupying forces by showing contempt for them, thereby attacking their self-concept as members of the "master-race."

Perhaps the most hopeful aspects of nonviolent methods lie in their effects on the participants themselves. Nonviolent campaigns have demonstrated that it is possible to create group standards powerful enough to hold ordinary persons to nonviolent courses of action despite extreme provocation. These group controls in turn strengthen internal controls against resort to violence (82). Groups practicing nonviolence, no less than those in battle, are motivated by strong allegiance to a guiding set of values and depend for their success on tight discipline, group solidarity, and strong charismatic leaders.

Group standards of nonviolence have also performed the feat of reversing the time-honored, stereotyped link between violence and courage. A major psychological determinant of the arms race seems to be the effort to overcome fears of weakness and helplessness (Section III, p. 383). Each side, by building more weapons, tries to reassure itself that it cannot be intimidated and equates willingness to resort to war with courage and honor.* For the nonviolent fighter, resort to violence is a sign of cowardice, and adherence to nonviolence is a demonstration of manliness, courage, and determination. Exclusive reliance on nonviolent techniques increases the sense of self-worth of their users; it may even afford a socially useful, indirect channel for discharge of aggression and hostility (79). This remarkable achievement may have great potential relevance for discovering how to overcome one of the major psychological drives toward war.

3. *Unilateral initiatives inviting reciprocation.* Some have suggested that international tension may in time be reduced through a series of graduated, unilateral acts that are intended to invite reciprocation by the opponent and so make possible even further tension-reducing steps,(24,84,85,86,)**. The aim of these actions would

* President Kennedy may have betokened a change in this pattern, at least on the part of the United States, when he said: "We do not need to use threats to prove that we are resolute"(83).

** Charles Osgood of the Institute of Communications Research at the University of Illinois has been among those actively engaged in promoting one such program. Some of the elements included in Osgood's program are (24):

1. The unilateral acts must be perceived by the opponent as reducing his external threat. (Possible methods: exchange of scientific information and

be to induce mutual trust by demonstrating to the enemy that we can be trusted, rather than by demanding that the enemy first convince us that he can be trusted. *To be effective, such unilateral acts would have to diminish the fears of the opponent without increasing the fears of the home population.* This action model is the reverse of the present nuclear arms race, in which graduated unilateral actions invite reciprocal tension-*increasing* behavior by both opponents.

This proposal is ingenious and rests on sound psychological principles. Nevertheless, there are at least two grounds for questioning whether unilateral acts can reduce tension when undertaken in a context of intense mutual fear and mistrust. First, since each side assumes that all actions of the other must be malevolently intended, an action that seemingly attempts to reduce tension might be regarded by an adversary as a ruse intended to lull it into a false sense of security. Thus the action might heighten tension rather than reduce it. Osgood argues that persistence in unilateral acts would eventually overcome the adversary's suspicions. Unfortunately, until reciprocation occurred, each unilateral act might increase the anxiety of the home population, making the next act more difficult.

This calls attention to the second doubt concerning such an approach: that moves or actions that appear to concede something to the opponent are apt to be felt by the home population, and

---

personnel, imposition of self-inspection, neutralization of territory, deactivation of bases, and so forth).

2. The unilateral acts must be accompanied by specific invitations to reciprocate.
3. Unilateral acts must be planned in sequence and continued over considerable periods regardless of reciprocation by the opponent and without requiring prior commitment to reciprocate.
4. Unilateral acts must be announced in advance and widely publicized to allied, neutral, and enemy countries as part of a consistent policy.
5. They must be carefully graduated in risk potential *so as not to endanger our "heartland" or reduce our fundamental capacity for retaliatory second strike.* This offers to the home population the psychological support for tension-reducing actions within tolerable limits of security. Thus the minimum capacity for effective deterrence would *not* be reduced by unilateral action, but further reduction, hopefully, would be arrived at through negotiation in the atmosphere of greater confidence and trust produced by the previous tension-reducing actions.

perceived by the opponent, as evidence of weakness. Therefore instead of reciprocating, the adversary might be more likely to respond by increasing the pressure in the hope of gaining further concessions. To avoid this, tension-reducing moves designed to evoke similar behavior by the opponent ought not to be undertaken at times of crisis or under pressure. As an example, the evacuation of obsolescent medium-range ballistic missile sites in Turkey subsequent to the Cuban crisis was said to have been delayed because the American government was concerned that such a move would be interpreted, not as a tension-relieving device, but as a *quid pro quo* to induce Russia to remove her missiles from Cuba and therefore as evidence of weakness and fear. Despite these weaknesses, Osgood's proposal has been a valuable stimulant to creative thinking in this difficult area.

Actions Taken by Two Parties in Conflict Management

1. *Competitive coexistence.* Opposing parties may mutually agree under a variety of circumstances to desist from active efforts at destroying each other. The power of each may grow to such proportions that victory of one over the other is no longer possible. The conflicts then settle into a chronic "cold war" in which each adversary, wherever possible, takes every opportunity to score against the opponent but abandons the effort to destroy, overwhelm, or subdue him. Such a pattern has an historical precedent in the form of coexistence between the major world religions. After seven centuries of futile and bloody violence, Christianity and Islam settled down to living side by side; even within Christianity itself, the coexistence of Protestantism and Catholicism is now taken for granted. The Ecumenical Council meetings in Rome in 1962 and 1963 further indicate that, given enough time and in the absence of violence, forces may be set into motion that will eventually tend to bring adversaries closer together.

Competitive coexistence is made possible by the realization that, as described above, not all competition need be a zero-sum game. Adversaries may compete without necessarily encompassing the destruction of either one. It is not easy for most people to tolerate acceptance of coexistence with a hostile party. Yet, there are survival advantages to techniques of competition in which both sides gain, rather than one side exclusively gaining at the other's expense or both sides losing totally, as would be the case in nuclear war. Intergroup conflicts and competition structured in this way often markedly strengthen each of the contending groups.

A competitive, win-lose orientation of parties in a conflict situation may make any compromise short of complete success virtually unacceptable, since it will be less than the maximum and hence evidence of weakness. Laboratory studies on the behavior of individuals in competitive situations suggest that the capacity to threaten injury to the opponent significantly increases the competitive orientation of both sides and consequently reduces the likelihood of their reaching a mutually satisfactory agreement [46].

Making clear the consequences of a failure to agree may often force a change in the competitive stands of both parties. For example, a strike may, over the course of time, make the high cost of unresolved disagreement painfully evident to both union and management. In the arena of international politics in the thermonuclear era, however, the danger exists that the adversaries may not come to such a realization until they have become irreversibly committed to acts of annihilation.

2. *Negotiation.* When one party to a disagreement possesses overwhelmingly superior power, it can dictate the outcome and the weaker party must be satisfied with whatever it can get. With an approach toward power equality between the parties, however, there is increasingly greater likelihood that demands by one upon the other will lead to threats on both sides to use whatever sanctions may be available, including violence. Unilateral solutions are then no longer possible. When trials of strength fail to settle the issue or are simply too costly to employ, negotiation or bargaining becomes the method of conducting the conflict.

Negotiation has been systematically studied by direct observation, simulated situations, and laboratory experiments. Game theory and statistical, mathematical, and other models have been employed to delineate the progression of developments in this form of nonviolent conflict resolution [87, 88].

In an initial phase each party generally attempts to gain acceptance of its own view by a widening range of maneuvers and is critical of the opposition. Later, as communication improves and the parties become better informed about each other and about the nature of the conflict, an ambivalent relationship develops between them. Finally, they begin to review alternatives and compromises and to gradually eliminate those that are not mutually acceptable until they reach some consensus on the points at issue.

Diesing (89) suggests that the applied psychology underlying successful negotiations includes the following principles:

> Avoidance of extreme weakness by either side, so as to prevent unilateral dictation by the opponent. At the same time, each side must establish clear limits to its own power, to reduce risks of a spiralling power race.
>
> Respect for the central power position of the other side, indicated, for example, by avoidance of threats to exterminate one's opponent.
>
> Identification of values, principles, and goals that can be shared, including procedure for conducting negotiations.
>
> Use of candor to a proper degree, accompanied by appropriate and restricted use of concealment, dissembling and bluffing, but with awareness of the crucial necessity for honesty in offering concessions to elicit counter-concessions.

The attainment of the kind of relationship that enables negotiations to proceed depends, among other things, upon the availability of adequate channels of communication, as discussed above (pp. 433-435). Their usefulness, however, appears to be a function of the degree of competitive orientation of the parties in conflict, i.e., the degree to which the desire to reach their own goal subordinates the desire to achieve agreement on a common goal. Some findings from laboratory experiments (90) suggest that the greater the competitive orientation of the parties, the less likely will they be to use such channels as do exist. Results are better, however, when communication is required rather than voluntary.

Some degree of mutual trust and respect appears to be crucial for the achievement of successful negotiations in union-management relations and, by inference, in international conflict as well (36). With it, opponents see each other as earnest and honest, even if in error, a broader range of concessions can be offered, a more comprehensive agreement can be obtained, and the resulting agreements can be more readily accepted as fair and warranting adherence.

However, the deadly paradox of the problem of trust in negotiation lies in the fact that the achievement of mutual trust is both the goal of the negotiations and the prerequisite for them. Being both the means and the end, trust produces, by its absence as well as by its presence, a circular situation. Trust enables agreement, agreement augments trust. This in turn broadens the area of negotiation and encourages further agreement. Contrariwise, a loss of trust provokes declaration of "bad faith," a resort to legalism, and a rise in skepticism about the opponent's intentions. With the appearance of suspiciousness, behavior tends to conform to expectations in a manner described earlier as the self-fulfilling prophecy, and trustworthiness becomes increasingly hard to establish or believe.

Another problem that complicates negotiations, especially in this age of mass media, is that of multiple audiences. The negotiator occupies a position somewhere between two audiences: (a) his opposition across the table, with whom he is trying to bargain; and (b) the silent but influential (and often far from homogeneous) party "over his shoulder," namely, the other members of the group he represents. He must consider each response and each offer through a triple perspective: how it looks to himself, to his adversary, and to his own constituency. Depending upon the issues at stake and the level of feeling developed in relation to them, the negotiator may be free in varying degrees from the need to account strictly and constantly to his constituency. He may have to couple offers at the table with reassurances to his constituency that they do not represent "appeasement" or "losing." Pressures upon the negotiator for continual evidences of success—or at least progress—may be so intense as to limit sharply the range of concession-making open to him. They may force him into such a rigid position that virtually no acceptable alternatives are possible. As indicated above (p. 409), efforts to bargain or compromise under such circumstances expose negotiators to charges of betrayal by some of their own compatriots (the "traitor trap").

The attempt to circumvent these difficulties by conducting negotiations in secret creates a different type of problem. Since secrecy enables negotiators to make "deals" behind the backs of their groups, and potentially at their expense, they breed distrust and threaten the negotiator with alienation from his group. Hence the widespread appeal of Woodrow Wilson's "open covenants openly arrived at" at the end of World War I. Knowing when to negotiate openly and when privately, therefore, requires extremely skillful judgment. A recent happy example of the exercise of this kind of judgment was the confidential correspondence between Kennedy and Khrushchev that culminated in the successful semipublic negotiations for a limited test ban.

Negotiations are influenced not only by the opposing power groups within each nation but also by nations that are not at the bargaining table. This has often been illustrated by the absence of Communist China at UN deliberations and in other negotiating situations.

Conflicting ideologies may create another important problem that complicates the negotiation process. When an issue becomes "a struggle over principle," it ceases to be negotiable since each side considers any substantial concession tantamount to total capitulation.

Closely related to the problem of ideology are differences in cultural or subcultural standards as to what is appropriate conduct in negotiations. "Negotiation mores" *(91)* establish a pattern of conceptions about negotiations that are accepted as "ground rules." Examples are the principle of proceeding from the specific to the general and the expectation that an opponent's concessions should be answered with counter-concessions. Unless both sides in a dispute adhere to similar negotiation mores—which is often not the case in disputes between unfriendly nations—the basis for establishing agreement about the very means for pursuing the negotiations is absent and itself becomes an issue. Thus disputes about the agenda, the manner of selecting the chairman, and the like become foci for power struggles, distracting time and energy from consideration of the substantive issues of the major conflict. Indeed, in some instances, the negotiating process itself may be pursued as a gratifying game for its own sake, thereby impeding progress toward its ostensible goals.

The very process of negotiating "procedural issues," however, has a legitimizing effect, because it tacitly demonstrates the faith of each party in orderly procedure. Furthermore, negotiations about procedure maintain contact between parties in conflict until they can move forward to substantive questions, although long-continued failure to resolve procedural issues ultimately may cast a demoralizing pall on the whole negotiation process.

Still another problem is presented by the conventional method of attempting to negotiate the toughest issue first, with the hope that it might then be easier to reach agreement upon subordinate issues. A conference agenda that includes subsidiary or even unassociated issues and preliminary negotiations about these can provide a "warm-up" period where the stakes are small and the chance of agreement is large. By leading to a sense of mutual understanding, success in reaching agreement on these issues often enhances the possibilities for successful negotiation on major issues.*

3. *Cooperation.* Cooperation between adversaries represents still another approach to conflict management that many people tend to reject emotionally. The possibility of collaborating with an opponent, particularly with an adversary whose fundamental ideology is profoundly contrary to one's own, appears at first glance to be utterly unrealistic. Yet, even in the midst of World Wars I and II *(70)* the opposing sides cooperated to some extent when their mutual interests were involved. Cooperation promotes satisfaction of the needs of both parties on a voluntary basis through the merging of common purposes. It differs from compromise in that neither party has to make an important sacrifice.

Cooperative activities can yield rewards that reinforce positive attitudes between adversaries and inhibit antagonistic ones. Particu-

* The agreement on nuclear testing achieved by the United States, Great Britain, and the Soviet Union is an example of an understanding reached on a limited issue. If it can be maintained, it may diminish mutual distrust and lead to successful negotiations on other issues.

larly effective are cooperative endeavors toward superordinate goals that both sides desire but cannot achieve alone.* A recent example of such cooperative activity is the research undertaken during the International Geophysical Year, which yielded data that all the participating countries wanted but none could achieve alone and from which all benefited. So successful was this joint undertaking that it has served as a model for cooperation in other international activities, such as the International Refugee Year and the Year of the Quiet Sun. Another example is the collaborative use by the United States and the Soviet Union of artificial satellites for long-range weather forecasting and for communication. Still another example of potential benefit to both sides is coöperation in the struggle to conquer space despite possible military overtones.

Shared goals and professional interests also can be a basis for collaborative activity. Disease control, mental health, population control, and control of starvation and poverty are targets of specialists in every country. These activities are probably stimulated by national rivalries as well as by altruistic motives. Nevertheless, they have the great advantage of directing these rivalries into nonviolent channels. At the same time they benefit human welfare and, to the extent that they are collaborative, improve the general atmosphere, thereby facilitating attempts at conflict control. This was the essential meaning of President Kennedy's "Peace Race" challenge before the United Nations in September, 1961.

Roles of Third Parties in Conflict Management

When two parties are deadlocked in a dispute, third parties may sometimes help to resolve the dilemma, even when the adversaries distrust each other. In most civilized cultures, the judiciary and

* Some years ago the Sherifs demonstrated the effectiveness of this mechanism by an ingenious social experiment in a boys' camp. Boys who did not know each other were made into two enemy groups through intensive team competitions in which much hostile feeling was deliberately aroused. The camp leaders then tried to resolve the mutual antagonism. Merely bringing the two groups together socially had no effect. When, however, several situations were created that presented threats to the entire camp and that could only be resolved by the cooperation of everyone (e.g., the camp water supply failed and the whole camp had to work together to restore it, or the camp truck was run into a ditch and the whole camp had to help pull it out), the enmity between the groups was markedly reduced(92).

its accompanying body of legal sanctions serve this function by ensuring that an agreement will be reached and enforced. In most instances the absence of such a third party at the level of international relations means that agreements in this area depend upon the development of some sort of trusting relationship between the parties themselves. In time, specific institutions may be developed or strengthened to surmount this problem and to augment the influence of international law in conflicts between nations. Notable possibilities include the World Court, the United Nations, and mediation committees established under the aegis of the UN. To be useful, of course, a third party must be perceived by each side as not committed to the other one, and both sides must have some confidence in it. The roles of third parties may be informal or formal.

1. *Informal use of third parties: the go-between.* An example of an unofficial third party is the go-between, whose function is to supply informal channels of communication between contending parties when formal channels have become blocked because the conflicting positions of the adversaries have become too rigid. Because his role is unofficial and his activities can always be disowned, the go-between makes possible the discovery of potential areas of agreement or compromise without loss of face or commitment by either side.

The go-between can be especially effective if the opposing sides recognize that he has the welfare of both at heart and if he can make constructive contributions to solution of the conflict. Such a go-between function is illustrated by the Pugwash Conferences on Science and World Affairs. The participants, being prominent scientists, have prestige in all countries; they are known to be concerned with improving the lot of all mankind, while their loyalty to their own nations is unquestioned. In addition, they bring specialized knowledge to bear on certain crucial areas of conflict, such as arms control and disarmament. Because the conferences have no official status, participants can be relatively flexible. The results of their deliberations are heard with respect by their home governments, who can, however, reject them without increasing tensions because of their unofficial nature. COSWA conferences have been credited with supplying much of the groundwork for the limited test-ban treaty.

A somewhat different example is afforded by the Quaker delegation at the UN, which serves as an unofficial channel of communication between deadlocked antagonists. The presence of this dedicated group of Americans also serves as a reminder of implicit cooperative tendencies in one of the parties to an international conflict that officially must often maintain apparently rigid and unyielding positions.

Another unofficial type of third-party intervention is illustrated by the peace teams in India, described above (p. 437), who strive by their intervention to prevent two-party conflicts from erupting into violence.

2. *Formal use of third parties: mediation and arbitration.* The official introduction of a third party into a two-party conflict may be illustrated by the use of a mediator or arbitrator in labor disputes. A mediator simply exerts his good offices to aid the parties in reaching a mutually acceptable resolution; an arbitrator offers a resolution that the parties have agreed in advance to accept. To be effective, the third party must be perceived by both sides as neutral, as functioning on the basis of reason rather than emotion, and as identifying with the rights and interests of *both* parties to the conflict. These attributes enable him to help the adversaries find paths that may lead to mutually satisfying results.

3. *Supranational organizations.* In an interchange of open letters[4] between Einstein and Freud, the latter, in discussing the relation between the right and might, expressed the view that wars will only be prevented with certainty if mankind forms a central authority with delegated power to pass judgment upon all conflicts of international interest.

Actually, this has already begun to take place upon a limited scale. The intense and rapid changes following the breakdown of former power centers, the disintegration of colonial empires, the revolution in underdeveloped areas with the rise of new nation states, and the remarkable development of rapid transportation and communication have all stimulated the growth of supranational organizations of many kinds. Conventions regulating postal rates, fishing rights, the use of Antarctica, telephonic and telegraphic cable connections, satellite functions, air and space travel rights, the use of international waters, disease quarantine, and many others are already in existence and reflect a steadily increasing recognition of the complex ways in which modern nations are interdependent.

The awareness that political and economic disputes between nations require something more than simple bilateral agreements or treaty alliances led to the creation first of the League of Nations and later of the United Nations. However, fears that a world organization would lead to serious loss of national sovereignty or to a tyrannical world government, have led to limiting these international organizations to liaison and parliamentary functions that are considerably short of the power of compelling agreement. Nevertheless, despite these limitations, the United Nations has already demonstrated its usefulness and has offered a preview of the kinds of functions that a more influential world government might perform.

Apart from its more obvious contributions to world peace in the form of its subsidiary organizations (WHO, UNESCO, and so forth) and in its interventions in military conflicts,* the United Nations has also provided a catalytic environment that makes possible many less obvious interactions between nations. Since the UN meets on neutral ground, national representatives can avoid uncomfortable issues of face and protocol and can meet in lounges or hallways for informal exchanges that may lay the groundwork for more official and public agreements. The setting of informality enables personal exploratory contacts between national representatives to be maximally effective. The availability of "neutral" nations may enable the organization to play a mediating role, both through informal channels and officially.

Although UN debates often seem irrelevant or mere "talk," their psychological value should not be underestimated, since they provide an outlet for national feelings of outrage, indignation, and disagreement and thus decrease pressures for more overt — and po-

* e.g., in Korea, Suez, the Congo, and Cyprus.

tentially more disastrous—action. Such "talk" also provides the means for working toward agreements.

The UN also exerts a moral pressure upon conflicting members to continue dealing with one another. This pressure, which tends to favor ultimate working through of disagreements, is not absolute, of course; various nations have "walked out" temporarily from the Assembly or the Security Council. But in each instance they have returned to confront their opponents again.

One of the more important functions that a supranational organization may provide is its symbolic function. Symbolically, such an organization may come to be perceived as the "good father" or "good authority." However, its success in fulfilling this benign and powerful role depends upon its having first earned the trust of people. Trust in this context is a function of widespread recognition that whatever the "parental" organization does, it does not intend to destroy or to permit others to destroy. A trustworthy international organization therefore would require the development of a police force that was strong enough to prevent other nations from destructive behavior, yet controlled enough to eschew a destructive role for itself.

Admittedly, such requirements seem difficult if not mutually contradictory. Without attempting to discuss the political or military feasibility of such a police force [93], we may comment on certain psychological aspects of this issue. It is conceivable, for example, that such an international body may not need to possess physical force of overwhelming magnitude—force big enough to control any nation on earth. When backed by legal sanctions, the mere symbol of authority may be enough to control deviant behavior. The unarmed bobbies of England are a case in point. What would seem to be as important as this symbolic factor, however, is the existence of some mechanism that would make it highly probable that the cause of justice would be served in any dispute and that the violators of international laws or agreements would be punished. Others have suggested that physical force actually may not be as valuable or effective for international policing and punishment as economic and other sanctions [94].

The acceptance of the authority of an international body could serve to stimulate inner behavorial controls, even as local or national authority symbols do. An external object standing for international law and order might thus have a controlling effect on national behavior, much as a red light controls the behavior of an individual motorist. The existence of a larger, benign power may contribute significantly to a more peaceful world order by symbolically indicating that anarchy and chaos will not result. This reassuring function of leadership may appear even in the absence of specific performance by the authority symbol (though ultimately the agency must show effective behavior if this reassurance-giving trust is to be maintained).

The development of a world organization capable of dealing with the potentially destructive behavior of deviant nations will undoubtedly require a period of world-wide education and repeated illustrations of the value and necessity of cooperative international effort. Eventually, this will mean giving up some degree of national sovereignty; but relinquishment of certain national options, such as conducting war, can only occur after many experiences with the advantages of international agreement have demonstrated that the risks involved in such relinquishment are outweighed by the increasingly grave hazards of not doing so.

VIII

SUMMARY AND CONCLUSIONS

We have endeavored in this report to discuss some socio-psychiatric factors bearing on the problem of war and peace in our nuclear age. It is our hope that our colleagues in the various behavorial sciences to whom this report is addressed will find it useful as an integrated condensation of a considerable body of relevant material. We hope also that the report may serve as a spur to urgently needed psychiatrically-oriented research into the many vital issues and unsolved questions in this area.

To recapitulate briefly:

War is a social institution; it is not inevitably rooted in the nature of man. Although war has traditionally served as an outlet for many basic human psychological needs, both aggressive and socially cohesive ones, the increasing mechanization and automation of modern warfare has rendered it less and less relevant to these needs. There are other social institutions and other means of conducting conflict between groups of people, or between nations, that can serve these psychological needs more adaptively in our modern world.

Many of the traditional stereotypes concerning the courage and manliness involved in the pursuit of war are psychologically questionable. As psychiatrists we know that the resort to violence is apt to stem not only from anger or feelings of strength but also from feelings of fear and inner weakness. It requires great strength and moral courage to carry on some forms of conflict without resorting to violence.

In addition to the objective political and ideological differences that divide East and West in the current struggle, there are a number of psychological factors that render more difficult the achievement of nonviolent solutions to this struggle. Some of these are:

(1) Psychological defense mechanisms, such as denial, emotional isolation, and habituation that enable large numbers of people to live in the shadow of imminent nuclear annihilation without searching for appropriate adaptive measures that might remove or reduce the awesome danger.

(2) The primitivizing effects of extreme fear or panic that can lead to impulsive or irrational behavior to ward off an immediate threat, without regard to the long-term consequences of such behavior.

(3) The increasing dehumanization, both of man and society, that depersonalizes the horrors of war and mass suffering and treats them as statistics. (We have dealt with this concept in considerable detail because we regard it as a serious and fundamental problem of our time.)

(4) Ethnocentric perceptual distortions, exaggerated nationalism, group identifications and pressures, and a basic human need to fit perceptions into one's pre-existent frame of reference. Inherent in these distortions, *which exist on both sides,* is the danger that they lead to stereotyped conceptions, both of one's self and of the adversary, hamper communication, and lead to mutual distrust and a biased perception of what is fair and reasonable.

(5) The fact that distorted perceptions and mutual distrust tend to provoke reciprocal behavior from the adversary, so that the mutual expectation that "the other side doesn't really want peace and can't be trusted" tends to become self-fulfilling.

(6) The fact that the above-mentioned psychological factors, in addition to political and military ones, exert a significant pressure upon political leaders, who are caught in a conflict between the things they have to say and do to maintain their power and prestige at home, and the taking of the kinds of initiative that might lead to a lessening of tension with the adversary.

We have discussed in detail some psychiatric aspects of two traditional approaches to nuclear war prevention: deterrence and civil defense. We have given reasons for concluding that although these approaches may be of some value with regard to immediate survival, in the long run neither one promotes the reduction of tension that is imperative before any genuine progress can be made in ending the costly and dangerous arms race.

In the final section of this report, we discuss some psychological aspects of alternatives to violence in the conduct of conflict and techniques that might lead to tension-reduction between national adversaries.

There are those who will argue that to consider such nonviolent alternatives represents "lack of realism," "starry-eyed idealism," and "lack of faith in the strength of our system." It seems to us, on the contrary, that the weight of evidence is that persons who continue to think in terms of military victory are reflecting precisely those attitudes. With the incredibly enormous nuclear destructive capacity that now exists on both sides in the East-West struggle, it is quite unrealistic to assume that either side can achieve traditional military victory. In a nuclear era any war may turn into a thermonuclear holocaust. It would seem to be the most starry-eyed kind of idealism to assume that if a nuclear war is fought, "our way of life" would be preserved for the tragic survivors of such a holocaust. And, finally, it seems to us that it represents a serious lack of faith in the strength and vitality of our democratic society to assume that we would not or could not survive in peaceful competition with the Communist countries. There are huge sources of untapped strength in the West that, given a world at peace, have an enormous potential for continued development.

We recognize, of course, that many other disciplines—political science, law, economics, the physical and biological sciences, and military science itself—are involved in the ultimate resolution of the complex problems we face. We realize also that the contribution of the behavorial sciences must be viewed in the total context of all these other considerations. But, as the preamble to the Constitution of UNESCO says, "Wars begin in the minds of men." Since this is so, the minds of men must also be capable of ending war. It is to this urgent goal that we dedicate this study.

REFERENCES

1. Lifton, R. J.: "Psychological Effects of the Atomic Bomb in Hiroshima; The Theme of Death," *Daedalus*, Journal of the American Academy of Arts and Sciences, Summer, 1963, pp. 462-497.
2. Aronow, S., Ervin, F., and Sidel, V.: THE FALLEN SKY: MEDICAL CONSEQUENCES OF THERMONUCLEAR WAR, Hill and Wang, New York, 1963, p. XIV.
3. Hobhouse, L. T., Wheeler, G. C., and Ginzberg, M.: THE MATERIAL CULTURE AND SOCIAL INSTITUTIONS OF THE SIMPLER PEOPLES, Chapin & Hall, London, 1915.
4. Freud, S.: COLLECTED PAPERS, Vol. V, London, 1950, p. 280 (in Essay "Why War"—correspondence with Einstein in 1932).
5. Dollads, J., Doob, L. W., Miller, N. E., Mowrer, O. H., and Sears, R. R.: FRUSTRATION AND AGGRESSION, Yale University Press, New Haven, 1939.
6. Scott, J. P.: AGGRESSION, University of Chicago Press, Chicago, 1958.
7. von Bertalanffy, L.: "Comments on Aggression," *Bulletin of the Menninger Clinic*, Vol. 22, March, 1958.
8. Osborn, F.: OUR PLUNDERED PLANET, Little Brown & Co., Boston, 1948.
9. Lorenz, K.: DAS SOGENANNTE BÖSE—ZUR NATURGESCHICHTE DER AGGRESSION, Verlag Dr. G. Borotha-Schoeler, Wien, 1963.
10. Lief, H.: "Contemporary Forms of Violence," in SCIENCE AND PSYCHOANALYSIS, J. Masserman, ed., Grune & Stratton, New York, 1963.
11. Marmor, J.: "War, Violence, and Human Nature," *Bulletin of the Atomic Scientists*, March, 1964, pp. 19-22.
12. Murphy, L.: THE WIDENING WORLD OF CHILDHOOD, Basic Books, New York, 1963, pp. 350-351.
13. James, W.: "The Moral Equivalents of War," in MEMORIES & STUDIES, Longmans, Green & Co., New York, 1911.
14. Glass, A. J.: "Observations upon the Epidemiology of Mental Illness in Troops during Warfare," in SYMPOSIUM ON PREVENTIVE AND SOCIAL PSYCHIATRY, Walter Reed Army Institute of Research, U. S. Government Printing Office, Washington, D. C., 1957.
15. Marshall, S. L. A.: MEN AGAINST FIRE, Wm. Morrow & Co., New York, 1947.
16. Hadley, A. T.: Quoted by Associated Press News Analyst James Marlowe, August 5, 1963.
17. Kennedy, J. F.: Address on the Nuclear Test Ban Treaty, July 27, 1963.
18. Adorno, T. W., et al: THE AUTHORITARIAN PERSONALITY, Harper and Brothers, New York, 1950.
19. Rokeach, M.: THE OPEN AND CLOSED MIND, Basic Books, New York, 1960.
20. Christiansen, B.: ATTITUDES TOWARDS FOREIGN AFFAIRS AS A FUNCTION OF PERSONALITY, Oslo University Press, Oslo, 1959.
21. Levinson, D.: "Authoritarian Personality and Foreign Policy," *Journal of Conflict Resolution*, Vol. I, pp. 37-47, 1957.
22. Menninger, R. W.: "Attitudes Toward International Crisis in Relation to Personality Structure," in HUMAN REACTIONS TO THE THREAT OF IMPENDING DISASTER, M. Greenblatt, G. H. Grosser, and H. Wechsler, eds. (in press).
23. Scott, W. A.: "International Ideology and Interpersonal Ideology," *Public Opinion Quarterly*, Vol. 24, pp. 419-435, 1960.

24. Osgood, C. E.: AN ALTERNATIVE TO WAR OR SURRENDER, University of Illinois Press, Urbana, Ill., 1962.
25. Goldstein, K.: THE ORGANISM, American Book Co., New York, 1939.
26. Personal Communication of Dr. M. Forman to Dr. P. Ottenberg, December 17, 1962.
27. Rappaport, A., and Singer, J. D.: "An Alternative to Slogans," *The Nation*, March 24, 1962, p. 248.
28. Engel, G.: PSYCHOLOGICAL DEVELOPMENT IN HEALTH AND DISEASE, W. B. Saunders, Philadelphia, 1962.
29. Szent-Gyorgyi, A.: "The Persistence of the Cave Man," *Saturday Review of Literature*, July 7, 1962.
30. Whorf, B.: LANGUAGE, THOUGHT AND REALITY, John Wiley & Sons, New York, 1956.
31. Levine, G. N., ed.: THE AMERICAN PUBLIC AND THE FALLOUT SHELTER ISSUE, A Nine-Community Survey, Bureau of Applied Social Research, Columbia University, New York, 1964 (mimeographed).
32. Koestler, A.: "On Disbelieving Atrocities," in THE YOGI AND THE COMMISSAR, The Macmillan Company, New York, 1945.
33. The term "ethnocentrism" was coined by W. G. Summer in 1906. Noted by Klineberg, O.: SOCIAL PSYCHOLOGY, Henry Holt & Co., New York, 1940.
34. ASCH, S. E.: SOCIAL PSYCHOLOGY, Prentice-Hall, New York, 1952.
35. Frankl-Brunswick, E.: in Adorno, op. *cit.*, pp. 461 ff.
36. Deutsch, M.: "Psychological Alternatives to War," *Journal of Social Issues*, Vol. 18, 1962, p. 103.
37. Bauer, R. A.: "The Communicator and the Audience," *Journal of Conflict Resolution*, Vol. 2, 1958, pp. 66-77.
38. Bauer, R. A.: "Problems of Perception and the Relation Between The United States and the Soviet Union," *Journal of Conflict Resolution*, Vol. V, September, 1961.
39. Krauskopf, K.: "Report on Russia: Geochemistry and Politics," *Science*, Vol. 134, 1961, pp. 539-542.
40. Bronfenbrenner, U.: "The Mirror Image in Soviet-American Relations: A Social Psychologist's Report," *Journal of Social Issues*, Vol. 17, 1961, pp. 46-47, 48.
41. Blake, R. R., and Mouton, J. S.: "The Intergroup Dynamics of Win-Lose Conflict and Problem-Solving Collaboration in Union-Management Relations," in INTERGROUP RELATIONS AND LEADERSHIP, M. Sherif, ed., John Wiley & Sons, New York, 1962, pp. 94-140.
42. Waskow, A.: THE LIMITS OF DEFENSE, Doubleday & Co., Garden City, New York, 1962.
43. Lippmann, W.: "Cuba and the Nuclear Risk," *The Atlantic Monthly*, February, 1963.
44. Singer, J. D.: DETERRENCE, ARMS CONTROL AND DISARMAMENT, Ohio State University Press, Columbus, 1962.
45. Michael, D. N.: "Psychopathology of Nuclear War," *Bulletin of the Atomic Scientists*, Vol. 18, May, 1962, pp. 28-29.
46. Deutsch, M. and Krauss, R. M.: "The Effect of Threat Upon Interpersonal Bargaining," *Journal of Abnormal and Social Psychology*, Vol. 61, 1960, pp. 181-189.
47. Singer, J. D.: "Arms Control and Beyond: A Review," *Journal of Conflict Resolution*, Vol. 5, September, 1961.

48. Frank, J. D.: "Breaking the Thought Barrier: Psychological Challenges of the Nuclear Age," *Psychiatry*, Vol. 23, 1960, pp. 245-266.
49. *Coffin Nails*, August 14, 1961. Published by Dick Fireman, 2223 East 68th Street, Chicago, Ill.
50. World Federation for Mental Health: MENTAL HEALTH IN INTERNATIONAL PERSPECTIVE, a review made in 1961 by an international and interprofessional study group, Vernon Lock, London, 1961.
51. Liederman, P. H., and Mendelson, J. H.: "Some Psychiatric Considerations in Planning for Defense Shelters," in THE FALLEN SKY: MEDICAL CONSEQUENCES OF THERMO-NUCLEAR WAR, Aronow, Ervin, and Sidel, eds. Hill and Wang, New York, 1963, pp. 42-54.
52. Air Force Manual 160-55, "Guidance for Implementing Human Reliability Program," February 28, 1962; also Air Force Regulations 35-9.
53. Kahn, H.: "The Arms Race and Some of Its Hazards," in ARMS CONTROL, DISARMAMENT, AND NATIONAL SECURITY, Donald G. Brennan, ed., Geo. Braziller, Inc., New York, 1961, pp. 89-121.
54. Milburn, T. W.: "The Concept of Deterrence: Some Logical and Psychological Considerations," *Journal of Social Issues*, Vol. 17, 1961, pp. 3-11.
55. Piel, G.: THE ILLUSION OF CIVIL DEFENSE, Scientific American, Inc., New York, 1961.
56. Stonier, T.: NUCLEAR DISASTER, Meridian Books, World Publishing Co., New York, 1964.
57. Bettelheim, B.: "Individualism and Mass Behavior in Extreme Situations," *Journal of Abnormal and Social Psychology*, Vol. 38, 1943, pp. 417-452.
58. Kahn, H.: ON THERMO-NUCLEAR WAR, Princeton University Press, Princeton, N. J., 1961.
59. Grinspoon, L.: "Fallout Shelters and Mental Health," *Resident Physician*, May, 1963.
60. Singer, J. D.: "Deterrence and Shelters," *Bulletin of the Atomic Scientists*, Vol. 17, October, 1961, pp. 310-315.
61. Waskow, A.: THE SHELTER-CENTERED SOCIETY, Peace Research Institute, Washington, D. C., 1962.
62. Baker, G. W., and Chapman, D. W., eds: MAN AND SOCIETY IN DISASTER, Basic Books, New York, 1962.
63. Erikson, E.: IDENTITY AND THE LIFE CYCLE, Psychological Issues, Monograph No. 1, 1959.
64. North, R. C., Hock, H. E. and Zinnes, D. A.: "The Integrative Functions of Conflict," *Journal of Conflict Resolution*, Vol. 4, 1960, pp. 355-374.
65. Caplan, G.: CONCEPTS OF MENTAL HEALTH AND CONSULTATION, Children's Bureau Publication No. 373, U. S. Government Printing Office, Washington, D.C. 1959.
66. Blood, R. O. "Resolving Family Conflicts," *Journal of Conflict Resolution*, Vol. 4, 1960, pp. 209-219.
67. Cavanagh, J. R.: "The Durable Incompatible Marriage," *Southern Medical Journal*, Vol. 55, 1962, pp. 396-400.
68. Houston, M., and Forman, R. B.: "The Durable Incompatible Marriage," Unpublished paper presented at the annual meeting of the American Psychiatric Association, May 10, 1961.
69. Rappaport, A.: "New Logic for the Test Ban," *The Nation*, April 1, 1961, pp. 280-284.
70. Schelling, T. C.: THE STRATEGY OF CONFLICT, Harvard University Press, Cambridge, 1960.

71. Newcomb, T. M.: "Autistic Hostility and Social Reality," *Human Relations*, Vol. 1, 1947, pp. 69-86.
72. Sharp, G.: "Creative Conflict in Politics," *The New Era in Home and School*, Vol. 43, 1962, p. 9.
73. Pool, I. de Sola: "Public Opinion and the Control of Armaments," in ARMS CONTROL, DISARMAMENT AND NATIONAL SECURITY, Donald G. Brennan, ed., Geo. Braziller, New York, 1961, pp. 333-346.
74. Wedge, B. M.: "National Perspectives and International Communications," *American Journal of Orthopsychiatry*, Vol. 33, 1963, pp. 209-210.
75. Watson, J., and Lippitt, R.: "Cross Cultural Experience as a Source of Attitude Change," *Journal of Conflict Resolution*, Vol. 2, 1958, pp. 61-66.
76. Wedge, B. M.: Personal Communication.
77. Colmen, J.: "Overview of Research in the Peace Corps," *American Journal of Orthopsychiatry*, Vol. 33, 1963, pp. 218-219.
78. Bondurant, J. V.: CONQUEST OF VIOLENCE: THE GANDHIAN PHILOSOPHY OF CONFLICT, Princeton University Press, Princeton, 1958.
79. Fishman, J. R., and Solomon F.: "Psychological Observations on the Student Sit-In Movement," in PROCEEDINGS OF THE THIRD WORLD CONGRESS OF PSYCHIATRY, University of Toronto Press, Toronto, 1962, pp. 1133-1138.
80. Fischer, L.: THE LIFE OF MAHATMA GANDHI, Harper and Brothers, New York, 1950, Chap. 31, pp. 263-275.
81. King, M. L.: STRIDE TOWARD FREEDOM, Harper, New York, 1958.
82. Wilmer, H. A.: SOCIAL PSYCHIATRY IN ACTION, C. C. Thomas, Springfield, 1958.
83. Kennedy, J. F.: TOWARD A STRATEGY OF PEACE, United States Arms Control and Disarmament Agent Publication 17, Washington, D.C., June 1963.
84. Ferry, W. H.: "Peace Through Disarmament," American Friends Service Committee, Philadelphia, 1961.
85. Szilard, L.: *New York Times*, December 3, 1961, p. 2.
86. Fromm, E.: "The Case for Unilateral Disarmament," in ARMS CONTROL, DISARMAMENT, AND NATIONAL SECURITY, Donald G. Brennan, ed., Geo. Braziller, New York, 1961, pp. 187-197.
87. Kuhn, H. W.: "Game Theory and Models of Negotiation," *Journal of Conflict Resolution*, Vol. 6, 1962, pp. 1-4.
88. Harsanyi, J. C.: "Bargaining in Ignorance of the Opponent's Utility Function," *Journal of Conflict Resolution*, Vol. 6, 1962, pp. 29-38.
89. Diesing, P.: "Bargaining Strategy and Union-Management Relationships," *Journal of Conflict Resolution*, Vol. 5, 1961, pp. 369-378.
90. Deutsch, M. and Krauss, R. M.: "Studies of Interpersonal Bargaining," *Journal of Conflict Resolution*, Vol. 6, 1962, pp. 52-76.
91. Ikle, F. C., and Leites, N.: "Political Negotiation as a Process of Modifying Utilities," *Journal of Conflict Resolution*, Vol. 6, 1962, pp. 19-28.
92. Sherif, M. et al: INTERGROUP CONFLICT AND COOPERATION: THE ROBBERS CAVE EXPERIMENTS, University of Oklahoma Press, Norman, Okla., 1961. See also Sherif, Muzafer, and Sherif, Carolyn: GROUPS IN HARMONY AND TENSION, Harper & Row, New York, 1963.
93. Wardlow, A.: "The Place of Hostility and Conflict in a Disarmed World," Paper delivered at the Academy of Psychoanalysis, Mid-Winter Meeting, Philadelphia, December 30, 1962.
94. Larson, A.: WHEN NATIONS DISAGREE, Louisiana State University Press, Baton Rouge, 1961.

STATEMENT OF PURPOSE

The GROUP FOR THE ADVANCEMENT OF PSYCHIATRY *has a membership of approximately 185 psychiatrists, organized in the form of a number of working committees which direct their efforts toward the study of various aspects of psychiatry and toward the application of this knowledge to the fields of mental health and human relations.*

Collaboration with specialists in other disciplines has been and is one of GAP's working principles. Since the formation of GAP in 1946 its members have worked closely with such other specialists as anthropologists, biologists, economists, statisticians, educators, lawyers, nurses, psychologists, sociologists, social workers, and experts in mass communication, philosophy, and semantics. GAP envisages a continuing program of work according to the following aims:

1. *To collect and appraise significant data in the field of psychiatry, mental health, and human relations;*
2. *To re-evaluate old concepts and to develop and test new ones;*
3. *To apply the knowledge thus obtained for the promotion of mental health in good human relations.*

GAP is an independent group and its reports represent the composite findings and opinions of its members only, guided by its many consultants.

MEMBERS AND COMMITTEES OF GAP

As of October 1, 1965.

Committee on Adolescence

Calvin Settlage, Ardmore, Pa., Chr.
Warren J. Gadpaille, Denver, Colo.
Mary O Neil Hawkins, New York
Edward J. Hornick, New York
Joseph J. Michaels, Belmont, Mass.
Joseph P. Noshpitz, Bethesda
Henry Wermer, Chestnut Hill, Mass.

Committee on Aging

Jack Weinberg, Chicago, Chr.
Robert N. Butler, Washington, D.C.
Alvin I. Goldfarb, New York
Lawrence Greenleigh, Los Angeles
Maurice E. Linden, Philadelphia
Prescott Thompson, Topeka
Montague Ullman, Brooklyn

Committee on Child Psychiatry

Suzanne vanAmerongen, Boston, Chr.
E. James Anthony, St. Louis
H. Donald Dunton, New York
John F. Kenward, Chicago
William S. Langford, New York
Dane G. Prugh, Denver, Colo.
Exie E. Welsch, New York

Committee on College Student

J. B. Wheelwright, San Francisco, Chr.
Robert L. Arnstein, New Haven
Harrison P. Eddy, New York
Alfred Flarsheim, Chicago
Alan Frank, Boulder, Colo.
Malkah Tolpin Notman, Brookline, Mass.
Earle Silber, Bethesda
Benson R. Snyder, Cambridge
Thomas Stauffer, Scarsdale, N.Y.

Committee on the Family

Israel Zwerling, New York, Chr.
Murray Bowen, Chevy Chase
David Mendell, Houston
Norman L. Paul, Lexington, Mass.
Joseph Satten, Topeka
John P. Spiegel, Cambridge

Committee on Governmental Agencies

Donald B. Peterson, Fulton, Mo., Chr.
William H. Anderson, Columbia, Mo.
Calvin S. Drayer, Philadelphia
Edward O. Harper, Cleveland
John E. Nardini, Washington, D.C.
Harold Rosen, Baltimore
Raymond Waggoner, Ann Arbor
Robert L. Williams, Gainesville

Committee on Hospitals

Lee G. Sewall, Perry Point, Md., Chr.
Walter E. Barton, Washington, D.C.
Morris E. Chafetz, Boston
Merrill Eaton, Omaha
James B. Funkhouser, Richmond, Va.
George W. Jackson, Little Rock
Francis J. O'Neill, Central Islip, N.Y.
Lucy D. Ozarin, Bethesda
Jack A. Wolford, Pittsburgh

Committee on International Relations

Mottram Torre, New Orleans, Chr.
Francis F. Barnes, Chevy Chase
Joseph T. English, Washington, D.C.
Louis C. English, Pomona, N.Y.
Robert L. Leopold, Philadelphia
John A. P. Millet, New York
Florence Powdermaker, Ridgefield, Conn.
Bertram Schaffner, New York
Bryant M. Wedge, Princeton, N.J.

Committee on Medical Education

Roy M. Whitman, Cincinnati, Chr.
Hugh T. Carmichael, Chicago
Robert S. Daniels, Chicago
Saul Harrison, Ann Arbor
David Hawkins, Chapel Hill
Herbert C. Modlin, Topeka
William L. Peltz, Philadelphia
David S. Sanders, New York
Elvin V. Semrad, Boston

Committee on Mental Retardation

Leo Madow, Philadelphia, Chr.
Howard V. Bair, Parsons, Kans.
Peter W. Bowman, Pownal, Me.
Stuart M. Finch, Ann Arbor
George Tarjan, Pomona, Calif.
Warren T. Vaughan, Jr., San Mateo, Calif.
Thomas G. Webster, Bethesda
Cecil L. Wittson, Omaha
Henry H. Work, Los Angeles

Committee on Preventive Psychiatry

Leonard J. Duhl, Bethesda, Chr.
Gerald Caplan, Boston
Jules V. Coleman, New Haven
Stephen Fleck, New Haven
Albert J. Glass, Oklahoma City
Benjamin Jeffries, Harper Woods, Mich.
Mary E. Mercer, Nyack, N.Y.
Marvin E. Perkins, New York
Harold M. Visotsky, Chicago
Stanley F. Yolles, Bethesda

Committee on Psychiatry in Industry
Spencer Bayles, Houston, Chr.
Matthew Brody, Brooklyn
Leonard E. Himler, Ann Arbor
Alan A. McLean, New York
Kenneth J. Munden, Memphis
Graham C. Taylor, Montreal
Harry H. Wagenham, Philadelphia

Committee on Psychiatry and Law
Gene L. Usdin, New Orleans, Chr.
Edward T. Auer, St. Louis
Bernard L. Diamond, Berkeley
John Donnelly, Hartford
Jay Katz, New Haven
Zigmond M. Lebensohn, Washington, D.C.
Andrew S. Watson, Ann Arbor

Committee on Psychiatry and Religion
Mortimer Ostow, New York, Chr.
Sidney Furst, New York
John W. Higgins, St. Louis
Stanley A. Leavy, New Haven
Earl A. Loomis, Jr., New York
Albert J. Lubin, Woodside, Calif.

Committee on Psychiatry and Social Work
Edward C. Frank, Louisville, Chr.
C. Knight Aldrich, Chicago
Maurice R. Friend, New York
John MacLeod, Cincinnati
John Nemiah, Boston
Eleanor A. Steele, Denver
Edward M. Weinshel, San Francisco

Committee on Psychopathology
Marvin Stein, New York, Chr.
Wagner H. Bridger, New York
Neil Burch, Houston
James H. Ewing, Media, Pa.
Daniel X. Freedman, New Haven
Milton Greenblatt, Boston
Paul E. Huston, Iowa City
P. Herbert Leiderman, Palo Alto, Calif.
George Ruff, Philadelphia
Charles Shagass, Iowa City
Albert J. Silverman, New Brunswick, N.J.

Committee on Public Education
Peter A. Martin, Detroit, Chr.
Leo H. Bartemeier, Baltimore
H. Waldo Bird, St. Louis
Daniel Blain, Philadelphia
Dana L. Farnsworth, Cambridge
Marion E. Kenworthy, New York
John P. Lambert, Katonah, N.Y.
William C. Menninger, Topeka
Mabel Ross, Washington, D.C.
Mathew Ross, Chestnut Hill, Mass.
Julius Schreiber, Washington, D.C.
Kent A. Zimmerman, Berkeley

Committee on Research
Robert Wallerstein, Stanford, Calif., Chr.
Grete Bibring, Boston
Stanley Eldred, Belmont, Mass.
Edwin F. Gildea, St. Louis
Louis A. Gottschalk, Cincinnati
Sheppard G. Kellam, Chicago
Gerald L. Klerman, Boston
Morris A. Lipton, Chapel Hill
Ralph R. Notman, Brookline, Mass.
Franz Reichsman, Brooklyn
Richard E. Renneker, Los Angeles
Alfred H. Stanton, Boston

Committee on Social Issues
Arthur A. Miller, Chicago, Chr.
Viola W. Bernard, New York
Robert Coles, Cambridge
Joel S. Handler, Chicago
Portia Bell Hume, Berkeley
Roy W. Menninger, Topeka
Perry Ottenberg, Philadelphia
Charles A. Pinderhughes, Boston

Committee on Therapeutic Care
Benjamin Simon, Boston, Chr.
Marvin L. Adland, Chevy Chase
Ian L. W. Clancey, Ottawa
Thomas E. Curtis, Chapel Hill
Robert W. Gibson, Towson, Md.
Harold A. Greenberg, Bethesda
Henry U. Grunebaum, Boston
Bernard H. Hall, Topeka
Melvin Sabshin, Chicago
Robert E. Switzer, Topeka

Committee on Therapy
Peter H. Knapp, Boston, Chr.
Henry W. Brosin, Pittsburgh
Harvey H. Corman, New York
Eugene Meyer, Baltimore
William C. Offenkrantz, Chicago
Albert E. Scheflen, Oaks, Pa.
Harley C. Shands, Brooklyn
Lucia E. Tower, Chicago

Contributing Members
Nathan W. Ackerman, New York
Carlos C. Alden, Jr., Buffalo
Kenneth E. Appel, Philadelphia
M. Royden C. Astley, Pittsburgh
Charlotte Babcock, Pittsburgh
Walter H. Baer, Peoria
Grace Baker, New York
Benjamin H. Balser, New York
Bernard Bandler, Boston
Alfred Paul Bay, Topeka
Anna R. Benjamin, Chicago
A. E. Bennett, Berkeley
Robert E. Bennett, Princeton, N. J.
Ivan C. Berlien, Miami
Sidney Berman, Washington, D.C.
Edward G. Billings, Denver
Carl A. L. Binger, Cambridge
Wilfred Bloomberg, Hartford

C. H. Hardin Branch, Salt Lake City
Eugene Brody, Baltimore
Ewald W. Busse, Durham
Dale C. Cameron, Washington, D.C.
Norman Cameron, New Haven
Ralph T. Collins, Rochester
Frank J. Curran, New York
Franklin G. Ebaugh, Denver
Leon Eisenberg, Baltimore
Joel Elkes, Baltimore
O. Spurgeon English, Philadelphia
Jack R. Ewalt, Boston
Jerome D. Frank, Baltimore
Lawrence Z. Freedman, Chicago
Thomas M. French, Chicago
Moses M. Frohlich, Ann Arbor
Daniel H. Funkenstein, Boston
George E. Gardner, Boston
J. S. Gottlieb, Detroit
Maurice H. Greenhill, New York
John H. Greist, Indianapolis
Roy R. Grinker, Chicago
Ernest M. Gruenberg, New York
Manfred S. Guttmacher, Baltimore
David A. Hamburg, Palo Alto, Calif.
Frederick R. Hanson, New York
Herbert I. Harris, Cambridge
Paul Haun, Trenton, N.J.
J. Cotter Hirschberg, Topeka
Roger William Howell, Ann Arbor
Joseph Hughes, Philadelphia
Robert W. Hyde, Boston
Lucie Jessner, Washington, D.C.
Irene M. Josselyn, Phoenix
Edward J. Kollar, Los Angeles
Othilda Krug, Cincinnati
Lawrence S. Kubie, Towson, Md.
Paul V. Lemkau, Baltimore
Maurice Levine, Cincinnati
David M. Levy, New York
Harold I. Lief, New Orleans
Robert J. Lifton, Woodbridge, Conn.
Erich Lindemann, Boston
Hyman S. Lippman, St. Paul
Reginald S. Lourie, Washington, D.C.
Alfred O. Ludwig, Boston
LeRoy M. A. Maeder, Philadelphia
Sidney G. Margolin, Denver
Judd Marmor, Beverly Hills
Helen V. McLean, Chicago
Karl Menninger, Topeka
James G. Miller, Ann Arbor
Angel N. Miranda, Hato Rey, P.R.
Russell R. Monroe, Baltimore
Don P. Morris, Dallas
Peter B. Neubauer, New York
Rudolph G. Novick, Des Plaines, Ill.
Humphry F. Osmond, Princeton, N.J.
Eveoleen Rexford, Boston
Lewis L. Robbins, Glen Oaks, N.Y.
J. Franklin Robinson, Wilkes Barre, Pa.
Philip Q. Roche, Philadelphia
Robert Roessler, Madison
Milton Rosenbaum, New York
W. Donald Ross, Cincinnati
William M. Shanahan, Denver
Harry C. Solomon, Boston
Benjamin M. Spock, Cleveland
Edward Stainbrook, Los Angeles
Brandt F. Steele, Denver
Rutherford B. Stevens, New York
M. A. Tarumianz, Wilmington, Del.
Lloyd J. Thompson, Chapel Hill
Harvey J. Tompkins, New York
Arthur V. Valenstein, Cambridge
Helen Stochen Wagenheim, Philadelphia
David Wright, Providence

Life Members

S. Spafford Ackerly, Louisville
Earl D. Bond, Philadelphia
William C. Menninger, Topeka
John R. Rees, London, England
Bruce Robinson, Culver, Ind.
Francis H. Sleeper, Augusta, Me.

Officers

President
Robert S. Garber
Carrier Clinic, Belle Mead, N.J.

Vice President
Herbert C. Modlin
Box 829, Topeka, Kans. 66601

Secretary-Treasurer
Malcolm J. Farrell
Box C, Waverley, Mass. 02178

Asst. Secretary-Treasurer
Paul E. Huston
500 Newton Road, Iowa City, Iowa